The Cerulean Soul

SRTD

STUDIES IN RELIGION, THEOLOGY, AND DISABILITY

SERIES EDITORS

Sarah J. Melcher
Xavier University, Cincinnati, Ohio

John Swinton
University of Aberdeen, Aberdeen, Scotland

Amos Yong
Fuller Theological Seminary, Pasadena, California

The Cerulean Soul

A Relational Theology of Depression

Peter J. Bellini

BAYLOR UNIVERSITY PRESS

Unless otherwise stated, Scripture quotations are from the New Revised Standard Version Bible, copyright 1989, Division of Christian Education of the National Council of the Churches of Christ in the United States of America. Used by permission. All rights reserved.

Cover Design by Kasey McBeath
Cover Image: *Melancholia Redeemed*, by Maria Bellini
Book Design by Baylor University Press

Library of Congress Cataloging-in-Publication Data

Names: Bellini, Peter J., author.
Title: The cerulean soul : a relational theology of depression / Peter J. Bellini.
Other titles: Studies in religion, theology, and disability
Description: Waco : Baylor University Press, 2021. | Series: Studies in religion, theology, and disability | Includes bibliographical references and index. | Summary: "Presents constructive theology of depression that brings philosophical and theological analysis into conversation with the current biomedical model"-- Provided by publisher.
Identifiers: LCCN 2021015555 (print) | LCCN 2021015556 (ebook) | ISBN 9781481310932 (hardcover) | ISBN 9781481314398 (pdf) | ISBN 9781481310956 (epub)
Subjects: LCSH: Depression, Mental--Religious aspects--Christianity. | Depressed persons. | Mental illness--Religious aspects--Christianity.
Classification: LCC BV4910.34 .B45 2021 (print) | LCC BV4910.34 (ebook) | DDC 248.8/625--dc23
LC record available at https://lccn.loc.gov/2021015555
LC ebook record available at https://lccn.loc.gov/2021015556

Printed in the United States of America on acid-free paper with a minimum of thirty percent recycled content.

Series Introduction

Studies in Religion, Theology, and Disability brings newly established and emerging scholars together to explore issues at the intersection of religion, theology, and disability. The series editors encourage theoretical engagement with secular disability studies while supporting the reexamination of established religious doctrine and practice. The series fosters research that takes account of the voices of people with disabilities and the voices of their family and friends.

The volumes in the series address issues and concerns of the global religious studies/theological studies academy. Authors come from a variety of religious traditions with diverse perspectives to reflect on the intersection of the study of religion/theology and the human experience of disability. This series is intentional about seeking out and publishing books that engage with disability in dialogue with Jewish, Christian, Buddhist, or other religious and philosophical perspectives.

Themes explored include religious life, ethics, doctrine, proclamation, liturgical practices, physical space, spirituality, and the interpretation of sacred texts through the lens of disability. Authors in the series are aware of conversation in the field of disability studies and bring that discussion to bear methodologically and theoretically in their analyses at the intersection of religion and disability.

Studies in Religion, Theology, and Disability reflects the following developments in the field: First, the emergence of disability studies as an interdisciplinary endeavor that has impacted theological studies, broadly defined.

More and more scholars are deploying disability perspectives in their work, and this applies also to those working in the theological academy. Second, there is a growing need for critical reflection on disability in world religions. While books from a Christian standpoint have dominated the discussion at the interface of religion and disability so far, Jewish, Muslim, Buddhist, and Hindu scholars, among those from other religious traditions, have begun to resource their own religious traditions to rethink disability in the twenty-first century. Third, passage of the Americans with Disabilities Act in the United States has raised the consciousness of the general public about the importance of critical reflection on disability in religious communities. General and intelligent lay readers are looking for scholarly discussions of religion and disability as these bring together and address two of the most important existential aspects of human lives. Fourth, the work of activists in the disability rights movement has mandated fresh critical reflection by religious practitioners and theologians. Persons with disabilities remain the group most disaffected from religious organizations. Fifth, government representatives in several countries have prioritized the greater social inclusion of persons with disabilities. Disability policy often proceeds based on core cultural and worldview assumptions that are religiously informed. Work at the interface of religion and disability thus could have much broader purchase—that is, in social, economic, political, and legal domains.

Under the general topic of thoughtful reflection on the religious understanding of disability, Studies in Religion, Theology, and Disability includes shorter, crisply argued volumes that articulate a bold vision within a field; longer scholarly monographs, more fully developed and meticulously documented, with the same goal of engaging wider conversations; textbooks that provide a state of the discussion at this intersection and chart constructive ways forward; and select edited volumes that achieve one or more of the preceding goals.

Contents

Part IV

A Trinitarian Theology of Melancholia

Preface

Cerulean comes from the Latin *caelum*, which means "sky" or "heaven." From the palette of nature's hues, cerulean is the azure or deep blue of the sky at its peak. The image drawn of the *cerulean soul* points to its profound and infinite capacity to hold space and time, even to touch heaven. Yet, in its depth, extension, and vastness, *cerulean* can express the expanse for alienation, loss, and melancholy, even depression. The cerulean soul has the capacity for depth, depravity, depression, and the divine. Our journey will explore these sites.

By trade, I am an academician, a professor in practical theology at a mainline Protestant denominational seminary. I primarily teach evangelization, church renewal, intercultural studies, and urban studies, and at times pastoral care and counseling when needed. I am an ordained minister in that same denomination. I have served in evangelistic and pastoral ministry for over thirty years in a variety of settings but mainly in urban contexts. In those settings, I observed many good people, often indigent, face mental health issues, though mental disorders do not discriminate. Many were without health insurance and were underdiagnosed and undertreated. Also, a higher than average number were addicted, and some in recovery. The two struggles, mental disorder and addiction, often coincided in the same persons. Around the same time, one of my children was diagnosed with several mental disorders and learning disabilities related to executive function. I assumed the role of lifelong caregiver and companion, alongside learning to be a father. Following, another family member was diagnosed with depression and anxiety, and I became their caregiver as well. And not long after, I went through a period of ministry burnout while planting a new church, managing a dying church, caregiving, and earning a Ph.D. Burnout for me, back in the early 2000s, involved a bout with anxiety and depression that lasted a couple of years but never relapsed. I learned much from these experiences that subsequently impacted my writing and ministry.

One of my lifelong goals as an interdisciplinary scholar and practitioner has been to develop a comprehensive and holistic approach to minister with persons who are challenged with mental health battles and to advocate for social awareness and change. Incorporating into that model the best that medical science and social restructuring have to provide was never in doubt. A theological rejection of the sciences can be tragic. Too often the church's remedies have exacerbated the challenges faced by persons with disabilities and disorder. The greater question for me has been how the church and its theology can be an asset and contribute constructively to the conversation. This book is my continuing attempt to answer that question.

It is no secret that in these matters the church has violated Hippocrates, let alone Christ, by not "doing no harm." Where theology has often misspoken for God and been guilty even of malpractice, can it be redeemed and reflect more clearly the God of radical mercy and love? I do not deny the dirty bathwater. However, I do not feel it necessary to throw out the invaluable resources of the Christian church and its theologies *in toto*. The indispensable riches of classical Christian theology rooted in the Trinity, the incarnation, and salvation in Christ have much to offer. I believe these irreplaceable treasures from the trusty storehouse of God's wisdom can be useful for us even today. Though this study is interdisciplinary in nature, it is primarily and unapologetically theological. More so, though conversant with a variety of theological voices, this work is especially tuned to the great tradition of the faith and interested in how it might shape an ancient problem in our contemporary context.

Amid the current myriad of perspectives on disabilities and mental disorder, theological perspectives are frequently dismissed as unscientific and thus disregarded. Further, among the polyphony of theological voices, the ancient ones are often deemed antiquated, irrelevant, insensitive, or even oppressive and hence neglected in contemporary conversations that may be asking different questions of a different world. Although in part true, this indictment is not the whole truth. Amid the increased advances and authority of the sciences, the church and its theologies have also been responsible for many of history's and today's transformative institutions, leaders, and efforts toward a more whole and just world. In recent history, we have been blessed by the likes of Dietrich Bonhoeffer, Dorothy Day, Martin Luther King Jr., Mother Teresa, Billy Graham, and Francis Collins, to name a few, along with countless hospitals, relief organizations, and other efforts that are on the front lines of working for compassion and justice. Many of these figures and institutions are rooted in the ancient faith of the church. Nonetheless, for all of the bright lights in the Christian tradition, there have been the misguided witnesses who have obscured the light of Christ. It remains no small task for religion, and specifically Christianity, to redeem itself from being the perpetrator of oppression and injustice toward the weak and vulnerable and also to stay steadfast and faithful to the timeless truth that has been delivered to its care.

In that light, I hope this work is redemptive and faithful to the task. Once again, I approach this study primarily as a practical theologian who has had scholarly, pedagogical, and pastoral interest and experience in mental health, healing, and wholeness. Some of that experience has gone into publications and classroom teaching, but primarily it has gone into pastoral care and counseling and an active healing prayer ministry in the church. This work reflects more of the research piece but is silently and heavily undergirded by my practical experience in counseling and praying for those who have faced mental health issues. While some critical disability theories condemn any attempt to ameliorate or heal (even eschatological healing) and interpret such gestures as power plays to strengthen existing ableness normativity and marginalization, I do not want to perpetuate or be an accomplice to oppression in any form but contend that the healing and restoration offered in Christ does neither. Any theory that censors our need for and access to God's redemptive love, restoration, and wholeness in Christ is incompatible with Christian teaching. In this regard, this work is unapologetically Christian and theological.

Although this work is part of a series that is in conversation with disability studies, I do not come as one trained in that particular field. Though aware of some of its major authors, texts, and theories, I am less conversant in the field than I am in the fields of theology, philosophy, and mental health. Thus, my main interlocutors are theological, philosophical, and medical and secondarily those in disability studies, though many of the frameworks, theories, and issues in disability studies overlap with the mental health field. Although the ADA classifies mental illness as a (psychiatric) disability, unfortunately, while disability and mental health are very compatible,[1] they have had an ambivalent relationship that focuses more on their incompatibilities than on their similarities. This work will refer to depression as both a mental disorder and a psychiatric disability. What is offered here is an interdisciplinary piece that prayerfully blends a harmony of clear and distinct sounds that lift up a theological voice of hope and healing for those in despair and those who care with them.

Peter Bellini | May 13, 2020
At home amid the COVID-19 pandemic

Acknowledgments

This book has stretched me in a way that none of my other writings have done. Interdisciplinary work can be tricky. It takes a far-reaching bandwidth to cover effectively the extensive fields, sources, and arguments that make for sound interdisciplinary research. One needs to identify the right intersection of fields that both addresses one's subject broadly and deeply and utilizes the best material from those fields to shape thick discourse. In addition to working out of fields that are the author's expertise, one needs to research peripheral disciplines in which one has some but less fluency and dexterity. One should have a smaller set of core disciplines that have been mastered, and another related set which the author has less mastery over but is growing in proficiency. Discovering the right combination takes much reading, reflecting, and discerning. This book works primarily out of the intersection of dogmatic theology, philosophy (ontology and epistemology), philosophical theology, philosophy of disease, and clinical psychology, with added discourse from the history of mental disorders, medical anthropology, and disability studies. My growing edges were in the history of mental disorders and disability studies, since these are not my fields of expertise.

It goes without saying that a work of this length and breadth owes much gratitude to those who have supported me in this endeavor. I would like to thank my family for the joy and strength that they give me. They are my day-to-day inspiration in all things. I thank them for being there to share blessings but also for sustaining me in lean times. Their patience and tolerance were golden, as they put up with me for endless hours lifelessly turned toward the keyboard with my back toward the world. My family has been with me through thick and thin. Thank you to my son, Aaronne, my daughter, Paola, my son-in-law, Zac, and my granddaughter, Costanza, and special thanks to my best friend, my wife, Mariuccia, who also provided the cover art. And thank you to my mother, Karyn, for your virtuous example. You all have been my life's breath.

I would like to thank Baylor University Press for giving me this opportunity to engage in conversation within the prestigious Studies in Religion, Theology, and Disability series. David Aycock and Cade Jarrell, interim director and editor at Baylor University Press, respectively, have been extremely helpful and supportive. I thank them for their tireless work and support that kept this project on the drawing board when outside circumstances made it seem unlikely. I want to thank series editors Sarah Melcher and John Swinton for their encouragement. Sarah, I appreciate the vote of confidence. I want to thank Amos Yong, one of the original series editors, for first approaching me with the prospect of tackling this project. I am thankful for the keen eyes of my copyeditors. I also want to thank Kasey McBeath for accepting my wife's cover art for the book. I would also like to thank my peer reviewers for their beneficial comments that helped to smooth out the text. Finally, special thanks to United Theological Seminary in Dayton, Ohio, where I serve as the Associate Professor in Evangelization in the Heisel Chair. United graciously granted me a sabbatical to complete the manuscript. Thank you, Dean David Watson and United faculty, staff, and trustees. Above all, praise Father, Son, and Holy Spirit!

PART I

INTRODUCTION TO MELANCHOLIA

1

Introduction

ERIC

Eric (not his real name) lived in the inner city. He came from a basically good and functional home. Eric always felt he was somewhat different from the other kids. He just did not seem to fit in, and he knew it. He spent much time alone, and the rest of his time seeking attention by acting up at home and at school. He found that other kids who were getting in trouble at school, for one reason or another, would give him the most attention. So he gravitated toward them and did what they did. He soon followed them and got in trouble at school and at home as they did. Early in elementary school, teachers began to track that he had learning disabilities. He was tested. An individualized education program (IEP) was put in place.

Eric had a family history of depression, OCD, and mood disorder on both sides of the family. The family suspected Eric had experienced some trauma as a child, but they could not figure out what, where, when, how, or by whom. They took him to a child psychologist to be evaluated. The diagnoses changed over the years—ADD, ADHD, bipolar, depression-anxiety, mood disorder, and so on. I am not sure whether they really ever knew exactly the correct diagnosis. He was treated with various psychiatric meds that were recommended at the time. Sometimes he felt better. Sometimes he felt worse. He went through frequent suicidal seasons.

I know Eric because I was his friend. As a pastor, I became a mentor to him. Eric wanted to know what was wrong with him and why he was not better after medication and therapy. He wanted to know why he was different. He wanted to know why God "made him this way." He wanted to know why he was bullied and beaten up in school even though he did everything the tough kids wanted him to do. The doctors told him he had a "chemical imbalance" and meds would help (a medical analysis). But his problem was not merely about chemicals. It was also about getting picked on and beaten up (a social analysis). The therapist gave him sound counsel and strategies, but he could not focus to process what he was hearing, and what he processed he could not remember or retain. His real problem was that the world around him was too fast, too complicated, insensitive, exclusive, painful, and not friendly. He could not keep up and be one of the "normal" kids.

Yes, there were mental disorders present. Yes, there were diagnoses and meds prescribed. Yes, there was counseling. Yes, there were IEPs and accommodations related to the Americans with Disabilities Act. But that was not all. There was more. Much more, and that is what this book is all about—more. Diagnoses, meds, counseling, accommodations . . . what we call a medical model and a social model of explanation and treatment were all given. But there was more. Much more. There was a boy. And above all, there was God. It would be God who would make all of the difference in that boy's life. I was blessed to be a part of his growth in God through-out his life. The meds, the counseling, and the accommodations helped, at times, and other times they did not seem to make much of a difference, especially when he wanted to end his life, which was frequently.

I was present in Eric's life, in all seasons, like a father, a mentor . . . a friend. In season and out of season, I shared God in Christ. When he was up and down, and when he could not take any more and had a plan to end it all, I was a friend who was there. I was there when he loved me. I was there when he hated me. Always accessible. Yes, I shared Christ. I spoke Christ. I "did" Christ (to the best of my ability). He shared his pain and doubt. He spoke of his faith and hope. The journey never seemed easy. At times he wanted out, and other times I wanted out. But above all I was present and open to him as Christ had been with me. I embraced Eric as Christ embraced me. That was my sanctification and Eric's. This book is about being in rela-tion with God, directly and through others. It is about being made holy by God's love and God's love alone. Eric can speak for himself, but this work reflects in part what I have learned from him.

Medical and social models, as well as other models, offer much, but we cannot leave out the divine. The theological must be present, as it was with Eric. All persons with disabilities or disorders and those without are rela-tional beings created and capable to receive and give the holy love of God in their own unique way. That is what a theological perspective has to offer.

This work attempts to do that. There are hard and deep questions to ask in the mental health field. I ask some of them and go to the root to try to answer them as thoroughly as I know how. The writing is unabashedly highly philosophical, theological, and technical because it is attempting to do the hard work and heavy lifting of laying the foundation for well-thought-out theology that deals with a very serious subject that often involves life or death. The subject matter ultimately is people (not disorders), people with psychiatric disabilities, and their humanity. This work seeks to lay a firm academic, theological foundation for other academics and professionals who educate those who care for persons like Eric or who directly care for persons like Eric. I desire that our work may be steadily grounded in God, who desires to work through us.

FELIX MELANCHOLIA?

> O felix culpa quae talem et tantum meruit habere redemptorem.
> [O blessed sin (literally, happy fault) which received as its reward so great and so good a redeemer.]
>
> Holy Saturday Latin Mass

> O goodness infinite, goodness immense!
> That all this good of evil shall produce,
> And evil turn to good; more wonderful
> Than that which by creation first brought forth
> Light out of darkness! Full of doubt I stand;
> Whether I should repent me now of sin
> By me done and occasioned, or rejoice
> Much more, that much more good thereof shall spring,
> To God more glory, more good will to men
> From God, and over wrath grace shall abound.
>
> *Paradise Lost* 12.461–478

Is depression a blessing, curse, neither, or both? Is depression some type of *felix melancholia*? Many of us are familiar with the theological term *felix culpa*. *Felix culpa*, meaning "happy fall," is the term in medieval theodicy used to speak of original or first sin in light of the incarnation and the good news of salvation in Jesus Christ. The understanding is that although the fall was a tragedy, it became a blessing because God came in the flesh to die on the cross for our restoration.[1] As Paul puts it in Romans 5:20, "Where sin abounds grace abounds more." The notion of *felix culpa*, proposed by such theologians as Augustine and Aquinas, attempts to reconcile the notions of freedom, sin, providence, and redemption in Roman Catholic theodicy. In the *Enchiridion* Augustine declares, "For God judged it better to bring good out of evil than not to permit any evil to exist."[2] Aquinas claims, "God allows evils to happen in order to bring a greater good therefrom."[3] God exists. Mental disorders exist. Why does God allow them, or why cannot God prevent them? *Felix melancholia* or happy (blessed) melancholy (depression) means that mental disorders, regardless of their etiology, whether they are attributed by some to God, the devil, the fall, an imperfect world, sin, poor choices, natural responses, part of the evolutionary process, social systems, genetics, neurochemistry, cognitive distortions, or any other source, can be part of God's overall redemption plan to bring forth eschatologically the new creation. Although this work wrestles with etiology, it is more interested in healing and wholeness. Does God embrace persons with mental disorders and incorporate them and their ailments into the larger story of salvation? Does any suggestion of "needing salvation" perhaps imply the harmful notion that we are somehow defective, insufficient, or inadequate? These are questions to be examined.

Traditional Christian theology has proclaimed that Christ has assumed our human condition that we may partake of the saving grace of God. Every person, regardless of state or condition, including mental disorders, is invited to the banquet table to partake of the kingdom of God. Though we all express difference and distinction in our beliefs, gender, ethnicity, sexuality, race, ability/disability, and socioeconomic background, as Galatians 3:28 implies, we all equally need the grace and salvation found in Jesus Christ. The grace of God touches each of us in our unique place and development and empowers us on our journey to wholeness and holiness. None of us are in a special class in this regard. We are all undone by sin and need salvation! As Hans Reinders has claimed, "One way or another, any view of disability as a special condition is to be criticized for being dependent on patterns of exclusion. Whether God has blessed you or punished you, in both cases you are set aside from his other creatures about whom such verdicts usually are not communicated. That is what is wrong with such views."[4] In this sense, the cult of normativity is undermined and the dichotomies of blessed and cursed, sinner and saint, abled and disabled, and ordered and disorder are supplanted.[5] We are all in need of God's grace, and no one is excluded. And the good news is all are freely given God's grace!

In the incarnation, God took our weakness and brokenness onto himself that he might restore humanity and the cosmos to God's eternal intention. The resurrection of Jesus Christ offers cosmic transfiguration to a disfigured world. No state is too far removed from God's redemption. The proposition of *felix melancholia* plays off of the term *felix culpa*, but it is not substituting *melancholia* for *culpa*. If it did, *melancholia* would be a type of *culpa*.

No, *melancholia* is not a type of *culpa* per se but connected to *felix*. Blessed depression. Together, *culpa* and *melancholia* make the term paradoxical. The comparison of *melancholia* with *culpa* is analogical, as *culpa* is usually not seen as a blessing, and neither is *melancholia*. And even in Christ, *melancholia* is not a blessing, but neither can *melancholia* prevent blessing. *Felix melancholia* denotes the possibility of blessing even in depression, because in Christ, God's saving power is made perfect in weakness (2 Cor. 12:9). Human weakness and constitutional poverty are not disqualifiers to struggles, benefits, or blessings as they often are in this world. Rather, they are receptors for the benefits and blessings of the kingdom of God extended by the grace of God. Neither are mental disorders or any condition markers that distinguish a "special" class of people based on our "ability" or lack of ability. Both conditions are measured in divine light and not our own judgment. We are not romanticizing or minimizing suffering in this life. The point is there is eschatological restoration found in Christ. In Christ, not only can human constitutional weakness and even the fall be a blessing, but also mental disorder, *melancholia*, can be a blessing because of the reality of resurrection and the emergence of a new creation. The driving premise of this work is that no human condition is marginalized or excluded from salvation. At the cross, human weakness becomes blessed because God also has become broken flesh that is blessed and offered for the life of the world as displayed at the eucharistic table of divine fellowship. All are invited to sit at the table and partake!

MELANCHOLIA AND THEOLOGY

This work is interdisciplinary in scope. Although it engages scientific and medical sources, it is primarily a philosophical and theological exploration that is historical and systematic in its approach. One would expect a work that theologically investigates the phenomenon of melancholia to define the term in all of its technical aspects. Accordingly, I use *melancholia* in various senses. First, I use it symbolically to address the entire species of depressive-anxiety disorders. A general use of the term provides facility for discourse, as we attempt to define also the various specific iterations of melancholia across time. Chapter 2 attempts this daunting task. However, it is essential to remember that although we would like a convenient, manageable, simple, uniform, and treatable definition, melancholia is a complex, pluriform, and multivalent phenomenon that is quite elusive to nail down, especially in terms of etiology and definition.[6] In fact, currently there is no one ultimate identifiable cause of melancholia, nor is there one unified theory that encompasses and connects all of the various explanations, from evolutionary to genetic to neurochemical to cognitive behavioral to psychosocial and so on.

To acknowledge the complexity of this phenomenon is not to ignore or reduce the significance of causation or avoid defining the malady. I will explore various theological efforts to identify causation. I will offer multiple hypotheses at both the popular and academic levels of interpretation, though none will ultimately satisfy any desire for a tidy, complete explanation. Historically, the Christian church has been known to attribute melancholia to God, the devil, the fall, an imperfect world, individual sin, and psychological causes. It is too easy to simply dismiss any or all of these or to accept blindly any or all of these explanations. Each case and its circumstances are unique, and at best causation may be partly revealed or not be revealed at all. I will critically engage a classical or historical typology that has entertained many of these speculations and make conclusions only insofar as they find theological resolution in Christ.[7] Ironically, it is often the case that recovery and healing may not be contingent on full or even satisfactory explanations of causation. People receive healing from treatments without exactly knowing why, such as the work of SSRIs, therapy, the placebo effect, and spontaneous remission. However, in this study, one binding correlation is made between how one defines a human person and how one defines the nature of depression. This connection incessantly emerges from the literature. A biological account of humanity will yield a biochemical understanding and treatment of depression. A semiotic account of humanity will yield a sociocultural understanding and treatment of depression. This connection serves as a hinge to my hypothesis, upon which my relational model turns. A relational anthropology and a theological exploration of the image of God and its relationship with the divine will be key to understanding a theological treatment of melancholia (chapters 3 and 4).

Theologically, melancholia is multivalent in terms of etiology and definition. Echoing Søren Kierkegaard and Paul Tillich, existential anxiety can be structural to the human condition and to freedom, serving as a catalyst for either faith or fear in our primary response to the divine and even in our human development. Grounded in our own contingent being, which is constituted out of *nihilo*/nothingness, our existence appears unstable. We fear an ontological implosion that would set off a series of chain reactions that evoke dread, despair, angst, depression, and meaninglessness. Our anxiety can be existential. Others believe our anxiety can be related to sin. With this view, melancholia can semiotically point to the aftermath of the fundamental alienation experienced by the autonomous *imago* that follows human choice to follow God or become its own god. Traditional Christian thinkers have also posited that melancholia can precede and even follow human lapse and further be instrumental in redemption. Chapters 5, 6, and 7 will explore the melancholic complex and some models from a theological and scriptural perspective.

Regardless of our predilection to reduce and manage depression, the results will be evident. The verdict is not unanimous in terms of pinpointing a single, uniform, or ultimate cause, nature, or purpose of melancholia. That is not to say that one, a combination of any, all, or none of the above speculative causes are not involved, relative to each unique case. Yet when one hastily identifies the elusive syndrome with any or none of these causes, one discovers many more related problems that are usually theological, ethical, and pastoral, and at times remain unsolved and can often exacerbate the problem and further stigmatize the condition. In terms of etiology, depressed persons live in the midst of this ambiguity, and so should the hermeneutics and the interpreters of depression. At times, the only valid firsthand account from experience is apophatic—silence and/or lament. In this work, my response is a secondhand account, a more detached safe, analytic reflection, which in one sense is a disqualifier. Yet its distance, as a critical, rational account, can be an asset as we seek some degree of objectivity. Taking a step back, we can see the proverbial forest for its trees. Though there are many angles to approach the nature of melancholia, one has to start somewhere. This work builds on theology, proposing the relational nature and treatment of melancholia in Christ.

Although this study will tackle some of the tough questions of etiology, it will focus even more on the theology and eschatology of mental disorder and God's response of healing in the resurrection. Chapters 8 and 9 will directly examine a theological response to melancholia as it relates to the *missio Dei*. The promise of hope and new life that is made possible in the resurrection is God's healing for the nations, regardless of the variety of speculative causes and definitions of mental disorder.

However we choose to examine the cause, definition, and treatment of melancholia, it remains the odyssey of its sojourners and bearers to define its logos for themselves in light of their struggle and their encounter with the resurrected One. Although not within the scope of this book, more attention needs to be paid directly to the firsthand accounts and theologies of those on this pilgrimage rather than merely our own thoughtful, theological, and pastoral responses, important as they may be. Because of the puzzling and complex nature of the matter, etiology, definition, and treatment, if they are to be found at all, are to be found primarily by those who sojourn through the valley of the shadow of death into new life in Christ. The theological and even pastoral task is to come alongside and to offer the gift of presence, comfort, and divine friendship, even the wisdom of healing. More so, the redemptive task is also for Christianity to educate itself, repent, and be equipped to better serve justly in an unjust world.

THE NATURE OF DEPRESSION

Depression is the leading cause of disability worldwide in terms of total years lost due to disability.[8] In 2015, depression cost the United States $210 billion dollars.[9] Depression is the leading cause of disability and suicide worldwide and is currently an epidemic. Not to diminish the magnitude of the current crisis, but this condition has also shadowed human history in some form from the dawn of civilization and the first human suffering. Although an unwanted assault upon the human soul, depression has been part and parcel of the human condition and can be thought of as a species of the genus of weakness (*astheneia*) and collateral suffering, regardless of etiological claims.

Depression, or melancholia, is a part of our limited frail, broken human condition, and possibly a necessary manifestation of our creatureliness. Like weakness and suffering, depression is universal, and in its various expressions can bring forth both destructive and creative ends. For a weak and broken humanity, Christ comes as God disfigured, that is, God in weakness and God crucified. In his disability, Christ shows us that the kingdom of God belongs to such as these. He identifies with our common human brokenness, which includes mental disorder, that we all may find a place at the cross and be transfigured in the image of Christ through the resurrection. No form is untouched by the stress of this life, and no form is exempt from the touch of God's love in Christ.

We readily acknowledge an imperfect humanity, even a moral lapse that touches us and fragments us all in a disjointed world. From the shards of brokenness emerge the various maladies and disorders from which no one is exempt. Yet what exactly or inexactly is depression, or melancholia? There are many resources that will be drawn upon in this work to answer this question, including historical, sociological, cultural, philosophical, psychological, critical, neuroscientific, and mainly medical. This study will explore many of these routes, with its chief aim to consider the problem theologically. Quite some time ago, I received a Ph.D. in intercultural studies, an interdisciplinary degree that focuses on different aspects of the science of mission. Part of my course of study and research focused on the social sciences, specifically cultural anthropology, and philosophical theology, and more specifically epistemology of theology. I had to be fluent in several dialects of research, though theology was my primary language. The methodology I utilize in the classroom as a seminary professor is also academically multilingual. While I primarily speak in the language of theology, the secondary dialects with which I articulate in the classroom are from the social sciences, the hard sciences, and philosophy. In the case of my research, writing, and teaching, I use all three of the dialects. Research in these academic dialects informs, shapes, and inspires my theological research. Yet all that these disciplines afford, and the yield is great, cannot substitute for theological inquiry. For the church, theology is our primary dialect and will be spoken chiefly in this text.

At the front end, this study utilizes interdisciplinary research in order to grasp the multivalence of melancholia and to examine critically the various models and frameworks that attempt to conceptualize the phenomenon. Interdisciplinary research also invites neglected fields such as theology into the conversation. We can explore how our theological resources complement, critique, or enhance current research and methods of treatment. Some of the driving questions behind our inquiry are, How does theology interpret melancholia? What is theology's response to the disorder? Does God suffer? How do Christ and the Holy Spirit minister to depressed persons, to caregivers, and to nondepressed persons? Also, how does a theological perspective serve as a corrective to existing models, and how can it be integrated with and work alongside other models of healing? How are we to understand melancholia theologically? What insight does theology offer in terms specifically of ministering healing? And ultimately, how can theologically informed insights and practices further inform an integrated model of mental health and treatment and our own education?

The goal here is not to examine all mental disorders, any number of mental disorders, mental disorders as a whole, or mental health in general, but to look at depression and its treatment as representative and symbolic of the issues across the mental health field and as a complex sign of creaturely or anthropological weakness, human suffering and struggle, meaning making, and cosmic disorder and order.

THEOLOGICAL ANTHROPOLOGY AND TYPES OF DEPRESSION

Current Enlightenment-based philosophical anthropology will be explored, specifically its correspondence with etiology and how it shapes an overall biomedical model of depression. It is at the anthropological level where the deficiency is often found. Theological input is lacking. Humanity is only considered in its materiality, excluding any nonmaterial dimensions to what it means to be human. The theological contribution that humanity is made in the image of God will be our basis for further anthropological considerations and its relation to depression. Examination of the *imago Dei* can yield rich results that transcend the standard rational-volitional model, opening the door to a relational notion of the image of God. The image of God as it stands in the context of creation, fall, and new creation will inform the emergence of mental disorder in terms of its relationship with God.

Various historical theological types that correspond to three relational states will be surveyed and critically analyzed as alternatives or at least as supplements to the current biomedical model. The three theological types are natural (creation), consequential (fall), and purgative (new creation) forms of depression. The natural or existential type, *type 1*, holds that the possibility of depression is natural to the human condition. Persons can be depressed because that is simply the nature of things. It's life. The consequential type, *type 2*, is that the possibility of depression can arise directly or indirectly as a result of the fall, the fallen world, and/or fallen human condition. Persons can be depressed because the world is fallen and out of order. The purgative type, *type 3*, or "the dark night of the soul," is the view that God uses depression as an agent of sanctification for those seeking union with God. Persons grow despondent in their pursuit of God, as God desires to further purify the faithful by a seeming absence. In this case, the dark night is intentional on God's part and used for our purgation from sin.

Some of these models involve prelapsarian and lapsarian dimensions. That is not to say that depression is univocally correlated with sin or that depression could not occur before Adam and Eve[10] in an evolutionary framework. Critical examination of these claims is warranted. Mainly, melancholia will be examined theologically, as a syndrome and sign of the human condition in all of its pluriform iterations, including so-called prelapsarian and lapsarian forms, as well as forms within the eschatological trajectory of redemption. The notion that depression is connected to (original) sin is frequently articulated by classic and even pop theologies. Likewise, it is countered that depression could have existed prior to and apart from sin. Hence, nonlapsarian, prelapsarian, and lapsarian hypotheses are considered. Even in an evolutionary scheme, it cannot be clearly determined whether hominids or other animals experienced depression twenty thousand years ago or prior to oral or written language. Depression has no objective test, and diagnosis is based on symptoms that are observed, subjectively experienced and reported. If an evolutionary scheme is accepted, then depression could have existed before Adam, but since observation and subjective experience, including self-consciousness and self-reflection conveyed through language, are the principal instruments of diagnosis, such knowledge is not available.[11] Thus, we will work with the biblical narrative of fall and redemption.

Depression is a complex with manifold iterations[12] within a larger milieu of the shadow side of the human condition. This complex has been interpreted contextually across space and time through a variety of frameworks that have sought to understand, rid, overcome, or cure the nature and influence of this complicated and elusive condition. Depression is complicated. Ontology, etiology, pathogenesis, typology, phenomenology, hermeneutics, symptomology, pharmacology, and functionality are not singular. In more familiar terms, we cannot merely say that depression stems solely from evolution, genetics, neurochemistry, sin, the devil, slothfulness, cognitive distortion, family environment, social injustice, boredom, or the depths of despair. It may be all of these, any of these, or none of these. Etiological and hermeneutical inquiries are complicated by multiple factors that work within a variety of theoretical frameworks that work within a range of semantic domains that work within a variety of historical and cultural contexts. All or any one of these frameworks and contexts are limited in their perspective. Finally, the redemptive model, offered in chapter 9, draws intentionally from the Trinity and Chalcedon and is a critical response to all three theological types reviewed in the middle chapters.

CONCLUSION

Depression is an all-consuming experience. It can inundate every aspect of one's life and manifest physically, mentally, emotionally, spiritually, relationally, and in other ways. The result is often a sense of multidimensional loss (connection with self, others, the world, and God) that paralyzes one's sense of agency. The will seems deactivated. Persons with melancholia can feel like their sense of self and their world are disintegrating. Nothing holds together. Life loses meaning, purpose, and direction. Further, one feels powerless to change one's predicament. The depressive condition feels like a deadly poison that voraciously eats away at every vestige of order, function, ability, connection, and faith that one has. Spiraling despair drives one to doubt self, one's faculties, reality, and even God. The theological case made in this work is that the holy love of God in Christ through the Spirit can create a new order amid cognitive chaos. God with us and in us can be the ontological anchor for persons with melancholia. We can find a transcendent mooring for self, our world, and our faith when all seems to be dissipating into nothingness. The transcendence of God becomes that Archimedean fixed point whereby God in Christ can dislodge us from the pit of despair and graciously move us forward into the hope of the future.

Christ was clothed in a body of weakness in order to identify with our human condition, that we might be clothed in him. As part of our broken human condition, melancholia is embodied by Christ in his cruciformity. He takes on the disfigured human condition and transfigures it into a new creation. Christ formed in us. Christoformity, informed by the subversive kingdom of God, redefines form and is intended to be the new form of all forms, for "abled" and "disabled." Persons who experience depression, anxiety, or other mental disorders in their weakness are being renewed by the Spirit daily. Society and the church are offered redemption from their prejudice and unjust acts of oppression against those with psychiatric disabilities. If anyone is in Christ—namely, the weak—we are a new creation.

2

Ontology of Melancholia

Definitions, Ontologies, and Anthropological Problems

INTRODUCTION

I begin by asking the ontological question, What is depression? I will crit-ically examine melancholia both historically and philosophically according to the latest models and theories in an attempt to answer this question. A survey of the latest definitions and ontologies will be analytically explored with an eye for theories that are nonreductive, explanatory (covering a wide bandwidth), and consonant with a theological approach to anthropol-ogy. Too often we have taken shortcuts and generalized in our conclusions. Reductive theories about humanity can result in reductive theories about depression. Broader research illustrates that there is a strong correlation between proposed models of mental disorder and their underlying theories of anthropology. This mantra will be repeated all throughout this book. Biological models tend to reflect a physicalist anthropology, while semiotic or cultural models tend to reflect a constructive or cultural anthropology. Historically, for example in the medieval period, theological interpreta-tions of mental disorder were more commonly found, as opposed to the biomedical interpretations posited today. The desert monastic notion of acedia within a Christian hamartiology was considered a valid etiologi-cal possibility when identifying mental disorder. In this case, a theologi-cal anthropology of the fall informed the interpretation of the nature of mental disorder. Currently, due to a predominant physicalist approach to philosophical anthropology, theological interpretations are rarely taken seriously in the scientific community.[1] How we view human nature impacts our understanding of mental health. Thus, this study will propose that a theanthropic relational anthropology has significant bearing on how we understand the theological nature and treatment of mental disorder.

DEFINING MELANCHOLIA, ITS COGNATES, AND THEIR BACKGROUND

Let us survey a few of the seminal texts from the history and philosophy of melancholia as we attempt to identify what is depression. Psychiatrist, physician, and author of the classic *Melancholia and Depression*, Stanley Jackson rightly claims, "In the terms *melancholia* and *depression* and their cognates, we have well over two millennia of the Western world's ways of referring to a goodly number of different dejected states."[2] Terms and definitions across time are innumerable and wide ranging. Historically, these terms at any particular time may have denoted a disease, a severe condition, a "cluster of symptoms," an unusual mood or emotional state, or a temperament of a particular character.[3] The language used to classify and define such states, and the states themselves, have varied across time and culture and are best understood both synchronically, as unique contextual expressions, as well as diachronically, with language that is distinct and yet broadly related to and built upon historical antecedents. As Wittgenstein helped us to understand, words and language in general are best understood in context. Simply, melancholia has manifested through a plethora of iterations over time, each contextually unique and yet more or less related to a general human condition of despondency.

A poignant diachronic question that gets to the heart of the matter is whether the melancholy of the premodern world is the same as the clinical depression of today. Jennifer Radden, specializing in philosophy of psychiatry, asserts, and I concur, that the current designation of *depression* does not refer to the same conditions that *melancholia* and *melancholy* did in the seventeenth and eighteenth centuries.[4] Depression is understood differently across time. Although there are similarities in terms of general features, such as a speculative biological component, sociocultural factors, and symptoms that warrant comparisons, "the conclusion that there is but one unchanging condition identified as *melancholia* in the past and renamed depression in our own era represents a troubling oversimplification."[5] This assertion stems from Radden's ontological analysis of melancholia over time and is tackled in the section below entitled "Ontology of Depression."[6] Consequently, any claim to a singular designation across time and space is a nonstarter when defining the complex instantiations of depression. Human despondency takes on distinctive forms and interpretations across cultures and across time. Examining a basic etymology of key terms within the semantic domain of depression can work as a starting point to unpack this loaded term both historically and ontologically.

Let us turn to the word itself, *melancholia*, and its definitions. *Melancholia* is a transliteration from two Greek words, *melas* (black) and *chole* (bile), brought together, μέλαινα χολή (*melaina chole*).[7] The term was translated into Latin as *atra bilis* and into English in the fourteenth century as *malencolye*. Later, the translation morphed to *melancoli* and *malencolie*. In the sixteenth century the word changed to *melancholie* and in the seventeenth century to *melancholy*.[8] In Jackson's estimation, these terms genealogically were all cognates of *melancholia*, which was defined variously across time.[9] Although the terms *melancholy* and *melancholia* may have functioned as synonyms for centuries, by the nineteenth century the homologous terms diverged to denoting distinct manifestations. *Melancholy* faithfully points to the normal human condition of occasional or poetic subjective suffering due to the slings and arrows of sadness and dejection to which the flesh is heir.[10] On the other hand, *melancholia* references the abnormal or pathological variant, anticipating the current usage of the idiom *depression*.[11]

Returning to Greek etymology, *melancholia* or *black bile / choler* (*melaina chole*) is one of the four humors along with yellow bile (choler), blood, and phlegm from the ancient Greek humoral theory as introduced by Hippocrates (460–c. 370 BCE) in the fifth century BCE. Hippocrates' theory was incorporated by Aristotle (384–322 BCE) and Galen (130–200 CE), physician to the emperor of Rome, whose work was foundational to Western medicine for centuries. Greek humoral theory formed the standard theory or basis of interpretation of depression up until the eighteenth century.[12] In Greek medical science, humoral theory as related to health and wholeness alleged that the four humors or fluids, later temperaments,[13] need to be in balance with each other, with the corresponding four Pythagorean elements (fire, air, earth, and water), with the four qualities of those elements (heat, cold, dry, and wet), and with the four related seasons. The imbalance of black bile, or the melancholic humor, was key to the "etiological factor" in melancholia.[14] Hence, the term *melancholia* was used to signify both the black bile humor itself and the imbalance of the humors, or disease, which manifested as fear, sorrow, despondency, or depression.[15]

Following the Greco-Roman humoral theory, the desert monastic tradition of Christianity examined mental disorder through hamartiological categories and ascetic spirituality. The tradition exemplified by the desert ascetics Evagrius Ponticus (345–399 CE) and John Cassian (360–433 CE) expanded the semantic domain of melancholia to the notion of *acedia* (idleness, boredom, slothfulness). Acedia was one of the eight (later seven) deadly sins that insidiously crept into the mind of the monk who was seeking to ascend the spiritual ladder of mystical union with the divine. In mid-ascent, the monk is thwarted by the "noonday demon" through *logismoi* (or passionate thoughts), falling into the pit of slothfulness and rendered ineffective. In Alina Feld's hermeneutics of depression, melancholy (as sadness) and acedia are viewed as two of the predominating hypostases of the genus that subsume all of its other iterations.[16] Synonyms for *acedia* include sloth, hypochondria, and boredom, while sadness, tristitia, mourning, and despair served as synonyms for melancholy. Both melancholy and acedia are assumed in the category of depression with a semantic range from "apathy, fatigue, pusillanimity, *taedium vitae*, spleen, ennui, depression, to even madness."[17] Contrary to usage in other historical periods, the entire medieval semantic range of melancholia is cast in a theological light as a condition brought about by moral lapse.

Subsequently, the ages of classical humanism and the Renaissance shifted the contextual focus of melancholia away from transcendent, religious, and moral categories to more immanent sensibilities. Instead of defining depression in theological terms, the Renaissance sought humanist terms. The Florentine Neoplatonism of Marsilio Ficino[18] (1433–1449) reclaimed the Aristotelian notion[19] that melancholia is attendant with genius and the heroic spirit through the Saturnine nature.[20] The term *melancholia* designated an areligious despondency in Elizabethan melancholy, characterized in Robert Burton's (1577–1640) classic *Anatomy of Melancholy* (1621) as causeless sadness and fear. Melancholic genius was later Romanticized in the eighteenth and nineteenth centuries as an aspect of the artistic or poetic charism in the so-called melancholy man heroic figure.[21] Depression figured as a muse. Finally, by the late nineteenth century the term *melancholia* gave way to the modern language of depression, as related to the biomedical disease model initiated in the work of pioneer psychiatrist Emil Kraepelin (1856–1926).[22]

Throughout the twentieth century, the biological disease model would advance correspondingly with the development and influence of the biological sciences, resulting in chemical treatments and a "medicalization" of the condition. Other currents tended to veer away from speculative biomedical etiology and directly treat empirical symptomology by addressing the underlying "core beliefs" that function as immediate correlates of depression. Various forms of cognitive therapy have taken this route. Modern cognitive approaches echo strategies implemented by the Stoics and later Immanuel Kant with faculty psychology. Innovators Aaron Beck (1921–),[23] with cognitive behavioral therapy, and Albert Ellis (1913–2007),[24] with rational emotive behavioral therapy, independently developed evidence-based strategies rooted in autodidactic cognitive restructuring for emotive and behavioral alignment. As of late this method has been coupled with techniques of mindfulness to reduce stress and symptoms. A symptom-based approach is also the prevailing epistemology in the *Diagnostic and Statistical Manual of Mental Disorders*, 5th edition (*DSM-5*).[25] However, in the *DSM-5* melancholia is no longer a distinct disorder but is a subtype of major depressive disorder. In melancholic depression, *melancholic* is a specifier for MDD, indicating features such as loss of pleasure or reaction to pleasurable stimuli.

THE MODERN TERM *DEPRESSION*

With the shift in nomenclature over the past century away from *melancholia*, *depression* has become the prevailing generic idiom used with major depressive disorder, occupying clinical currency as its predominant pathological iteration. The term *depression* is derived from the "Latin *de* (down from) and *premere* (to press), and *deprimere* (to press down)."[26] The Latin terms *depressare* and *depremere*[27] (also to press) convey "to be pressed down (in spirits)," or *depressio*. In terms of historical usage, *depression* seems to be more of a modern coinage. Robert Burton, who suffered from the malady and wrote his epic *Anatomy* in part to keep "busy to avoid melancholy,"[28] hardly mentions the term *depression* in his colossal 1383-page compendium. It was poet, essayist, and lexicographer Samuel Johnson (1709–1784), who read Burton's *Anatomy* and was also a lifelong sufferer from depression, who used the term *depression* more frequently as denoting a "pressing down of the mind."[29]

Surprisingly, prior to the nineteenth century, the term would rarely be used taxonomically as a formal diagnostic category. Jackson recognized that "the nineteenth century witnessed an increasingly frequent use of *depression* and its cognates in literary contexts to mean 'depression of spirits,' 'melancholia,' and 'melancholy' . . . and also in 'descriptive accounts of melancholic disorders to denote affect or mood.'"[30] *Depression* eventually became more frequently employed in the mid-nineteenth century as a synonym for *melancholia* in medical texts and dictionaries, like those of Wilhelm Griesinger and Daniel Hack Tuke.[31]

In the late nineteenth century, Emil Kraepelin, who is often claimed as the father of modern psychiatry, sought to ground the field in modern science, as opposed to humoral theory or other precritical notions. His advances anticipated the modern biomedical model. Kraepelin identified depression as a disease with biological correlations, specifically brain pathology. He is recognized as one of the first to employ the term *depression* clinically. Although he did use the term *melancholia*, he also employed the nomenclature of depression alongside insanity (*depressive insanity*), paranoia (*depressive form*), and mania (*manic-depressive*), under which he subsumed all mood disorders, and in essence subsumed and consumed all iterations of melancholia.[32] American psychiatrist Adolf Meyer (1866–1950), who was a contemporary of Kraepelin and Sigmund Freud (1956–1939), argued that the category of depression as a clinical term should replace that of melancholia and introduced the designation more formally.[33] By the late nineteenth century, *depression* had replaced *melancholia* and functioned as the primary clinical idiom for the syndrome, anticipating clinical and legal standardization in the genealogy of DSMs.

The *DSM-5*, published by the American Psychiatric Association, is the gold standard instrument in the United States for taxonomy, classification, and diagnosis of mental disorders, providing a psychiatric lingua franca of standardization in the field. The epistemological method of the *DSM-5* is an empirically grounded descriptivism,[34] rather than a causally or etiologically based one, relying on definitions and descriptions of clinical features of disorders as a shared reference for the industry in the United States. The *DSM-5*'s global counterpart, produced by the World Health Organization (WHO), is the *International Statistical Classification of Diseases and Related Health Problems* (*ICD-10*), which classifies and diagnoses mental disorders and broader health issues. In both manuals, depression is defined primarily by symptomatology subjectively reported, although signs that are observable by others and that are objectively reported are employed as well.[35] The DSM's epistemology and sociocultural location indubitably circumscribe its contextual influence on the classification and diagnosis of disorders, as would those of any instrument.

USE OF *MELANCHOLIA* IN THIS TEXT

A nosology, or the enterprise of naming, defining, and classifying diseases and disorders, of depression or *melancholia* and its cognates is a daunting task, to say the least. In the title and throughout the text, I employ the term *melancholia* as a genus, or general taxonomic category, and more out of convenience to provide wide-ranging, shared language, or a linguistic placeholder, for the facility of discourse rather than claiming at first any specific or precise meaning. Although the designation *melancholia* has carried over time both generic and specific connotations, its overall import is both historical and substantial and functions loosely to communicate the real and elusive condition of depression.[36] *Melancholia* will be used in this book both in its general/representative and particular historical designations. The context will determine which is being used.

Melancholia in the larger taxonomic sense will function as a genre or general term to categorize all of the manifestations and instantiations of the human condition, defined in a variety of ways but often summed up as a disorder of despondency in body, mood, mind, and behavior throughout time and space. In this usage, *melancholia* becomes an umbrella term for the genus that incorporates all of its diachronic iterations and related contextual species. *Melancholia*, in this way, serves as a convenient construct for discourse to facilitate analysis and conversation. The premise in using *melancholia* in a representative and symbolic sense is that the human condition of despondency is not named, theorized, expressed, or realized in precisely the same manner across time and space in terms of manifestation, semiotics, hermeneutics, nosology, etiology, pathogenesis, symptomology, or regimen/treatment. Thus, a widely familiar term is warranted to function in discourse.[37] Finally, along with its general use, the term will also be used specifically as an iteration of depression from a particular period in time, such as the eighteenth-century notion of melancholia as charism.

PROBING FOR AN ONTOLOGY OF DEPRESSION

After this brief survey of the historical development of depression, the ontological question of depression remains open. "What is depression?" as John Swinton asks in his article "Theology or Therapy? In What Sense Does Depression Exist?"[38] Is the notion of depression related to a real, objective disease, or is such a notion reified with this claim? Is depression a thing, a definable entity? Is it like other diseases, such as cancer, that can be tested and identified? Is depression rooted in a malfunctioning of the brain, that is, the "felt effects of an underlying dysfunctional state of the brain which has caused, and so causally explains, the felt symptoms and more readily observed signs?"[39] Or is the malady social in origin, a form of conflict and oppression elicited by a variety of contextual forces acting upon the subject, experienced symptomatically? Is depression a construct that is informed by multiple value-laden factors that are biological, psychological, and/or social? Further, and most importantly, is depression theological? If so, what contribution can theology make to answering the question of depression? Proposed answers are often negotiated between the tension of biological and sociocultural hermeneutics, correlating with a particular philosophical anthropology. As contending medical and social models dominate mental health, so likewise do their cognates dominate disabilities studies in general.[40] The field is forever working out the tension between medical and social influences on disability. As William Gaventa states, "There is no nondebated, static, universal, or objective definition of disability."[41] We may not be able to answer unequivocally the ontological question of depression, or even mental disorders, but addressing the question allows us to begin to discover limitations and inadequacies in our research, definition, and treatment of the subject. We may find current models of depression and their link to certain philosophical anthropologies wanting, as such notions of what it means to be human often restrict any "unscientific" analysis or influence from theological inquiry.[42]

As highlighted above, a brief, cursory analysis of mental disorder and depression reveals the heterogeneity of the melancholia idiom. Historically, depression has been construed as humoral imbalance,[43] acedia[44] or moral idleness, natural affect gone awry and becoming fear and sadness,[45] saturnine creative genius,[46] ennui,[47] meaninglessness,[48] mourning over loss,[49] and absurdity and entropy internalized,[50] among other, more modern biomedical iterations. More recently the question has been asked whether depression is a disease, a disorder,[51] a syndrome,[52] cognitive distortion,[53] evolutionary maladaptation,[54] a semiotic problem,[55] social conditioning,[56] a harmful dysfunction,[57] an aberration in brain structure and function, or a marketable commodity for the pharmaceutical industry.[58] These and many other claims have been made to identify the elusive phenomenon of depression. The diversity of definitions and analyses of melancholia are in part a logical outcome of the respective theoretical frameworks from which they are derived. Thus, there are biomedical, psychological, social constructive, semiotic, evolutionary, and other models available that reflect their respective epistemologies and anthropologies.

It is revealing to explore briefly an ontology and epistemology of depression. Philosophical influences are embedded wittingly or unwittingly in every theory or model of depression. Aristotle, among others, is often credited with the apocryphal statement, "If we ought to philosophize, we ought to philosophize, and if we ought not to philosophize, we ought to philosophize." Exploring the philosophical roots behind our constructs of depression is needed. Philosophers of science can plot disease on a continuum of realism-antirealism on three different levels: ontological, semantic, and epistemological. On one end of the spectrum would be scientific realism, with critical realism somewhere in the middle, followed by constructive empiricism, instrumentalism, and on the other end any variant of idealism.[59]

The *ontological* question asks whether the reality, in this case depression, is mind independent (external reality) or dependent (idealism). The *semantic* question, which pertains to the relationship between reality and language, asks whether the scientific statements made about observable and unobservable realities have a literal meaning and can be taken as true or false (semantic realism), or whether such statements function in some other nonliteral way, especially regarding unobservables, as in instrumentalism and constructive empiricism. Constructive empiricism and instrumentalism are agnostic as to unobservable reality and claims about it. On the other hand, instrumentalism asserts that the meaning of sentences about observable reality functions pragmatically as a useful tool (an instrument) for predicting phenomena but not literal in terms of empirical adequacy. However, in terms of observable reality, constructive empiricism holds that scientific claims are semantically literal in terms of empirical adequacy.[60]

Finally, the *epistemological* question asks whether the scientific claims we make about the world (observable or unobservable) constitute real knowledge or not. In other words, can we have knowledge of an external mind-independent world? Translated into our discussion, is or are there a disease entity or entities causal to depression, or is depression more sociocultural in origin? Is depression a product of neurobiology, computationally understood, is it cultural, or is it something in the middle? Can we know the truth about scientific claims concerning such a relationship? Finally, does this entail real knowledge of disease and depression? Answers to these questions are thoroughly debated by specialists in the interdisciplinary field of philosophy of disease and are beyond the scope of this text. However, the inquiry brings to light what is to be debated and what is at stake. There is no room for convenient reductions. For our purposes, we can examine a broad sketch of some of the prevailing opinions in lieu of the claims staked between scientific realism (usually biological) and antirealism (usually constructive), with attention paid to tendencies toward reductionism and explanatory power.

OUR AIM IN EXAMINING ONTOLOGIES OF DEPRESSION

A topography of ontologies for mental disorder and depression, according to Lawlor, can be laid out between the principal polarizing positions of various biological objectivist theories and constructivist theories, usually cultural constructivist theories.[61] Is depression biological, in regard to etiology, specifically neurochemical, or is the syndrome a value-laden, sociocultural construct or something in between? Are we creatures of chemistry or creatures of culture? Nature or nurture? Several models will be reviewed. In critiquing these models, our intention is to veer away from reductionism on either end of the spectrum (objectivism or interpretivism), which may reduce the model's explanatory power to cover depression's elusive etiology and symptomology. Reductionistic theories can carry over into an oversimplified view of what it means to be human, that is, a reductive physicalist notion that views humans as merely biological material beings, as opposed to constructivist or even theological notions. A guiding hypothesis in this work is that theories of depression mirror theories of anthropology. In other words, we interpret depression in terms of how we ontologically define humanity, either on one end as physical beings or on the other end as cultural beings. What about the ancient claim that we are spiritual beings, beings bent toward transcendence? The problem becomes that our philosophical anthropologies may turn up wanting, especially if they do not account for or at least reference immateriality or our relationship with the divine. The goal of this chapter is not to identify or construct an ontology of depression on purely philosophical or scientific grounds or both. One aim, though, is to examine existing models and identify or develop a model that can allow for a theological contribution that addresses the problem of depression. Thus, in searching for a model that can accommodate theological input, we are looking for a flexible, integrative model that is broad, nonreductive, and open to transcendent causal mechanisms, such as the divine, and yet can incorporate the valid findings of existing models, such as in the biological, social, and psychological models.

VARIOUS ONTOLOGIES OF DEPRESSION

Jennifer Radden's own breakdown of key ontologies of depression is divided into causal (biological and psychological) and descriptive models (based on clusters of observable symptoms, e.g., *DSM-5*).[62] Biological theories are mainly tied to causal models of disease that explain how the signs and symptoms of the syndrome are generated. These models hold some form of realism (on ontological, epistemological, and semantic levels), usually *entity* realism expressed in a real disorder that is addressed by biological psychiatry.[63] The criticism leveled at entity realism is basically that no biological etiology has ever been identified for mental disorders. Simply, science has never located the biological agent that directly causes depression, though neural correlates may be identified. Also, a strict biological explanation does not account for empirical cultural factors.

On the other hand, a descriptivist ontology, found in the *DSM-5*, deviates from causal explanations and steers toward an attempt at a "shared discourse" in the field, classifying clusters based on observable signs and symptoms derived from "psychological, bodily, and behavioral traits."[64] Significance is placed on classification and categorization based on observable phenomena, not on etiology. The descriptive ontology of the *DSM-5* also attempts to recognize factors in cultural formation[65] and its impact on the experience of illness.[66]

Yet it is not surprising that the genealogy of DSMs has always endured harsh criticism of all sorts, some warranted, including reductionism, lack of reliability, overdiagnosis,[67] and ethnocentrism, among a host of other concerns. Beginning early in the 1960s, psychiatric nosology, as reflected in the

DSM, had been under fire with the stinging critique of the field of psychiatry in general delivered by Thomas Szasz, who claimed the entire enterprise was a fabrication. Szasz alleged that the psychiatric industry and its creation and classification of mental disorder and treatments were a construct via legislation and medicalization.[68] In his seminal work *The Age of Melancholy*, which identifies the social origins of depression, Dan Blazer rightfully laments the recent obstruction of social psychiatry, the medicalization of mental health, and the misdirected localization of disorder in the autonomous biological individual.[69] He pinpoints the gross neglect of recognizing the social forces impacting mental health. Social factors influencing mental disorder, including poverty, sex, gender, and racism, are surely understated and need further consideration for a fully orbed diagnosis and treatment.[70] Often social constructs, limitations, and stigmas related to psychiatric disability create as much as if not more disability than the impairments themselves. As a result, there are many who hold strictly to the social construction of disability and disorder, believing they are created in toto. Recently, there have been needed social (Brown and Harris),[71] cultural (Kleinman and Good), and political-economic[72] appraisals of the field. We note that their work incorporates various social models of disability. In its most radical forms, the model understands disability as something created by society's oppressive structures, laws, policies, and practices that restricts persons with neurodevelopmental disorders, which are not pathological or problematic in themselves. The neurodiversity movement, which uses the social model, claims that "our concept of mental illness should be revised to reflect the diverse forms of cognition that humans are capable of without stigmatizing individuals that are statistically non-normal."[73]

These reactions are challenges to supplement or supplant the biomedical model, enhance descriptive models, and incorporate key contextual factors in the construal of mental disorders. Even the DSM through its fifth edition has recently responded to many of these challenges and currently operates more out of a biopsychosocial approach rather than a purely biomedical framework. In this sense, the biological aspect is treated by pharmacology, while the psychosocial aspect of the disorder is treated by therapy and the social dimension is addressed through laws, policies, and practices. Constructivist efforts have provided needed social critiques and added to the overall explanatory power of our modeling. But we need to be aware of easy reductions motivated by ideology. The dismissal or denial of the biological either ontologically or causally, although in vogue across the soft sciences and pop cultural opinion, would be shortsighted, irresponsible, and disastrous. If anything, depression is at least somatic and psychosomatic.

In spite of the vast improvements in the treatment of depression, there are still growing challenges in understanding the nature of this disorder and care for persons. As we feel the increasing impact of globalization and unprecedented growing diaspora movements, the reality and influence of culture become more acute in defining, diagnosing, and treating mental disorders. Regarding cultural impact on disease, Arthur Kleinman, among others in anthropological medicine and cross-cultural psychiatry, has reconstructed theories of depression cross-culturally, developing them out of an interpretive cultural anthropology. Kleinman's work with the somatization of depression as experienced in Chinese culture led him to recognize that not all illness is defined and experienced the same. Rather than conceptualizing and suffering depression through mental and emotional states of despondency and sadness, persons in Chinese culture tended to experience depression through bodily pain, such as in the lower back.[74] Illness is at first a culturally interpretive experience made by the client in terms of perceived symptomology. The clinician proceeds to reinterpret the narrative in terms of signs of a particular disease as directed by a particular framework of pathology.[75] Thus, "diagnosis is a semiotic act."[76]

Ultimately, a culturally constructivist perspective views medicine itself as a cultural and subsequently a semiotic construct. For Kleinman, "*disease* refers to a malfunctioning of biological and/or physiological processes, while the term *illness* refers to the psychological experience and meaning of a perceived disease."[77] Thus, as a medical anthropologist working out of the interpretive school, Kleinman bifurcates *disease* and *illness* along the lines of the biological etic (external/outsider) perspective and the cultural emic (internal/insider) perspective. Although Kleinman relies heavily on the semiotics of illness and seems intentionally nebulous as to whether the notion of disease is to be construed etiologically, descriptively, or agnostically,[78] he nonetheless acknowledges that "the biological component of clinical depression is important and cannot be disregarded."[79] Thus, the tension between biological and cultural approaches continues.[80]

Though Kleinman, in passing, tips his hat to biology, it may just be a perfunctory gesture. Kleinman's colleague at Harvard in medical anthropology Byron Good claims that Kleinman holds to a culturally constructive view of disease that is not grounded ontologically in nature as an entity but in meaning via signs that give shape to an explanatory model,[81] that is, "the social production of disease," "the cultural construction of illness," and "the clinical construction of reality."[82] Disease is understood as medical semiotics and hermeneutics, as even the self and the world are also understood in the same way. Good elaborates his own position on the clinical construction of reality,[83] "arguing that medicine formulates the human body and disease in a culturally distinctive fashion," while biology is not external but is a symbolic form within culture and constructed by culture.[84] Hence a semiotic anthropology lends to a semiotic approach to mental disorder.[85]

What are the problems with the conclusion that humanity and disease are constructed by semiotic representation, besides the issue of realism versus antirealism? One practical problem is communication. Lawlor, as well as Good,[86] recognizes the dilemma with cross-cultural translatability between semiotic worlds, which by a constructivist definition are incommensurable. One is never translating apples for apples. Hence, Lawlor claims that one cannot have cross-cultural discourse without some notion of the universal, which seems to be the innate aporia with cultural anthropology and relativism and the main point of tension with any natural or biological model.[87] The WHO, through its management of the *International Classification of Disease and Related Health Problems* (*ICD*), attempts a global perspective accounting for cultural diversity but is still vastly influenced by Western nosology and struggles to find a universal cross-cultural framework of clinical utility and global applicability to identify and treat mental disorders.[88] The inability to find a valid, acceptable ground for universal concepts and meaning, language, and translatability is a perennial problem for frameworks that tend to place extensive ontological and epistemic weight on the matrix of culture, fostering cultural solipsism or even nihilism.[89] Thus, reducing anthropology and ontology of depression to either neurobiology or culture becomes problematic.

A deeper look at the ontological landscape of depression reveals that the ebb and flow from theory to theory oscillates between biology and culture. Unlike Kleinman and the constructivists, professor of psychiatry Stanley Jackson declines separating "disease" from "illness" but nonetheless recognizes that historically the philosophical nature of depression has been bifurcated. He divides disease into "ontological theories of disease," such as entity realism (disease as a physical entity), and "physiological theories," more related to structural realism, which theorizes real relations rather than existent disease entities. Physiological theories attempt to identify "bodily reactions and deviations from the norm in response to a pathogenic agent" with standards of norms and deviations varying across culture that are thus value laden.[90]

On the contrary, objective naturalist views, such as entity realism, as opposed to physiological, value-laden normative models established by social standards, attempt to identify health and disease based on biological facts from statistically normal functioning systems that are determined by their ability to survive and reproduce.[91] Christopher Boorse is responsible for the Biostatistical Theory of Health (BST), one of the leading theories of naturalism. The BST seeks to move away from the evaluative, relative constructivist view and toward a more objective account of disease based on properly functioning biological mechanisms and processes as indicated by what is statistically typical for a reference class in question, such as middle-aged white females.[92] Critiques of this and other versions of naturalism attempt to demonstrate how all models, processes, and categories, such as reference classes, are evaluative and not objective. Through these examples, it is clear that the tension between any objective and constructive features or between entire models is the recurrent, problematic conflict within epistemological realism as to whether one can know mind-independent reality, or whether knowledge is always context bound, and what the nature is of that reality—chemical or cultural or both. In any case, we end up with a reductionism that does not fully explain the greater reality. Either the chemical or the cultural component is left out, and in all cases there is no consideration of transcendent, spiritual, or theological factors.

Some propose a way forward, at least between the aporia "biology versus culture," through a middle ground between these two poles. Professor Jerome Wakefield constructs a hybrid model that integrates both objective scientific accounts with value-laden sociopolitical accounts of mental disorder.[93] Wakefield's depression as "harmful dysfunction" similarly operates with an objective biological/physiological component of dysfunction working alongside a subjective cultural construction of harm or deprivation of well-being. Dysfunction is deviation from the normative, natural function of a causal mechanism that no longer performs as it was intended by natural selection through evolution and is deemed harmful by social standards.[94] Critiques[95] of this position, however, cite the existence of spandrels and vestigial parts as defeaters since they represent disorder without dysfunction or evolutionary malfunction.[96]

THE MODEL OF CRITICAL REALISM

One strategy to overcoming a reductive polarization of the biological and the cultural was offered by the Austrian philosopher of science Karl Popper (1902–1994) in his "three worlds" model of reality.[97] Simply, he proposes that things can coexist in three distinct worlds without reducing any one to the other. The first world is a physical world, consisting of physical energy and all things material. The second world is consciousness, comprising the mental or psychological world. The third world is the product of the human mind and action, such as language, theories, equations, formulas, works of art, products of culture and custom, and other human constructions. For

Popper, the three worlds are not mutually exclusive but coexist. Any given reality can occur at three levels of observation and experience. For example, a novel such as *The Sound and the Fury* can exist as a physical paperback in world one, as a psychological encounter in the mind of both Faulkner and the reader in world two, and as a literary product written by the author in world three. Using Popper's three worlds, we can overcome the tendency to polarize and reduce mental disorder to either a biological or sociocultural phenomena by acknowledging that it can exist in multiple worlds as biological, though that neurological work has yet to be developed conclusively; psychological, in the inner experience of the individual; sociocultural, in terms of its semiotic expression and hermeneutics; and even theological, in terms of our relationship with God, which is the goal of this book.

Another similar way forward philosophically can be found in another *via media*, multilevel approach to the problem. Critical realism[98] affirms both a mind-independent reality and the social process of science that produces value-laden, contextual, though nondeductive, analogical models of reality. For example, critical realist philosopher Roy Bhaskar (1944–2014) affirms three domains of reality, the real (causal mechanisms and structures), the actual (events or what actually happens due to causation), and the empirical (what is observed).[99] The real is mind independent. The actual is contextual, and the empirical is value laden. Any given reality can be tracked in all three domains, defeating any reductive, objectivist, or constructivist accounts of reality.

In a further application, some Christian missiologies incorporate critical realism to overcome the impasse between scientific realism and constructivism, while integrating theology as well. Christian missiologists and cultural anthropologists have long wrestled with the problem of cultural relativism and the difficulty of translating the gospel message through critical contextualization. Some have found a way forward through various forms of critical realism that allow for an external transcultural reality that is critically engaged and understood in terms of contextually mediated explanatory models.[100] Missiologically, such a system holds together the external, supracultural truth of divine revelation with contextual, local theologies that are understood and interpreted through culture-specific forms and semiotics. In this way, reductive extremes through a positivist, commonsense realism or a constructivist approach are avoided, and the integrity of multiple levels of reality, including the theological, are validated through an interdisciplinary critical realist approach.

When applying critical realism to a theory of mental disorder, "it is not reality which is deemed to be socially constructed (the axiomatic radical constructionist position), rather it is our theories of reality, and the methodological priorities we deploy to investigate it. Our theories and methods are shaped by social forces and informed by interests."[101] Critical realism affirms the empirical and contextual nature of the experience of illness and symptoms, and yet recognizes the real causal mechanisms that may be involved—though we are reminded in the case of depression that there are no biomarkers or conclusive identification of any neurobiological etiology, and thus etiology and ultimate causal mechanisms remain theoretical and speculative. Such a critical realist position "respects empirical findings about the reality of misery and its multiple determinants but does not collapse into the naive realism of medical naturalism. It accepts causal arguments but remains sensitive to the relationship between empirical methods and pre-empirical (e.g., professional) interests and social forces."[102] Critical realism offers a philosophical framework that accommodates a variety of levels of reality, including the theological, and has even been adapted and integrated by various Christian scholars and theologians, including T. F. Torrance, Alister McGrath, and N. T. Wright, as well as by scientist theologians, such as Ian Barbour, Arthur Peacocke, and John Polkinghorne. Scottish theologian and renowned disability scholar John Swinton also works from a type of critical realist epistemology when approaching spirituality and mental health.[103] His view holds to both an external world and constructed forms that mediate that world as well as the significance of our relationship with God in interpreting meaning while facing mental health problems.[104] A critical realist move permits us to incorporate a theological angle on the problem that can be integrated at some other point in time within a larger approach that would involve biological, psychological, and sociocultural perspectives.

Depression is a heterogeneous disorder, a complex, with multiple factors. It works within a variety of historical and cultural contexts that view it through multiple theoretical frameworks (biological, psychological, sociocultural, and even theological), which in turn express the phenomenon through a range of semantic domains.[105] A critical realism model that incorporates emergence can accommodate such vast terrain. Applying critical realism and the notion of emergence at a lower level, knowledge of neural correlates and neurological pathogenesis for depression is still in early development. However, we can hypothesize lower-level upward causation from neurons up to neurophysiology, biology, psychology, and then the sociological and then higher-level downward causation from the sociocultural and even theological back onto the psychological and so forth. Further, we do not know the real and ultimate generating mechanism of the phenomenon in terms of identifying the ultimate ontological reality of depression, what it is, whether genetic, chemical, traumatic, environmental, or even theological, and so on.

It is essential to remember that correlation is not causation. We know these are contributing factors to the phenomenon, but we ultimately do not know ultimate etiology. In latter chapters, however, we will hypothesize about theological mechanisms.

Critical realism examines mental disorder as a complex system that is shaped and occurs on a variety of emerging levels, including the neurobiological, psychological, sociocultural, and even theological. Mental disorders, such as depression, become emergent realities of consciousness and qualia. Thus, our ontological model, a critical realist one, integrates multiple levels of influence with an aim toward the theological. A theological perspective assumes that we are spiritual creatures, transcendent beings, persons in relation to God. A further inquiry into philosophical anthropology needs to be explored as we consider the validity of depression as theological.

PART II

THEOLOGICAL ANTHROPOLOGY

3

Models of Theological Anthropology and Depression

PHILOSOPHY OF MIND AND PHILOSOPHICAL ANTHROPOLOGY

Our journey has led us from exploring the nature of depression to the nature of humanity. We cannot comprehend the nature of depression without understanding how it is registered anthropologically. A nexus has been drawn between theoretical frameworks of depression and related philosophical anthropologies. Construals of mental disorder are influenced by the ways we define the nature of humanity, which are often reductive. A reductive physicalist anthropology conceives of depression in biochemical terms and is treated similarly. A constraining approach to the human person may have parallel consequences, resulting in a constrained approach to treatment, one that may be unduly controlled externally by the market and internally by overestimating the capacity and value of rationality and autonomy to the exclusion of contextual factors. Such factors as environment, socioeconomics and poverty, family systems, culture, race and ethnicity, as well as philosophical and theological concerns, are often not accounted for in the modern biomedical model.

Proceeding forward, we need to examine more critically the existing relationship between the ontology and epistemology of depression and philosophical anthropology. Until the Enlightenment, philosophical anthropology for the most part had been dominated by some form of dualism involving material and immaterial substances, from Plato to Descartes. Theories of melancholia correspondingly were located in bodily humors and/or psychological states or even in moral states as related to the immaterial soul. With the increase of the development of the hard sciences and our epistemic reliance on them since the Enlightenment project, the shift has been toward a physicalist (either nonreductive or reductive, usually reductive), hyperrational, and positivist (evolutionary) view of the human person. These anthropologies have their correlating theories of disorder, usually to the exclusion of theological consideration.[1]

The options are dizzying. Currently, such concerns occupy the field of philosophy of mind.[2] Perspectives vastly range from eliminative materialism[3] to physicalism (reductive or nonreductive)[4] to property dualism[5] to substance dualism[6] to panpsychism,[7] with some version of physicalism occupying the predominant view in scholarly scientific and philosophical circles. Few of these options in today's research would consider the human person in any immaterial sense, let alone in relationship with an immaterial God. Nonetheless, any version that holds to some variant of an immaterial substance could potentially argue for mind and even soul and thus create space for transcendence, the divine, and a theological anthropology. An ontology of consciousness that identifies human experience as immaterial or even an interaction of two substances (material and immaterial) can correlate such experience with an immaterial theological anthropology. Further, an immaterial theological anthropology will account for depression similarly in terms of immateriality. In any case, by hypothetically considering the immateriality of human experience, we carve out space to consider further the possibility of human persons, at least in part, as immaterial, even theological, beings. This conclusion is also undergirded by Scripture. We noted that biblical language utilizes terms that point to our material (embodiment) and immaterial (spirit, soul, mind) orientation and relation to both creation and the divine.

There are other options for nonphysical reality as well. Although not claiming immaterial substance like soul or spirit for the human person, some versions of nonreductive physicalism also account for nonphysical properties, such as mind. In this case mind is a supervenient property of the brain, followed by the strong emergence of consciousness and first-person human experience that is dependent upon but not explained by physical substance. In that case, depression, like any other experience, becomes emerging first-person qualia from a neurological substrate. Depression becomes an emerging bio-cognitive-emotional illness with a certain emerging conscious quality of symptoms and suffering. Some theologians, such as Philip Clayton[8] and Amos Yong,[9] would expand this notion of strong emergence to include even the emergence of spirit and religious or transcendent experiences. Spirit emerges from transcending consciousness. Such a bold move brings the divine into the orbit of an empirical theological anthropology, opening the door for a theology of depression that is conversant with neurophilosophy. Although there are various possibilities, the reductive physicalist model is in currency and dominates the field, thus demanding our attention.

LIMITATIONS IN A REDUCTIVE PHYSICALIST ANTHROPOLOGY

The modernist biomedical model of mental disorders and depression is premised on a philosophical anthropology that is troubled, to say the least, precisely in its limitations. The model inherited an Enlightenment understanding of humanity and the self. This anthropology in its foundation or consequences is intertwined with an inflated rationality, reductive materialism, radical libertarian autonomy, unchecked consumerism, and a particularly limited substantive account of humanity, usually monistic reductive physicalism. A strong materialist worldview simply eliminates all nonmaterial outsiders. Transcendent and immaterial aspects of the universe and the human person are often discounted as mythic wish fulfillment of a bygone era or an uncritical, juvenile projection. Categories like soul/spirit (either emergent property or substance) or heaven and hell are readily dismissed and explained away or eliminated as the material universe, secular society, and the human person become an ever-closing and imploding, rationally disenchanted system.[10] These limitations lead to philosophical and social concerns that bear theological ramifications, which usually involve negating God's existence and activity in the world. Reductive physicalism fundamentally relies on strong natural causation. Philosophically, a closed, self-sufficient (causal closure) natural system of reality restricts any admission of the divine, divine agency, or divine action in the universe and in the life of a person. Strong physical causal closure claims that all events are physical, all physical events are physical effects, and all physical effects have sufficient physical causes.[11] Such stricture makes no room for the divine and reduces mind, consciousness, free will, and subjectivity to types of physical events with sufficient physical causes. In a self-originating and sustaining universe that seemingly demonstrates causal closure, immaterial causes or forces are unnecessary, per Ockham's razor. Left to reductive physicalism, we are perhaps left with atheism and a godless humanity.

As mentioned above, there are other options. There are versions of the nonreductive physicalist position that allow for emerging mental and spiritual properties that are supervenient upon physical substance and causes but also allow for downward causation from these properties. This position frequently conceives of the divine panentheistically, meaning the world is somehow within God, while God is not identical with the world (pantheism) but exceeds the world. Panentheism, for some, overcomes the problem of theism and causal closure. The theory allows for the existence, agency, and action of God as an emergent property within the world process, though at the cost of a traditional Christian view of God and creation.[12] Although the nonreductive physicalist and substance dualist positions make room for the divine, these positions are not accepted by much of the scientific community. Hence, we need to posit, rather than prove, the existence, agency, and action of God as postfoundationalist basic beliefs on our way toward a theological anthropology. Such an assumption is not without reason.

We posit this claim not based on traditional epistemological foundationalism,[13] which would require an unrealistic Cartesian degree and burden of proof that few other disciplines require to justify a belief. Though postfoundational, our assertion can demonstrate the rationality of our basic theistic belief if needed. However, we are not forced to commit at this time to an emergent panentheism or substance dualism, though both would be permissible, the former on scientific grounds and the latter perhaps on the grounds of Christian tradition interpreting Scripture. We take an epistemological pause. Many of these philosophical decisions are not necessary in order to stake a theological claim at this point and can be considered following. Our theological beliefs are not contingent on any particular philosophy of mind. In terms of proving the existence of the divine, epistemology does not precede ontology. We do not need a tautological, incorrigible foundation of proof of God before we can establish or even experience the existence of God. God's existence is an irreducible nonderivative that is not deduced or irrefutably inferred through argumentation but is a postfoundational, basic theological a priori belief.[14] Suprarational belief in the numinous is immediately, directly, and innately presented and established through God's self-revelation to God's creation. Its function is that we who are theological beings made in the image of God can participate and commune with the divine.[15] The revelation of God's existence is known innately, immediately, directly, and self-evidently as a basic belief that arises through the proper function of our spiritual senses. The further rationality of such a belief is subsequently confirmed through other evidences and arguments cumulatively considered but is not necessary to its establishment as an incorrigible foundation.[16] Simply for the scope and purpose of this work, we are asserting the existence of God and the agency and action of God in creation and our relationship with him.[17] The fact of God's existence and action in the universe affirms that there is more to reality than matter and that the Creator is active in our world.[18] This assertion is necessary to examine the theological nature of our relationship with the divine and a theological approach to mental disorder.

OTHER CRITIQUES OF REDUCTIVE PHYSICALISM

Having unpacked some of the philosophical limitations of an Enlightenment anthropology, we can move on to a few social limitations. The modern construct of the autonomous individual may have functionally run its course. The fallacy of the autonomous individual is the myth that the modern, self-constructed individual is a quasi-sovereign, self-sufficient, self-referential, libertarian polis that grants itself the space, the right, and the freedom to actualize and fulfill its own purpose without the need to reference the other or the divine.[19] This overly optimistic myth is coupled with a positivist evolutionary narrative as well that views the individual as adapting and developing for better fitness in a changing environment, including the overcoming of challenges, even (mental) disorder. An advanced capitalist society markets this fitness incentive to another level, engendering the cultural commodification of a commercial materialist *eudaemonia* as the goal of an evolutionary trajectory of our advancement. Our culture's commercial *eudaemonia*, a secular pseudo-salvation, is the right to happiness, over against merely the pursuit of happiness, which readily leads to a culture of narcissism[20] and the "triumph of the therapeutic" as a means to recover happiness when thwarted by despondency.[21] Western commodified *eudaemonia* is the core promise of the myth of the American Dream, the "evangel" of U.S. civil religion, which promises to supply every demand for happiness determined by the autonomous individual, often to the exclusion of moral correlation or consequence.

In terms of the right to pursue happiness and its relation to the market, the modern hyperindividual becomes a rational-choice consumer driven by the commodification of commercial happiness, as indicated by the tyranny of immediate sensation and symptom. Such a vision flies in the face of those whose agency is either not present or disabled by society's restrictions on physical and mental impairments. The fundamental fallacies are threefold. The first assumption is that such aimless consumption of *eudaemonic* experiences will not have moral consequences.[22] The second is that any inability to attain the goal of happiness is the result of a mental disorder and can be cured with therapy and medication.[23] The third is that the autonomous individual exists and is self-generating, self-sustaining, and meant to be self-serving without responsibility to the other.[24] Critiques and prophetic judgments leveled against the notion of a brave new world enlightened by autonomous rational beings that have evolved beyond good and evil and transcended their collective guilt of theocide are abundant.[25] Over the past century, disability,[26] existentialist,[27] and postmodern[28] thinkers have long reacted to and exposed the limitation and bankruptcy of such rationalist accounts and utopias that have denied and repressed their own internal contradictions. When honestly confronted with our own naked existence, we are haunted by a dystopia of the irrational, the absurd, the angst and alienation that characterize the shadow side of humanity (*Homo absurdus*) and reality.

Such polemics arise not just from the humanities but also from the sciences. Sociologist of religion Peter Berger[29] long prophesied the extinction of religion and the rule of the secular at the hands of science. Later he experienced a theological turn and recanted his former claims. He conceded that our valid inner longings and impulses amid secular entropy are signs pointing toward transcendence. Secularization can lead to sacralization.[30] The seemingly innate spiritual and religious predilections within the human person are also momentarily capturing the attention of the hard sciences as well. The neuroscience of religion or neurotheology, what at first appears to be a contradiction of terms, is a growing movement that seeks to comprehend the neural correlates of religious belief, experience, and practice.[31] In some cases claims are even made for the neural correlates of transcendence and spirituality, even a proto-consciousness and hardwiring for religious belief.[32] These trends are hardly proof of or even arguments for the existence of God, which is not required in this discourse. However, they are signs that we may be incurably religious, often presupposing faith in many of our so-called scientific commitments.[33] As some phenomenologists, existentialists, and others have taken a theological turn[34] to overcome the limitations of modernity, perhaps so should we in our investigation of the nature of mental disorder and depression. For humanity as a maker of transcendent or sacred meaning, religion is universal, structural, perennial, necessary, and inseparable from human endeavors. Religion claims to construct a well-ordered society that sufficiently addresses the key existential questions of life and so functionally serves a greater purpose. If we are creatures that seek and make meaning theologically, then we need not only to be aware of such predilections but to consider intentionally how theology can resource other concerns such as the mental health question.

THEOLOGICAL ANTHROPOLOGY AND THE *IMAGO DEI*

Our concern in this text is not to develop a full-blown theological model of depression that would eliminate existing nontheological models. The hope is that the theological framework constructed here could inform and supplement the deficiencies found in the biomedical model and be integrated into a larger holistic approach. The goal is to offer a theological corrective aimed at a faulty anthropology. The strategy of such a corrective is simple: attempt to round out and fill in the features that are conspicuously absent, inadequate, or insufficient in the biomedical model in terms of theology. Further, we need to critique our theology, which has often excluded persons with disabilities. What contribution can theology make to understanding and treating depression? How can we frame depression through the lens of theology? How does a theological contribution integrate and supplement existing models? These questions guide our exploration.

Humanity as a theological species, *Homo theologicus*, created in the *imago Dei* and in relation with God, is a common assertive ground to begin a theological anthropology. We will explore various options of the *imago Dei*. As created beings, we are contingent and dependent on God for our existence and ongoing life. In the *imago Dei*, we are not only *Homo sapiens* (sapient or wise), or rational creatures, we are also *Homo adorans* and *Homo liturgicus*, creatures in relation with the divine that worship and serve God. In utilizing classical theology of the great tradition, we know that we are also creatures that have fallen short of God's glory. We are encumbered by depravity and weakness, which impact all that we do, and are in need of redemption, which is found in Jesus Christ. On our journey from creation to fall to new creation, we are subject to all the natural shocks to which the flesh is heir, including the despair that awakens us from our fallen condition and the ensuing dark night that calls us into God's more perfect light.

We are reminded that anthropological commitments are telling when constructing an ontology of depression. Physicalist views of the human person lend toward a biological notion of mental disorder. Constructivist views of the human person that are cultural and semiotic lend toward a cultural construction of mental disorder. Moving away from reductionism, we noted that a critical realist view of the human person has better explanatory power covering greater ground, interpreting mental disorder as biological, social, psychological, and even theological. Critical realism and emergence allow for multiple levels of reality and causality to be at work, including theological mechanisms. Our task in a theology of depression begins with an analysis of a theological contribution to the human person that can inform how we think about mental disorder by resourcing Scripture and the great tradition. This study does not provide the space for a comprehensive theological anthropology. Nonetheless, some essential considerations can be useful. The *imago Dei* lends itself as a logical starting point in traditional theological anthropology. The Christian tradition, for the better part, has universally defined humanity, at least in part, in terms of the image of God. We will briefly examine the following models of the *imago Dei* and their relation to mental disorder: substantive, structural, functional (mediating power), and a proposed *imago Christi* relational or participatory model. We will also investigate these models of the *imago Dei* in light of agency and disability. Critical analyses will lend toward a proposal that addresses sufficiently not only theological concerns but also disability concerns as well, which are of equal or greater concern.

IMAGO DEI AS SUBSTANTIVE

As we begin to examine the three predominant models of the image of God, let us begin with some definitions. We define *imago* as copy, representation, or theologically as *analogia*.[35] There are a few ways to look at analogy. There is analogy of substance (being), or who or what are we. Analogy of structure (attribution) identifies what we have, and analogy of function (mission) labels what we do. When speaking of "substance" we are addressing ontology or the fundamental nature of being. What constitutes being or human being? What is the underlying, fundamental, irreducible, constitutive element, entity, or substance (Latin *substantia*: *sub*, under; and *stare*, to be or to stand) standing under or undergirding human nature? Much of this language and methodology is philosophical in its nature and historical development. We have examined the ontology of the human person in light of the classic mind-body problem. We have inquired into this problem through philosophy of mind and will continue to pursue the subject through a theological lens. Turning to Scripture, holy writ seems to suggest a theological anthropology of holism. Scripture addresses the entire human person over against any partite view of substances or attributes comprising the human person. However, biblical speculation on trichotomy (spirit, soul, and body, e.g., 1 Thess. 5:23), dichotomy (body and soul/spirit, e.g., Rom. 8), or monism (living soul, Gen. 2:7), which defines the ontological or constitutional problem of what is the human person, is similar to the problem we tackled with the philosophy of mind. Anthropological terminology is extensive and varying in Scripture: for example, *nephesh* (Heb: soul, life), *leb* (Heb: heart), *ruach* (breath, spirit), *basar* (Heb: flesh), *soma* (Gk: body), *psyche* (Gk: soul, natural life, self), *kardia* (Gk: heart), *nous* (Gk: mind), *pneuma* (Gk: spirit), *sarx* (Gk: flesh). However, these distinctions in context do not seem to point to any form of faculty psychology or partitioning of the human person in terms of substances or distinctive parts. It does seem to point to, at the least, an immaterial orientation (soul, mind, spirit) that we have toward the divine. Whatever we are, we are at least embodied immaterial beings. We have both a physical and spiritual orientation. The various anthropological terms connect us to both physical and spiritual realities in terms of experience and relationship. We are related to and commune with both creation and the divine. The biblical language reflects an integrated, holistic understanding of the entire person as fully embodied conscious self within creation, especially in the call of sinful humanity to salvation.[36]

However, if we are looking to Scripture to direct our sights to a singular anthropology, holy writ is not conclusive and does not seem to promote a sole or specific theory of ontology of human nature, beyond the holism of the human person directed relationally toward creation and God. Neither is our modern framing of the question addressed and answered by Scripture.[37] Our modern metaphysical and anthropological debate around substance/ essence versus process or constructive approaches is anachronistic and out-side of the Scripture writers' concerns.[38] Our indecision at this point is not to say that Scripture cannot inform a theological anthropology, but merely that the exegetical and hermeneutical work needed cannot be reduced so sim-plistically and a much more nuanced and detailed undertaking would be needed, which is beyond this work.[39] At this point, it seems Scripture points to a holistic integrative view of the human person over against any one sub-stantive or partite model. Additionally, the scriptural context for the variety of anthropological terminology, for example, *flesh*, *spirit*, or *soul*, is usually in relation to salvation, rather than an analysis of human nature.[40]

Moving from Scripture to history and the great tradition of the Christian faith, we further probe how historically we have defined human nature. Prior to the writing of the New Testament, we find the roots of the substantial-structural view of human nature in Plato (428/427 BCE–348/347 BCE) and Aristotle (385 BCE–323 BCE). Plato held basically a substance dualism of immortal soul and mortal body, while Aristotle proposed the hylomorphism or composite unity of being as body, or matter, and soul, or particular form. The views of these metaphysical giants echoed throughout the history of phi-losophy as well as through the great tradition within Christianity. Plato held that the immortal soul is imprisoned within the mortal body and seeks to be released back to its eternal form or ideal.[41] He located the soul or mind in the brain, inheriting the encephalic theory from Hippocrates.[42] Aristotle claimed human nature as an individual substance made up of the soul and the body, with the former as the *form* of the latter. He located the soul in the heart, a cardiovascular view inherited from Empedocles,[43] but defined the human person as primarily a "rational animal."[44] Both Plato and Aristotle understood the soul as rational in nature.[45] Many in the Christian tradition have built upon this definition, as well as upon a developing Logos tradition[46] and later Logos Christology.[47] Rationality became one of the primary features that defined the human person. Boethius (480–524 CE), and later Thomas

Aquinas (1225–1274),[48] who was dependent on Boethius, defined the human person as "naturae rationalis individua substantia" (an individual substance of a rational nature).[49] Later, the Platonic tradition was inherited by René Descartes (1596–1650). Descartes' substance dualism of *res cogitans* (thinking/mental substance) and *res extensa* (extended/physical substance)[50] translates into a modified version of the human body-soul dualism. With this duplex, the soul is eternal and able to live outside of the body, which of course became a mainstay of theological anthropology into the twentieth century.[51]

The classic definition of human personhood as rational being has often been used by these same thinkers to deem those with "less" rationality as less than human and lower on the great chain of being. Defining human nature solely or primarily through rationality becomes heavily problematic on numerous grounds. Not only has much of the Western Christian tradition utilized this definition, but it has also linked it with our understanding of the triune persons. The two immanent divine processions are through the divine intellect and will. Comparatively, humanity is conceived as rational and volitional. First, we affirm the traditional characteristics of human person defined by the modes of intellect and will and their antecedents and ground in the *processio* of the immanent Trinity. However, we note that the *processio* is a procession of persons (the Son and the Spirit) who are defined relationally in terms of their eternal origin in the Father. The modes of intellect and will (*modum intellectus* and *modum voluntatis*) proceed in the context of relationship. Second, in qualifying the nature and relative place of reason, we are not supplanting it. We recognize that the *processio* of the Logos is God's internal reflective self-knowledge, more precisely wisdom. We also acknowledge that in Christ the Logos and the rational soul/image (*logikon*) are fully present in one person. We are affirming the rational nature of human being, though its definition is constructed at some level. However it is defined, the faculty of reason is integrated with volition and other attributes, and these are situated relationally.

Even in affirming historically the weighty place proffered to human reason, we are forced to reckon that rationality is a slippery term to define. Whose rationality?[52] What determines rationality? What type of rationality are we using as the measure?[53] Is human reason pure reason in the type Kant opposed? Is reason fallen, and to what extent? Are reason and rationality generated autonomously apart from God? Is reason instrumental, socioculturally constructed, or foundational? If rationality is a universal attribute that would measure humanity, then universal agreement as to what determines rationality becomes unequivocally problematic. As Heather and Kenneth Keith have painstakingly shown us, measuring humanity based solely, primarily, or as an end on rationality or intelligence[54] becomes dangerous when we apply such an anthropology to the humanity of those with disabilities or disorders. Persons who are deemed less rational owing to disabilities or disorders can potentially be deemed less than human and have less value in the eyes of society.[55] Such a conclusion may foster discrimination, human rights violations, and even genocide in the eyes of the "rational" public.[56] What type of and how much rationality does one need to demonstrate in order to qualify as human and worthy of life?[57] Simply, those who cannot demonstrate a certain acumen and level of rationality are not deemed human or worthy of life. Such faulty inferences open the door to revisiting the whole misguided venture of social Darwinism and ensuing ethnocentrism, racism, eugenics, genetic engineering, sterilization, and even genocide. This critique is not to eliminate reason from the definition of human nature but to limit it from functioning as an end in itself. Reason cannot function as the sole or primary marker to measure humanity, a rationale for marginalization and dehumanization, or as its own autonomous ground and hypostasis.[58] Thus, we are leaving the precise nature of rationality open at this point but stressing it cannot be the ground for defining what is human. However we define reason, it must be in relation to other factors that bear on rational functionality within the human person. Some of those features and conditions are highlighted by science, philosophy, theology, and disability studies.

Does reason, especially our nihilistic Western brand of it, deserve the preeminent place we assign it when determining human personhood? Let us shift our attention to current neuroscience and the biology of reason. Elevating and centralizing reason within the human person may prove to be not only inhumane but also scientifically erroneous. The rigorous work of neuroscientists such as Antonio Damasio (1944–) surprisingly reveals that Cartesian mind-body dualism (the disembodied mind and the notion that the mind can exist apart from the body) and the related primacy of human reason do not hold up. Rather, we as humans are not so much defined as purely rational beings (the *cogito*) but more so emotional beings that reason. We are beings who are (exist) before we think.[59] Reason is a secondary faculty. A priority is placed on *being* over the *cogito*, along with the import and integration of emotion and feeling that are needed to support human rationality. In terms of delineating a particular faculty that would define the human person, Damasio locates the center of activity in the organism (the body) itself, viewing us as somatic conscious beings.[60] Clear designating lines between reason, the brain, emotion, and the body cannot be drawn. Reason is not an independent substance or even faculty or property that works autonomously or purely. Thus, there is no single defining faculty or site that undergirds the human person, but rather the entire integrated activity of the somatic conscious self is what makes up who we are, as Scripture suggests. Therefore, any subsequent affirmation of reason in the human person needs to be made contextually in light of the greater whole. There are no scientific grounds for the hegemony of reason in the human person.

Thus far we have examined the faculty of reason from the legacy of Platonic psychology to neuroscience and its limitations as the defining feature of human nature. Other aspects of Plato's notion of the soul (will and appetites/ emotions) along with its rational component are developed over time, as well.[61] The significance of the will is seen in the voluntarism (the divine will and human freedom) that dominated late Scholasticism (Scotus and Ockham) and is reprised in the Reformation with Luther (the bondage of the will) and Arminius (grace-empowered libertarian free will). In philosophy Hobbes (will as action without impediment), Schopenhauer (will to live), Nietzsche (will to power), Freud (will to pleasure), James (will to believe), and Foucault (power is knowledge) develop the import of volition and even freedom in defining the human person. However, in theological terms, the will is primarily understood to some degree or another as bound by sin and not a faculty that is fully free.[62]

On the other hand, we also note the development of the emotions and religious experience in characterizing human nature even grounding theological methodology.[63] The emotional self in some traditions is condemned, while in others it is affirmed. With desert ascetic monasticism (Pseudo-Dionysius, Evagrius, John Cassian) and later traditions of Catholic mysticism and quietism (Ignatius, Teresa, St. John, Molinos, Guyon, Fenelon) earthly affections are to be overcome. The anchorite or mystic begins to ascend the divine ladder through *apatheia*. The senses are purged of the affections toward the sensual world and the mind purged of cognitions toward the intelligible world en route to illumination and union with God and thus the transformation and deification of the passions.

While the Enlightenment, on rational grounds, further sought to subdue "unruly and distorted" passions under the dominion of reason, Pietism countered with its emphasis on religious experience fueled by renewed religious affections and their significance in confirming the veracity of the Christian doctrine of justification through authentic conversion. Theologically, Friedrich Schleiermacher (1768–1864) exemplifies this methodological shift from grounding Christian faith in rational assent to the primacy of "pious self-consciousness," one's creaturely dependence and experience of self, world, and the *mysterium tremendum*.[64] The Lutheran Pietism of Johann Arndt (1555–1621), Philip Jacob Spener (1635–1705), and Augustus Hermann Francke (1663–1727), the Moravianism of Nikolaus von Zinzendorf

(1700–1760), and the Quakerism of George Fox (1624–1691) also emphasized the validating authority of religious experience over against dry, rational assent to a mere propositional orthodoxy. The quest for experiential
religion specifically in terms of the new birth fueled the Great Awakening
on both continents under the leadership of Jonathan Edwards (1703–1758),
George Whitefield (1714–1770), and John Wesley (1703–1791), the founder
of Methodism. At the core of this movement was the recognition that true
conversion, including conversion of religious affections, involved a thorough
repentance and amending of sinful ways and a spiritual rebirth. The entire
person is transformed, including one's spiritual senses, which are awakened
to experience the divine.[65] Early Methodism would go on to seed the Holiness
and healing movements of the nineteenth century, which in turn were significant in launching the subsequent Pentecostal-charismatic movement, which
influenced the renewalist Christianity of the global South shift.[66] Many of
these movements, in recognizing the significance of religious affections for
the theological self, reintroduced not only validating power of religious experience but also the need for intentional, rigorous dogmatic pneumatology
that could discern and ground such experience.

The rational, volitional, and emotive domains of the human person
each have had to do the heavy lifting for the *imago Dei* tradition. Although
these attributes are noted in Scripture and throughout the Christian tradition and are in a sense *vestigia trinitatis*, no single justified substantive view
of the *imago Dei* holds under scrutiny, even in Scripture. Historically, the
imago as primarily rational has been the most touted but also has faced the
most just criticism from the disability community. We will examine such
criticism later in the chapter.[67] Again, it is worth repeating that a pressing
commitment to any specific philosophy of mind is not sought after in this
work. It was noted above that both emergent property dualism and interactive substance dualism are feasible options to explore, although the latter is
often disregarded as an option in light of current neurophilosophy and other
neurosciences. These fields tend to see the self as not a mental or physical
entity but rather as self-reference (empirical-self model), that is, an integrated neurological reflection and representation of the brain's own data
and patterns and structures of processing.[68]

IMAGO DEI AS STRUCTURAL

The predominant and most historically enduring model of the *imago Dei*
has been the structural or attributive model. With this model, attributes of
God are mirrored, or at the least represented in some measure, in human
nature, providing the capacity for compatibility. Thus, throughout history

we have concluded that human beings are personal, spiritual, transcendent, rational, moral, relational, volitional, emotional, and creative because in some greater way God is as well. We also recognize that some of these designations have also excluded persons with disabilities.[69] The understanding has been that human nature was crafted or structured with the capacity to reflect God's attributes, most notably rationality and righteousness, which are prerequisites to relating to God. As humans we are creatures that are gifted with reason and moral agency to choose and reflect the righteousness of God. The structural model grounded in Genesis 1:26 conceives human nature "in the image of God" and "after the likeness of God." "Image" (*tselem*) and "likeness" (*demuth*) connote "reason" and "righteousness," respectively. Structurally, human nature has the capacity to reason, choose morally, and reflect the divine attributes of God's reason or rationality and righteousness. The structural view is related to the substantive view and is often viewed in light of it, as illustrated above in our focus on the rational substance of human nature. Historically, the substantive view has maintained that the "substance" of reason has been persistently central to defining human nature over against the rest of creation. Again, the problem arises when reason and will are scored in degree and development along a continuum that proportionally measures the degree and development of humanity, leaving those with disabilities and disorders in a subhuman category of some sort. The reason and righteousness attributive approach to human nature is heavy on ability and performance both intellectual and moral. Those suffering with disabilities and disorders are often thought to underachieve in these areas because of their impairment, or the impairment is viewed as judgment for a supposed personal or genetic failure.

Rationality and volition are multivalent phenomena that are slippery to standardize when used as a baseline to qualify "what is human." The definition, demonstration, and performance of human faculties vary in expression and are not uniform, static, or monosyllabic. Hence, definitions and levels of function should not be standardized in terms of labeling what is human. In assessing performance levels, our standards of what qualifies as "functional" or "normal" are contextual, cultural, or even biased, as many of these norms are socially constructed and suspect.

Further, our modernist tendency to measure, quantify, and evaluate would tempt us to do likewise with the questions, "What does it mean to be human?" and "How much ability would qualify one to be human or to earn the right to live?" The debate continues as to whether disabilities are prelapsarian or postlapsarian human conditions or even related to the fall. But in any case, an understanding of the *imago* based on ability still creates the same problem of standard, measurement, and value. A loophole would remain for a "might makes right" standard to measure and evaluate the weak. In the case of might, the truth of the matter is that only the Almighty can be the one who establishes the measure for humanity. And God has chosen the weak and foolish things of this world to bring forth salvation. Again, this is not to say that rationality or volition do not play a significant role in our human experience and thus should not be included in an understanding of the *imago*, but it is to say that space needs to be made for the differentiation of the human person (including those with psychiatric disability) in all of its loci. We will specifically be calling attention to the relational aspects of the *imago Dei* that are christologically defined.

Let us return to our scriptural and historical evaluation of the *imago Dei*. The common shorthand definition for the *imago Dei* has been "image" and "likeness." The "image and likeness" are frequently correlated with "reason and righteousness." However, the connection is derived more from patristic tradition than from Scripture itself and its five references to the *imago Dei* (Gen. 1:26-27; 5:1; 9:6; 1 Cor. 11:7; Jas. 3:9).[70] Biblical scholars, contrary to a majority of early Christian tradition, disagree that the two Hebrew words signify two different meanings, in this case the attributive designations of reason and righteousness.[71] Conversely, scholars agree that the terms, though having a broad semantic range, are related and are virtually synonymous.[72] What they cannot agree on is what they exactly mean. Inferences about "image and likeness" vary and point to notions of resemblance, copy, or similitude in relation to an earthly representation of divine royalty, dominion, or companionship. Although the verdict is still out, the consensus seems to be that the terms, whatever they may mean, are not ontological but functional in nature.

In Pauline theology, human reason and righteousness are insufficient for grounding the human person. Our righteousness falls short of God's righteousness. We are called by faith to seek instead the righteousness of God in Christ, which is a gift from above. Likewise, we are exhorted to redirect the use of our rational faculties. The mind of the *sarx* becomes a mind engaged in vice, such as pride (1 Cor. 8:1). A mind focused on the *sarx* is death, but the mind controlled by the Spirit bears the fruit of virtue, such as life and peace.[73] Exercise of the rational faculty is to be surrendered in service to the work of the sanctifying Spirit in order to cultivate intellectual virtues, such as humility, wisdom, and obedience. Thus, Paul commands us to be renewed in our minds and put on the new creation in Christ, who reflects the true righteous and holy image of God (Eph. 4:22-24). The *imago Dei* is not pointing inwardly to us but outwardly to God in Christ.

So, where does the notion that the *imago Dei* signifies reason and righteousness break into the Christian tradition? As referenced above, the notion to define human nature in terms of rationality has its roots in Greek thinking from the pre-Socratics (e.g., Heraclitus, 535 BCE–475 BCE, and the logos), to Plato and Aristotle[74] to the Stoics (universal Logos and *logos spermatikos*—rational seed) and in the Hellenized Judaism's Logos tradition (Philo, 20 BCE–50 CE) and in early Logos Christology represented by Justin Martyr (c. 150 CE), Irenaeus (130–202 CE), and Athanasius (296–373 CE). The *imago* or the logos in the human soul is conceived as an earthly copy of the divine archetypal Logos. The nexus made between "image and likeness" and rationality and righteousness is allegedly first made by Irenaeus, though some claim Irenaeus did not intend to separate the two terms.[75] The rationality-righteousness interpretation has been inherited by the vast stream of Christian tradition for the next 1,500 years, including Clement of Alexandria (150–215 CE), Athanasius, Gregory of Nyssa (335–394 CE), Cyril of Jerusalem (313–386 CE), Augustine (354–430 CE), Maximus the Confessor (580–662 CE), and Thomas Aquinas up until the Reformation, according to Grenz.[76] Citing *Against Heresies*, Grenz contends Irenaeus also originated the notion that the image (reason and will) is retained though altered postlapse, while the likeness, or original righteousness, is lost.[77] However, Irenaeus did not believe that humanity was made righteous or holy in a perfect or finished sense but as a starting point. The full and true image of God is found in Christ. Christ is the image of God, and that image is to be recapitulated in all of creation, the *telos* of all things including the image of God (Christ) eschatologically revealed in humanity.[78]

Clement of Alexandria (150–215 CE) likewise differentiates *image* from *likeness* in Adam and his potential to grow in righteousness. He also understood that the attributes were truly realized only in Christ, the image of God.[79] Differing from Irenaeus, Clement, owing to Greek philosophical influence, gave reason a prominent place. His understanding of sin, moral agency and action, and the *imago* are all informed by his idea of reason. Further, he defines *likeness* soteriologically in terms of a life controlled by the dictates of a purified reason.[80] Similarly, we discover this same interpretive thread with slight variation throughout the tradition in Athanasius, Gregory of Nyssa, Cyril of Jerusalem, Augustine, Maximus,[81] and Aquinas. The *imago* signifies the rational soul (*logikon*), and *likeness* points to the righteousness of God as an incipient state. *Likeness* can also signify the moral development of a person who is growing in the image of Christ.[82] Augustine, drawing on the apostle Paul, deeply emphasized this latter corollary that the *imago* is renewed in Christ through the knowledge and love of God. The built-in capacity to participate in the divine image in the knowledge and love of God (*vestigia trinitatis*) is restored in Christ.[83] Thomas Aquinas, known most prominently for extending the Aristotelian notion of humanity as a rational animal, likewise builds on Augustine and the capacity and restoration of the *imago* in the knowledge and love of God via the immanent Trinitarian processions of knowledge (Logos) and love (the Spirit). From the early church fathers to Aquinas the *imago Dei* is defined structurally and specifically as reason.[84] The structural view predominated Christian theological anthropology up until the Reformation, when a more relational view began to emerge and gain ground. Grenz contends that although the Reformation with its stress on depravity and its impact on the image and likeness of humanity shifted its emphasis from a structural to a relational view, the structural view remained influential up until the twentieth century.[85]

A clear conclusion from Christian tradition is that any attempt to discard a rational component from one's notion of human experience would be shortsighted, and I would add futile and disastrous. There is grave disagreement as to what is intended by "rational" and to what extent if any it should be the measure of our humanity. The human experiment, however, has made at least one thing evident: it has painstakingly spent an exorbitant amount of time and energy utilizing all of its available resources to know itself, the universe, and the God of the universe and to justify that knowledge with the same available resources. One goal in this work is to redefine reason from being its own autonomous ground and hypostasis to its limited instrumental and relational location as a faculty conjunctive with human volition directed toward God and others. Any position that holds human faculties or their operation as a prerequisite to being human and further claims that some intellectually disabled persons do not have such faculties needs to be refuted. If one were to contend that persons who empirically demonstrate no rational-volitional faculties still maintain those faculties in some transcendent way, then such a position, though not without its problems, could still be technically considered. Later in the chapter I will examine such cases. The *imago Dei* in many cases involves a rational attribute but is not exhausted in this attribute. Based on its performative and exclusive nature, reason should not be given primacy when defining the human person. Other options need to be further considered.

IMAGO DEI AS FUNCTIONAL

Another common framing of the *imago Dei* within the Christian tradition has been as functional or missional. The functional view claims that the terms "image and likeness" from Genesis 1:26 refer to God's purpose for creating humanity. God created *adam* in his image representatively and functionally to carry out a specific calling in the world, a missional model.[86] Assigned functions vary across interpreters but can be summarized as "divine counterpart," specifically in terms of agency, dominion, and rulership[87] and functioning as a divine mediation of power through human agency.[88] The functional sense of the *imago* is that human agency carries out God's will and establishes God's rule or kingdom in the social order. With echoes from an ancient Near East (ANE) worldview, the Lord, in Genesis chapter 1, bestows humanity with the call and mission to represent the divine will in the world. The functional view has had some historical precedent but has lately gained ground through biblical studies and exegesis of Genesis chapter 1.[89] Middleton's work best exemplifies an attempt from biblical studies to define the *imago Dei*. His exhaustive exegetical effort is a linguistic-syntactical, rhetorical, and social study of the *imago Dei* in light of the first chapter of Genesis and its ANE background and parallels. He proposes a "royal-functional" reading. Middleton claims that "the *imago Dei* refers to humanity's office and role as God's earthly delegates, whose terrestrial task is analogous to that of the heavenly court." The task is the "exercise of power over the earth and its nonhuman creatures" "organizing human society or culture" through an alternative, nonviolent, subversive democratization of power. The proposed view is counter to ANE (absolute) narratives and to current (violent) sociopolitical orders.[90]

Christological implications of Middleton's work would seem to permit space for the kingdom of God's order and rule to operate through Christ and subsequently the church and spread throughout the world eschatologically.[91] However, the church does not have a good track record in handling temporal power, usually converting it into a type of politically realized millennial eschatology. Christ rules the world through the church. The Christ and culture quandary has been worked out time and again since Niebuhr,[92] but the problems are enduring. The immediate challenge of early Christianity along this trajectory was Constantinianism. There is always a colossal conflict of interest when ecclesial power aligns with secular, corrupt power, as the history of the Western church, the modern nation-state, and colonization well attests.[93] The anthropocentric notion that the purpose of the *imago Dei* is to mediate power on the earth on behalf of the divine, though it seems exegetically correct in Middleton and yet theologically unchecked,[94] strikes hard against our better intuition and the lessons of history. Human depravity has not been kind to the church wielding power, specifically as it has been administered against the weak, the marginalized, and those with disabilities.[95]

There are other obvious concerns to level against a functional *imago* that is fashioned to mediate divine authority. An instrumental, political *imago* establishes a power or warfare a priori. The image of God would presuppose control as its reason for being. A Nietzschean will to power becomes transcendental and definitive of human doing and being. All human decisions would presuppose divine fiat. The consequence is that all human agency and activity would be given the divine right to power. Surely an apocalyptic war of the worlds. Not only is such a principle inconceivable as a universal rule for all humanity (Kant), but a functional model of might makes right and survival of the fittest is also outright incompatible with the humane treatment of persons. Persons who experience disability and disorder would suffer the most. Society rewards function with power and further disables those who do not function according to its norms. The connection between functionality and power touches on the very injustice that is wielded against persons with disabilities. The result can be viewed in terms of equal access to quality of life. The ICF model[96] of the WHO attempts a just account and analysis of all of the variables in both medical and social models of function and disability. The model defines disablement and functioning in relation to health condition (disease or disorder), body functions and structure, activity (execution of a task), participation (in a life situation), and the environmental and personal factors experienced by the individual. The WHO classifications delineate between the disorder/disease, its resulting impairment (functional loss), disability (activity limitations), and handicap (social disadvantage).[97]

Mental disorders that are caused or exacerbated by social factors and are untreated can result in cognitive-emotional disability. Disability can limit the quality and productivity of life. The burden of the disorder in terms of loss of health and function can be devastating. Years lived with disability (YLD) are combined with years of life lost (YLL) to arrive at the disability-adjusted life years (DALYs). This formula is used by the WHO to measure the burden of the disorder. Disability that results in years of life lost leads to social disadvantage, for example, in obtaining or sustaining employment. Multiple and balanced factors contribute to the analysis and response to disability. If the image of God is measured by functionality, then persons with disabilities are at a grave disadvantage. Thus, definitions of the nature of personhood that are strictly and solely functional are debilitating and exacerbate marginalization and dehumanization by creating an ableist normativity.[98]

Our lust for power needs to be addressed. Prophetically, postmodern hermeneutics have justly toppled the foundations of such sociopolitical power and performance-based hegemonies.[99] Many of these theories have been adopted by disability studies and have intersected with other areas like race and gender. Nonetheless, postmodern responses to deconstruct modern power as logocentric constructs, and even ecclesiocentric power plays, have not resulted in redeemed notions of power. Postmodern and neocritical sub-versions have proven unable to transcend their own critique, falling victim to the fallacy of self-reference.[100] Violence breeds violence. Power vacuums are filled with power structures that may vary in form but remain the same in substance. Oppressor and oppressed binaries remain but with different players performing the same roles. Violent, oppressive totalizing regimes are toppled by other violent, oppressive totalizing regimes. Power as the ultimate a priori can only lead to further oppression and violence. The true reign of the Prince of Peace subverts and redefines the terms of power in a radical way unparalleled in human thought. The Almighty lays aside power and privilege. The Messiah becomes a suffering servant, but not a victim, for the least of these. His sacrifice empowers the last to be made first. Christ resides on the margins and undergirds and empowers the weak, so that they can be strong in him. Similarly, he calls us to do likewise. Lead by sacrificial serving. So we affirm the kingdom of God. We affirm the rule and reign of Christ through the power and authority of the Spirit. We affirm his rule in and through the church. But this kingdom subverts power from power over to power undergirding and serving people. If any impulse of a functional *imago* is to be reappropriated, it needs to be as Christ's mission of sacrificial service.

THEOLOGICAL ANTHROPOLOGY AND DISABILITY

As we examined traditional theological sites that have defined the image of God, we noted that the tradition has shown little awareness or inclusion of disabilities in its definitions of the human person. By elevating human reason, will, and achievement, substantial, attributive, and functional defi-nitions often marginalize and dehumanize persons with disabilities. In unpacking the meaning of the *imago Dei*, we need to know how that mean-ing informs disabilities and how it is informed by disabilities. How do dis-ability and theological anthropology mutually inform each other? Each of these areas of disability has its own specific contexts and questions. How we define humanity in general would be the same for all disabilities. Otherwise, we would have multiple and even conflicting definitions of human person-hood. We may even erroneously conclude that there are different types of humans, which instinctively is wrongheaded.

Although our fundamental consideration of an *imago*-based anthro-pology remains the same for all disabilities (physical, intellectual, psychiat-ric), our insights will be applied to a theology of depression in particular.[101] However, in order to address psychiatric disabilities, we must consider first "profound intellectual disabilities." Profound intellectual disabilities estab-lish our baseline for theological anthropology. Why? Some persons with profound intellectual disabilities do not appear to have agency. This is problematic because a significant contribution to our philosophical anthropologies involves agency. As a result, they have been frequently kept out of the disability conversation. We need to deal with agency as the baseline of anthropology. Unlike with physical and mental disabilities, there are some cases of intellectual disability in which persons seemingly have no empirical agency. As far as experience presents, such persons do not seem to be operating rational or volitional faculties and have no sense of consciousness or a constructed self to do so, whereas in physical and psychiatric disabilities there is usually some sense or degree of agency, uniquely defined. We are assuming that mental disorder does not nullify human agency in toto. The *Diagnostic and Statistical Manual of Mental Disorders*, 4th edition,[102] states that mental disorder can result in "an important loss of freedom," though it is relative and in degree. Mental disorders can, to various degrees, intermittently and temporarily undermine rational and volitional agency. This problem is not only psychological but can also become a moral and legal issue in terms of attributability, accountability, and responsibility. Is someone with impaired freedom responsible? Forensic psychiatrist Gerben Meynen, and I concur, contends that the connection between mental disorders and a compromise of freedom is imprecise[103] and thus inconclusive. The verdict is still out.

For those with mental disorders, free will can be compromised, but, as a divine gift, it cannot be annihilated. Still, it remains unclear in which way it is compromised.[104] Agency and free will are not synonymous: the latter is a subset of the former. The free will I am assuming for persons with mental disorders, in terms of originating rational choice, is in the least occasional, circumstantial, and in degree but nonetheless present. Free will is not absent or incapacitated permanently.[105] With psychiatric disability and compromised free will, the etiology of the problem has not been ultimately found to be organic. For example, the problem is not located in the brain through a known neural correlation, and thus not debilitating, unlike in some profound intellectual disabilities (e.g., Hans Reinders' friend Kelly discussed below). Conditions that compromise or undermine free will in persons with mental disorders, like addiction, psychotic states, kleptomania, Tourette's, and so on, can be treated, and agency is potentially recoverable. Also, with some mental health conditions, catatonia can be comorbid. Catatonic states, though, usually last only for a time and are not permanent.[106] Even though persons with mental disorders may experience tough outer restrictions (negative freedom) from society and even inner restrictions due to the mental disorder, no person with mental disorders "can lose personal freedom completely because she is the active agent in her lifeworld."[107]

The potency of the faculties with mental disorder is congenitally and naturally present but intermittently and temporarily compromised. For example, a person who has OCD and is compelled to behave a certain way, and cannot act otherwise, can take psychiatric medication and receive clinical therapy and potentially recover their free will to some degree. They do not thoroughly and permanently lose agency.[108] However, when considering a theological approach to depression, compromised rational-volitional faculties need to be taken into account when discussing salvation, agency, and living the Christian life as a person with psychiatric disabilities.

Let us return to our discussion about nonagency and some intellectual disabilities. We considered that agency remains a qualified capacity for persons with physical and psychiatric disabilities but not with all intellectual disabilities. Disability studies traditionally works at the level of agency and empowerment. Persons with disabilities, along with those who advocate for them, seek to liberate that agency, allowing for self-actualization and self-representation. The premise is that persons are agentive rather than nonagentive. Agency is usually the case in physical and psychiatric disabilities and in most intellectual disabilities. What about persons who do not empirically demonstrate agency? Does our theological anthropology, which is usually capacity based, have a place at the table of humanity for these persons?

PIDS, AGENCY, AND BEING HUMAN

Should our definition of the image of God be grounded in human agency? This question is tackled by theologian Hans Reinders in his seminal text *Receiving the Gift of Friendship: Profound Disability, Theological Anthropology, and Ethics*. Reinders makes a clear distinction between nonagency in some persons with intellectual disabilities and agency in persons with physical and psychiatric disabilities. How can we define humanity, specifically in terms of the *imago Dei*, in a way that will be valid and inclusive for all persons, expressly those with "profound intellectual disabilities" (PIDs)? Reinders will be our primary interlocutor in this essential conversation. He painstakingly examines how this problem has been addressed by the disability rights movement and Roman Catholic moral theology. His claim is that the models that these groups offer do not consider, are exclusive of, or are irrelevant to persons with PIDs. Reinders offers us Kelly as an example. Kelly is a friend of Reinders, who is "a *micro-encephalic*" woman in whom "a significant part of the normal human brain is missing."[109] Upon first visiting Kelly, Reinders' conclusion was that Kelly did not seem to have purposive agency, self-consciousness, a notion of selfhood, or any rational-volitional capacity, at least by standard definitions or in any way that is empirical. What struck Reinders was that according to most definitions of human personhood, Kelly would not be human.[110]

The standard capacity-, faculty-, or agency-based approach to defining humanity or the image of God falls grievously short. Kelly simply fails to meet the criteria and "qualifications" to be human according to such measures. Persons, like Kelly, with PIDs are often without purposive agency, unlike those with other disabilities. While persons with physical disabilities, some milder intellectual disabilities, and psychiatric disabilities assume and function with some degree of agency, the same is not the case for persons with PIDs. Thus, our definitions and models tend to be exclusive and create a "hierarchy of disability."[111] Reinders notes, and we concur, that "disabled people are not the problem; the problem is a society that discriminates against them."[112] We, along with Reinders, recognize that Kelly is "one of us," as Reinders puts it, but we fail to understand how without further oppressing people with PIDs. Reinders' fair critique is leveled against the disability rights movement and Roman Catholic moral theology.

HANS REINDERS, THE DISABILITY RIGHTS MOVEMENT, AND ROMAN CATHOLIC MORAL THEOLOGY

The disability rights movement should be lauded for its many advances. The movement strives to eliminate social stigmas and obstructions that limit persons with various impairments. Through legislation, policy, and practice, it empowers human agency, provides equal access for all persons, and enables them to represent and express themselves as equal liberal citizens in society. The movement views disability as a negative, restricting, and unjustified response by society against persons who express human diversity through physical impairments. The problem, in this case, is not human diversity but society's oppressive constraints.[113] Empowerment for self-determination as a sociopolitical act of liberation is one of the chief goals of the disability rights movement. Reinders applauds all that the movement has advocated and achieved. Yet he recognizes that for persons with PIDs, social justice, equal rights and access, and self-actualization and representation are not enough. How does one exercise self-determination when "in many cases, developing 'selfhood' is the problem rather than the solution."[114] Reinders retorts, "The logic of the social model excludes considering the relevance of physical conditions of impairment." Defining human beings by their potential for self-representation in society presupposes some degree of human agency. Removing the disabling semiotics and systems of society can achieve much. But these liberating measures primarily benefit those who have agency that is recoverable. Some physical impairments, like Kelly's, will simply not be impacted by such a model.

As it stands, the anthropological model offered by the disability rights movement creates a hierarchy of disability with PIDs remaining at the bottom. We concur with Reinders that a hierarchy of disability reflects a hierarchy of cultural moral values that in turn reflects deeper assumptions about humanity and what we value: "namely, that selfhood and purposive agency are crucial to what makes our lives human in the first place."[115] We short-sightedly define human personhood and rank human value based on human capacity and achievement. Privileged functions of the neocortex that allow for self-consciousness, self-construction, reasoning, and volition are assumed to define humanity and set the goal for purposive agency. For the disability rights movement, that goal is self-representation, equality, and liberal citizenship. The problem is that persons with some PIDs are excluded from this threefold goal because they do not have the same starting point of agency. As a result, they cannot attain the same goals. The starting point and goal hence need to change. We cannot begin with agency and, on the basis of agency, then end with equality.

Reinders continues by critiquing similar complications with Roman Catholic moral theology, which in his estimation has an acceptable starting point but falters on its goal, or *telos*. Drawing from Aristotelian-Thomistic tradition, which identifies a human based on generation of species, Roman Catholic moral theology recognizes that "human life is identified by human parentage."[116] Founded on Aristotle's rule that "man is born from man," the tradition makes space for all persons to be included and valued as human as its starting point. But what is connoted by the designation *human*? Reinders' reading is that within the Aristotelian-Thomistic tradition *human* means having the capacity for reason and volition. The problem with this definition is its *telos* for what it means to be human. Roman Catholic moral philosophy defines human actualization or its *telos* as exercising the intrinsic capacities of intellect and will that are in potency for a human to fulfill their true nature and final end in moral perfection. This *entelechy* of human faculties is the greatest good, the good life, or the purpose of human life.

For Reinders, the problem with this definition is that a person only properly fulfills their *telos* as a human when they develop their intellectual and volitional faculties to their intended potential and moral goal.[117] Reinders notes that some persons with PIDs do not possess the agency for intellect and will and do not qualify as truly human under those terms. Roman Catholic moral theology begins well by including all persons as human due to their origin or genesis from another human. Yet, for Reinders, it has failed to identify all persons as human when it identifies them according to the development of the rational-volitional soul.[118] In this respect, there is no space for Kelly to live the good life as a human being. At best, she fits into Aristotle's category of "marginal cases." For example, consider "perfect apples" and less-than-perfect apples or "marginal apples." A case for marginal apples would unfold something like this. Since all apples are apples, even if an apple's growth and quality are underdeveloped and it is less than appealing in terms of its size, color, and taste, it is still an apple. The apple begins as an apple without a doubt, since it came from an apple seed that came from an apple. However, the apple "underachieves" in its goal to be a perfect apple, and the same is true for persons who do not attain their *telos* of development.[119] Some apples are better than others. This subdivision of good and bad apples is transferred to human beings. Some persons are more human than others because they can do more and achieve better than others. Some persons are even defective owing to their lack of innate capabilities. The problems with these anthropological models are clear. They are exclusive and at best create subdivisions as to who is human.[120] In a limited space, I have simplified but hopefully represented Reinders' basic arguments faithfully.

HUMANITY AS RELATIONAL BEING

We concur with Reinders. The image of God should be inclusive of all persons, including Kelly and others like her. Reinders solves the problem by removing human agency or capacity from any starting point in defining what is human.[121] That seems like a rational and humane move considering what we have critiqued of other agentive models, though this move is not without its difficulties, which we will untangle below.

For Reinders, "being human is properly understood in terms of a relationship with God," and that relationship is unconditional, a gift.[122] Reinders at first considers Barth's view of relationality[123] but thinks it still "presupposes the concept of the human being as individual rational substance." Ultimately, he goes with Bishop Zizioulas' Trinitarian concept of relational being.[124] Zizioulas' is a highly debated position. Reinders acknowledges as much and addresses the issue. Zizioulas claims that the Cappadocian fathers argued that "the *being of God himself* was identified with the three persons of the Trinity."[125] In this case, controversially, God's being resides in the hypostasis rather than in the *ousia*.[126] For Zizioulas, "the ontology of *hypostasis* was understood in terms of the relational category of existence"—being and being in relation are synonymous.[127] With this move, Reinders claims that being human does not rest in its ontology or its natural faculties but in its participation in the triune communion of Father, Son, and Holy Spirit. Being human is given and not found in purposive agency.[128] Anthropology must follow theology.

The triune God exists as being in communion, and so we exist as we participate in that communion. We concur. Personhood both human and divine is relational. So, for Reinders, human personhood stems from its relationship with the triune God. Triune being is in the free act of the personhood of the Father in relation with the persons of the Son and the Spirit. Reinders moves us away from a capacity-based image of God in a relational direction. All persons are defined by the gifts of humanity and love, which are unconditionally given by God. Reinders will use this definition as a ground for the purpose of all persons, which is to be chosen for loving friendship by God and others. In the next chapter, in accord with Reinders, we will pick up on the relational notion of the image of God. We will also examine more of Zizioulas' understanding of relational being.

PROBLEMS WITH EXCLUDING AGENCY
FROM HUMAN EXPERIENCE

At this point, we want to return to our main reason for examining Reinders' text. Reinders leveled a blistering critique against theological anthropologies that are based on human agency. They exclude persons like Kelly who have a PID. What does a definition of the human personhood look like that will include all persons like Kelly without relegating anyone to second-class status or creating a subdivision in anthropology? And more so, how can the *telos* of all human persons based on such a definition be both universal and inclusive of all persons? Reinders begins by removing any understanding of humanity based on their intrinsic capacities. Thus, he excludes the traditional rational-volitional notion from his idea of human personhood. His notion of humanity does not come from legislation, sociopolitical constructs, or from human beings themselves, but extrinsically, ecstatically, and unconditionally from God. Human personhood begins with divine agency rather than human agency.[129] Our humanity comes as a gift from a loving God, not based on human constructs, capacities, or performance. Likewise, our humanity is fulfilled similarly by God, as he chooses us in friendship to partake of the good life, which is receiving friendship. We do not choose him, but he chooses us. Similarly, we are called to embrace and befriend those with PIDs as both ours and their fulfillment of being.[130]

Much of Reinders' thesis we also embrace. We are defined relationally by the image of God in Christ for the purpose of being in a loving and saving relationship with the triune God. However, what do we do with the rational-volitional attributes of the human person if they do not define us? Unfortunately, Reinders does not leave us much direction for what to do with the intellect, the will, or any of the differing human capacities. He briefly alludes to Zizioulas' distinction between "person" and "personality," in which "person" references relational being and "personality" designates the psychological and moral qualities possessed by individual human beings.[131] I presume he would locate our rational-volitional faculties in "personality," though he does not specifically state it. "Personhood" is what all humans are unconditionally, and, I presume, "personality" is contingent, relative, and differentiated in all persons. These are my conjectures. Reinders does not develop the position and leaves us with little to work with concerning human faculties. He does not offer any strategy as to how faculties fit into human ontology or experience, or how they relate to personhood.

In entirely removing human faculties from the definition of being human, he provides no robust alternative for those who exercise agency to account for, explain, or register their rational-volitional experiences in human terms. These attributes are reduced to nonhuman functions. Also, if being chosen as a friend is "the" *telos* for human life, then what becomes of all of our other pursuits, specifically those that involve employing human faculties? What defines us as human must apply to us all. Did Reinders create the anthropological subdivision he sought to avoid when he removed faculties from the human equation? Did he further the subdivision when he designated that the purpose for persons with PIDs is to be befriended and for those without to befriend? Befriending would also involve agency, which has been excluded from his working definition of human. In excluding human capacities like reason and volition from what it means to be human and not giving an alternative account for these human experiences, has Reinders marginalized over 95 percent of the population, or was it simply not in the scope of his work?[132] In either case, making such a seismic subversive move requires some alternative account of agency for the sake of the explanatory power of his own argument. His groundbreaking thesis opens the door to more questions and problems that we do not need to address here but should be considered in the future.

In his thoughtful and compassionate tome, I do not believe Reinders intends to eliminate the faculty-derived experiences (qualia) from what it means to be human or from our experience as humans, which would be philosophically and morally problematic. Such a move would render the experiences of many meaningless, irrelevant, without moral consequences, and virtually impossible. I cannot separate my humanity from my reason, emotions, will, or any other faculty or vice versa. First-person qualia define me significantly. However, in accord with Reinders, we want to be clear that our humanity is a priori to our agency. It is presupposed when operating our faculties. We agree with Reinders that those faculties are not the experience of all persons and should not define our a priori humanity. That move comes from divine agency. God alone freely and lovingly chooses us in creation and in salvation. Our humanity is a gift given and is sustained by the Spirit of God and not by our doing. All of that said, it still remains what we are do with human faculties.

MIGUEL ROMERO: AQUINAS ON HUMAN AGENCY AND *AMENTIA*

As we attempt to respond to Reinders, we want to ask first whether Reinders' reading of Aquinas and the human rational soul is a fair one. In terms of the *imago Dei* and human faculties, what is a way forward? Miguel Romero, in his essay "Aquinas on the *Corporis Infirmitas*," proposes Aquinas' view on intellectual disability (*amentia*—mindlessness; one not present in one's mind). Romero's work is, in part, a response to Reinders' reading of Aquinas.[133] We will look at Romero's response to Reinders. Aquinas' hylomorphic *anima forma corporis* (the soul is the form of the body), according to Reinders, contends that the rational-volitional faculties in potency define what the human is and is to become through their actualization. Persons like Kelly do not have the cerebral apparatus to qualify for pursuit of that version of the good life. Contrarily, Romero reasserts that Aquinas does identify a human as a rational soul. However, that designation does not refer primarily to cognitive operations like intelligence or reason but to the image of God.[134] Also, such accidental characteristics like intelligence or reason do not qualify one for "species membership."[135] Opposing Reinders, Romero states, "To claim as Aquinas does, that the 'rational soul is the principle of human nature' is very different from the (false) claim which identifies the capacity for discursive reason or purposive action as constitutive of human nature and personhood."[136] The rational soul, which is the image of God, in its rationality is always capable of knowing and loving God and cannot be incapacitated in doing so. The reason is that capacity is not located in a bodily organ, like the brain, which would "reduce human nature to a corporeal operation."[137] Although the external sensory powers are of the body, the rational soul is also needed for the operation of intellection.[138] Reason is not a mere function of the body or the brain.

Further, according to Romero, Aquinas holds that those with corporeal infirmities, such as the *amens* (*amentia*), retain the image of God and the rational-volitional faculties, which are incorruptible.[139] These capacities are constitutive of the rational soul. They are imperishable and not to be excluded from a definition of the image of God. Corporeal infirmity, according to Aquinas, is not a constitutive limitation but an operative limitation, a key distinction.[140] A person may experience impairment, a privation of good function inherited from Adamic sin and not one's own according to Aquinas, and the body may be restricted in its expressive interface with the immaterial soul. Nevertheless, the rational soul's breach with the person's material properties due to an impairment does not negate or impede its connection and communication with the triune God.[141] Thus, the *telos* for all persons, including those with *amentia*, can still be fulfilled without creating subdivisions in anthropology.[142] Romero indicates that Aquinas understands the situation of the impaired as somewhat similar to, though different from as well, the condition of fallen humanity and its broken relationship with the Creator. The "orderly operation of the soul in relation to the human body" is impaired. The powers of the body and soul are retained but disordered. Nonetheless, one is still human. The capacity to know and love God is not destroyed but can be restored by baptismal grace and fully healed eschatologically.[143]

With the Aristotelian-Thomist hylomorphism, the human person is a composite of immaterial (immortal soul) and material (physical body) created by God and is intimately in relations with God (natural, spiritual, beatific).[144] The immaterial properties of intellect and will, though "configured to cooperate with the body," also can operate with limits independent of the body.[145] The *amens'* capacity to know and love God is not ultimately "hindered" in "her active imaging of God (which is an immaterial operation of the rational soul), nor is she prevented (as we shall see) from participating in the supernatural life."[146] According to Romero, "Aquinas maintains that *amentia* cannot keep a human creature from responding to God's grace, nor is the condition able to impair the *amens* in the realization of her ultimate good."[147] Romero continues, "No degree of dysfunction or disorder of the normal internal sensory operations proper to the human creature can ultimately impair the self-communicating intercourse between God and the image of God, which is our capacity for participation in the life of God through Christ."[148] For Aquinas, the divine agency of sanctification in baptism and communion further enhances the person's supernatural communication with God, "according to the economy of divine grace."[149] Thus, God fulfills his eternal purpose to love and sanctify all persons, regardless of their temporal condition. Romero remains agnostic as to the specific nature of the communication that transpires through the nonempirical agency (not biologically expressed) of the *amens*. Specifically, the grace communicated through the sacraments ultimately remains a mystery.[150] This silent sanctified discourse is not heard by Aquinas or Romero and may not be heard by Kelly as well. We cannot know, but presumably it is heard by God. Is the Thomist model unfair to Kelly? Does exemption from sin and its suffering, as one who is nonagentive, balance the equation? It would seem there is no sin for the nonagentive. The conditions of possible experience of temptation and sin are not there. To one who knows not whether it is sin, it is not sin. Is this the boon, curse, or neither of nonagency? This too remains unknown, though considered. Regardless, persons with PIDs prophetically correct our Pelagianism. Salvation is a gift from God and not from ourselves.

A WAY FORWARD

Thus, both Reinders and Romero arrive at an inclusive theological anthropology but through different paths. Reinders is clear that capacity cannot be included in a model of the *imago Dei*, and Romero insists it cannot be excluded. Aquinas' model validates persons without agency and allows for the human experiences of persons without PIDs. Yet phenomenologically not much can be known or experienced by persons with some PIDs. According to Romero, still, they are not excluded from the *telos* of sanctification nor eschatological healing, possibly giving Aquinas' view more explanatory power. In either case, the verdict is not clearly resolved, and issues remain. One has to either remove human agency from our definition of the image of God (Reinders) and still explain human faculties or retain it in a Thomist model but qualify it for those with PIDs (Romero).

Let us briefly tackle the human faculty problem. If human faculties are not universal but a relative part of my personality (presumably Reinders), then they remain a vital component of my personal and human development. My agency may not determine whether I am human or determine my human value. But it does participate in determining what type of human I am currently and will become. If not, then my life as a human (I can know no other life) becomes irrelevant. My thought-life is meaningless if the actions that flow from my thoughts are not connected to my being human and what type of human I become. I can break every command of God and not have it impact my humanity or what I have become as a human. In accord with Reinders, I am still a human with infinite value in the eyes of God. Nonetheless, it is evident that I have misused my gifts, favor, and humanity for evil. I have become one who has not loved as God loves. I have not loved God and neighbor. I have not done unto to others as I would want done to me. The different attributes and gifts of reason and will are used by God to allow me to become what he has planned for me. My rational-volitional faculties are intimately connected with the type of human I become. They cannot be extracted from my human becoming. Surely Reinders did not intend these consequences, but he does not account for these problems either.

Reinders rightfully sought an "extrinsic" source and meaning to ground what is human. We affirm extrinsically grounding humanity in divine agency rather than human agency. Human agency and faculties cannot define human qua human. Relational being initiated by God transcends human agency. Human faculties are not a sufficient reason for being (raison d'être). Our existence is a gift from God that expresses his unconditional love, which is the sufficient reason for our being. Human existence, which points to relational participatory being, is a priori to agency. Attributes, such as reason and volition, are secondary and instrumental to relational being.

Reinders claims our faculties are intrinsic and hence a faulty ground for our humanity. Is anything we possess truly intrinsic? Even our agency and its related faculties are gifts from God. We are not our own. Our faculties are not properly our own. All is gift. So, in a sense, our capacities are not ultimately intrinsic (contra Reinders). For those with disabilities and mental disorders, God's initial, gratuitous, and unconditional motion toward us in creation, in the sacrament, and in our ongoing sanctification all is a gift from beginning to end. Without divine movement, we cannot move in any sense. Agentive and nonagentive, God freely grants unconditional existence and love to both alike. Yet, in terms of capacity, we are all different in terms of gifts and calling. Our differences express but do not ground our humanity. Those gifted with agency respond as so gifted. Both agentive and nonagentive are human and remain human under any conditions. Both are loved and valued the same.

Regardless of either of the two paths (Reinders or Romero) represented in these arguments, faculties such as human reason need to be decentered, relocated, and redefined so that they are not given disqualifying or qualifying power regarding the humanity of all persons. The impact of the fall on the human faculties and the disordered glory we have placed on them are inordinate. Deconstruction involving decentering, relocating, and redefining them is scriptural and warranted. Relocation is the path we will take without having to commit necessarily or dogmatically to either Aquinas or Reinders in this matter.

4

The Relational Image of God

JESUS CHRIST IS THE *IMAGO DEI*

In the previous chapter, we noted two problems with any theological anthropology that is grounded solely on a substantive, structural, or functional model of the *imago Dei*. First, capacity-based models can be exclusive, especially of persons with PIDs. Some models simply function as weapons of power that can be employed to further oppress disabled persons and need to be overhauled in toto. The second is overemphasis on certain features of human nature, while other vital aspects are left out. We are left with inhumane reductionism. As Vladimir Lossky noted, hypostasis, or person, includes but cannot be reduced to a nature or its properties.[1] Phenomenologically, the human person is in excess of what appears. Even in its contingency, existence exceeds its own nature and cannot be reduced. The parts do not add up to the sum. The human person exudes externality and transcendence, pointing outside and beyond itself. There is more than meets the eye. Employing the category of saturated phenomena of Jean-Luc Marion, we note that the overload or excess of givenness in the phenomenon of the human person saturates our gaze and transcends our categorical and intentional limits.[2] Boundaries can become tricky. The problem is exacerbated when constructing a theological anthropology around the features of rationality, ability and performance, or moral achievement. We are tempted to qualify and disqualify persons based on attainments and metrics. These oversights stem more from an Enlightenment notion of the autonomous individual and positivist ableism than from a scripturally informed *imago Christi*. An anthropology that borrows predominantly from philosophy and science is often closed to transcendence. Theological resources are not permitted. The results can be a deflationary theology and a dehumanizing anthropology.[3]

The problem with either overemphasis or reductionism is exemplified in stressing exclusively the rational, specifically in its performance mode, the moral, or the functional images. The human person exceeds but does not deny or reduce their nature and properties. As noted, traditional structural accounts of the *imago Dei* have repeatedly construed "image and likeness" in terms of "reason and righteousness." Human attributes are gifts that express our diversity as persons. However, they are not a priori to our humanity but a posteriori. Our humanity is a gift from God that is given in creation and fulfilled in sanctification. In our measured attempt to decenter and redefine some of the key claims of structural and functional models, we are claiming that these assertions should not be defining or central and thus totalize the account of human nature. Alone, they offer only an atomistic account of who we are. Instead, these attributes are part of a much broader, complex, differentiated, relational, and theological picture of the human person. These attributes and functions are brought in and under Christ for kingdom service. Rather than glorified, our faculties are humbled. They were created to serve within a larger participatory relationship that ontologically highlights the dissimilarity of these human features to the divine, uncreated being.[4] But in reality, attributes are often idealized to hyperbolic proportions within a theology of glory that features human achievement over against virtues, such as epistemic humility and poverty of spirit. As a counterbalance, we will be examining the *imago Dei* as a relational or participatory framework, as informed theologically by the incarnation. Along the way, traditional loci of theological anthropology, such as substantial, attributive, and functional dimensions, will be redefined and relocated within a relational incarnational framework. Their operation is instrumental and relational. Union with Christ, incorporation into *familitas* (daughter/sonship), and *theosis* are the way faculties render their service.

We recall that how we define human nature will shape how we define depression. It does not seem feasible to separate the experience of a mental disorder from the experience of our embodied consciousness. As long as there is the former, there will be the latter expressing the former. The two are intertwined: the nature of humanity and the nature of depression. Consciousness is a precondition for experiencing depression. Unlike PIDs, mental disorders usually involve consciousness, experience, and some degree of rational-volitional agency. Although these do not define humanity a priori, they are usually part of the experience of persons with mental disorders. We have opted to recenter and reorder traditional aspects, attributes, and functions of the human person around a relational *imago Dei* to create accessibility to diverse human experiences for all people.

Many of the models and frameworks that we reviewed have mistakenly stressed one anthropological feature over another (reason, will, function, etc.). Yet, in their error, they have unwittingly stumbled across the proper way forward. Each model has linked its single *imago* feature to Jesus Christ. Christ, in fulfilling that selective feature, fulfills the image of God. Each one points to Jesus Christ as the true icon of God. Jesus Christ, the incarnation as the true *imago Dei*, serves as the common denominator in all of the perspectives that we have reviewed. The *imago Christi* functions as the point of departure and the *telos* for the human person. In this way our theological anthropology is inexorably linked to Christology and soteriology.

We are defined in terms of Christ. He becomes the beginning and end of our salvation. The Athanasian idiom that claims that "God became human that we may become like God" provides a guideline that defines the image of God in Christ and how it shapes the *via salutis*. The image of God in Christ is revealed to us through him that we may become like him. The proposal is that the image of God in Christ, the incarnation, is understood relationally—a hypostatic union between God and humanity. The incarnation defines who Christ is and why he came (to save us). Further, the incarnation defines our image in creation and redemption, our genesis and our end. The relational framework for the *imago Christi* is characterized as *identificational* (in creation) and *soteriological* (in redemption). The identificational aspect highlights created being in its differentiation, dependence, and weakness. The nature of created, contingent being is differentiated from and fully dependent on uncreated being. Following the fall, the image of God is intact but disfigured, disordered, and in need of redemption. The whole human person, reason and will, is depravedly affected and adverse to the will of God. Through the incarnation, Christ identifies with the dependence and weakness of our humanity to the fullest extent, even our sin (2 Cor. 5:21). Christ took on the human condition, our weakness, and our sin to become an offering for humanity in order to renew the fallen image of God. This dimension is the soteriological aspect of the incarnation. Christ identifies with our humanity, even our hamartiological disfigurement and disorder. The aim is to heal and save us in our brokenness through the love of the Spirit that adopts us as God's children and transforms us in the *imago Christi*. Hence, we observe the relational model of the image of God in Christ in three modes: *creation, fall,* and *new creation*. A theological typology of mental disorders emerges: *natural, consequential,* and *purgative* types. These three modes and three types will drive much of our discussion in the middle chapters of this book.

THE *IMAGO CHRISTI*, TRINITY, AND THE FAMILY OF GOD

Thus far, we have critiqued an *imago Dei* from below and have relocated it in Christ from both above and below. We have defined the image of God in Christocentric rather than Adamic terms. Jesus Christ, the incarnation, is the true *eikon* of God. While *adam* is made in the image of God, all that is inchoate and intended in Adam, which failed, is realized in Christ. With the fall, the image of God remains and is still good based on its created nature. However, the image is no longer shaped by holiness and righteous and thus is disfigured and disordered but redeemable. Human disorder is not inherent or ontological but hamartiological, which is a vital distinction. The fall does not render humanity ontologically defective but alters its intended course for *theosis*. Our impairments and our mental health conditions do not disqualify us as human, nor do they label us as defective. However, our universal identification in Adam includes us with all persons. We need a Savior!

Our claim to universal spiritual "disorder" does not mean that all suffer disability (physical, intellectual, or psychiatric).[5] It also does not mean that the metaphorical use of disorder and disability related to various unfortunate human circumstances, like being left handed, uncoordinated, or unemployed, is equated with the disability experienced by persons with physical, intellectual, or psychiatric impairments. In this particular sense, all people do not have disabilities, though at some point in our lives up to 50 percent of us may acquire one. Notwithstanding, one day we all will also face death, which is total disability in this world. We do not want to reduce, minimize, appropriate (which is to misappropriate), or devalue the experience of persons with disabilities as we include all persons in God's grace and salvation. The common "spiritual" disability we share is that we innately do not possess the righteousness of God, nor do we have the innate ability to attain it. We all need righteousness to be given to us as a gift in Christ. However, our shared spiritual brokenness, though a figure employed here, is not equated to or synonymous with, and does not reduce, the physical, intellectual, and psychiatric disabilities experienced by persons.

Our work will attempt to parse these distinctions when needed. Some of the remainder of this work will not treat those with mental health conditions differently from those without. In one sense, they are treated together, as those who are broken and have been offered grace and salvation. Although salvation in Christ is provided universally and uniformly in Christ (his atoning death and bodily resurrection), it is manifested, appropriated, and effected uniquely in each person relative to their biopsychosocial and hamartiological context. The same love and grace of God works uniquely in each life. This work focuses on what salvation looks like for those who have depression.

Following the fall, the image of God in Adam (in each of us) is being restored according to the image of God in Christ (*imago Christi*), a new creation. The *imago Christi* is not only the soteriological *telos* of the image of God in *adam*, but it is also the archetype from which it was originally conceived. The term *image* hearkens to the second person of the Trinity. In the *processio*, the Father eternally generates the Son or image (an eternal subsistent relation). The *processio* of the image, immanently, is also causal and definitive of the *missio*, economically. This is the inherent connection between the processions and the missions. The *processio* is revealed in the *missio* as the Son takes on human form to reveal the divine image to humanity. The mission is to transform humanity in the divine image (*imago Christi*). In prolepsis, Jesus Christ is the image of God from the foundations of the world, in the creation of *adam*, and in the new creation. From all eternity, the *imago Dei* is defined as Jesus Christ and realized in us by the love and power of the sanctifying Spirit of God.

Jesus Christ, the God-man (*Theanthropos*), has revealed the true *imago Dei*, from eternity. He is the invisible image made visible. Jesus Christ, as the incarnation, defines the *imago Dei*. Christology defines anthropology. Here, we are using God's own incarnational terms to give substance and shape to the image. To understand the *imago*, we need to understand the theanthropic hypostatic relationship in Christ and the interpersonal relationship between the Father and the only begotten Son within the one *ousia* (divine nature). The persons of the Father and the Son, as indicated by their names, are constituted relationally. The Father of eternal origin generates the Son. The only begotten Son is eternally generated from the Father. The relation defines the identity of the Son (filiation) and the Father (paternity). The Son is generated from the Father. The Word proceeds from within the divine nature, as a thought would proceed from the mind that thinks reflectively about itself. The Word then is a procession of knowledge from God to God. From the bond of the Father and Son proceeds the Spirit, the procession of love. For us, that does not signify the intellect and will to power, as it has throughout history. The processions received economically signify that we know the love of God.

The nature of the processions is significant because it discloses the missions of the Son and the Spirit. The processions of the Son and Spirit reveal the knowledge and love of God within the immanent relations of the Trinity. They are also causal and definitive of the *missio Christi* and *missio Spiritus*. The Father sent the Son by the Spirit to become human. In so doing, we may know the love of the Father and be incorporated into God's family by baptism, as daughters and sons reborn in the image of God in Christ. In this sense, the *imago Christi* is identificational. God took on our nature and identified with our disfigured, disabled, and disordered condition. He descended to become truly human as a particular Jewish man at a particular time and place, first-century Palestine. He also became truly human emblematically for the race. He chose to assume the humblest construal of the term *human*, a suffering slave, poor, despised, and rejected (Isa. 53). Christ further identified with our sin as the Lamb of God and was sentenced to death by the powers of this world. The person of Christ is truly divine and truly human ontologically and existentially. The image present in the hypostatic union is divine, but it is also the truest form of our humanity in all of its weakness, dependence, and *nihil* (nothingness). Christ embodies the full *diastemic* essence of our created being, which distinguishes us from uncreated being. The union reaches the fullness of our ontological difference. It touches the extent of our humanity, even in our hyperhuman conditions. Hyperhuman experiences reveal our extreme, true weakness and frailty. They disclose our camouflage and pretense to demi-divinity.[6] The function of the *imago Christi* is to identify with the entirety of our condition, so as to transport and transform us into divine likeness, forever approaching God, a crescendo toward infinity.[7]

The ontological difference[8] here is not only between uncreated and created being but also between the One whose existence and essence are synonymous and creaturely being whose existence and essence are not identical. The Logos bridges that chasm and is joined with the creaturely difference of becoming (acting from potency). The Almighty is united with our humanity in the person of Jesus Christ, who identifies with our *nihil*, our frame of dust. Further, he who did not know sin became sin for us. He embraced our impoverished and impaired moral image that we might be redeemed. God, the Almighty, is hypostatically joined with embodied weakness to touch our humanity that we may touch his divinity. We behold his divinity in the *imago Christi*, the archetype of our sanctification. Jesus Christ, the Son of God, is the *imago Dei*, and so it follows that the nature of that image is familial, indicated by *Son*, a term defined relationally with the Father.

Also, the image is relational in Christ's union with our humanity through the incarnation. The purpose of the Father's relation with us through the Son and the Spirit is soteriological and doxological that we may become the *familitas* of God and bring glory to God. Here, there is no medical or sociocultural register that defines or measures us as human, abled or disabled. Christ is both definition and measure. In sum, we are defining, at least in part, the image of God in Christ, relationally, specifically a family relationship. This familial relation *en Christo* depicts the image of God as equal access for all humanity to become one family with God. All are equal, and all are invited!

In terms of the de facto universal inequities, prejudices, and oppression that exist among persons and systems, let it be unequivocally reaffirmed and firmly stated that the image of God in Christ based on creation and fully realized in salvation is the theologically universal ground and rule for equality (value, freedom, rights, opportunity, protection, etc.) of all persons regardless of race, ethnicity, ability, sex, gender, age, health, status, and so on and is the basis for our theological anthropology and all of the theories, laws, policies, and practices that stem from it that pertain to all humanity.

THE RELATIONAL IMAGE OF GOD

Let us delve further into Scripture and unpack what we mean by the image of God in Christ. The New Testament undeniably affirms a Christocentric construal of the *imago Dei*.[9] Christ as the glory and image of God is cited directly in 2 Corinthians 4:4-6; Colossians 1:15-20; and Hebrews 1:1-4. The Greek translation for the Hebrew *tselem* is *eikon* and denotes not only a copy of an archetype but also a participation[10] in its nature as well.[11] Further, the fullness (*pleroma*) of the original dwells within the *eikon* (Col. 2:9), and the copy is even equated with the original in these scriptural contexts.[12] The creed proclaims, "God from God, light from light." The light of God's own glory is revealed in the face of Christ, who as light from light is the *eikon* of God. In seeing the visible Christ, one then sees the invisible Father in his "nature and being" (John 1:14; 2 Cor. 4:4-6; Col. 1:15).[13] The image of God's glory, light inaccessible, is an attribute that God cannot share with *adam*, though made in the *imago Dei*. In the Old Testament, Moses could not directly behold the *kabod* but only its wake (Exod. 33:23). Even the tabernacle and the temple would only provisionally house its shadow until the glory was fully embodied in the one who is the true icon. No one before had beheld the image of divine glory but the only begotten Son. He declares the invisible and unseen *doxa* as its shines from his face reflecting the Father (John 1:14, 18). The relationship of image to the original is Son to Father (Sonship) and Spirit to Son and Father (*familitas*) and becomes "the archetype of the image in mankind [*sic*]."[14]

Again, in stressing relationality, we are reminded that the divine persons are identified distinctly by relations. The Son is constituted by a subsistent relation to the Father. Further, in becoming human, the Son reveals the image as relational, reflecting the glory of the Father, while also identifying with our full humanity. Aquinas is unequivocal that the Son is the image of the Father. St. Thomas claims *image* is a proper name for the Son, and it is a relation (a relative opposition to what is imaged).[15] Of course, created human persons and divine uncreated persons are not univocal terms, and so the relational nature of person is analogical and different for both types, human and divine. Unlike uncreated being, relations of created being are accidental. For the persons of the Trinity, the relations are subsistent and constitute the person, while the relations among created beings and with God are contingent and accidental. Relation does not univocally define a human person in the same way it defines divine persons. The subsistent relations of divine persons are not accidental but within the divine essence. Created beings and their relationships are not necessary. Technically, a person can still be a human being, though unfulfilled, without or outside of their human relationships. However, in God, even though our relational existence is accidental and not necessary, we would not exist without participating in his existence. Nonetheless, the point is that between humanity and the divine, the *imago Dei* is relational in nature.[16]

In centering on the relational dynamic of the image of God, we recognize that this move is not to the exclusion of the various attributes that also shape human experience. The Christian tradition has identified God's attributes analogically reflected in human nature, though again these designations have not always been accommodating to all people. Thus, a traditional working definition of *person* often will fall short for all persons.[17] However, we are relocating human functions, when present, in a larger relational dynamic of daughter/sonship facilitated by the love of the sanctifying Spirit of God.

Theologians like Augustine[18] and Maximus[19] identified vestiges of the *imago Trinitatis*[20] in the human soul, reason, and will. Yet these processions of knowledge and will/love are relational. The triune God is a *perichoresis* of loving relations between the distinct persons in divine unity. This mutual love also extends to relations with humanity. We are called to be the family (*familitas*) of God and participate in divine Sonship through the perfecting love of the Spirit.[21] The *telos* of being created and renewed in the *imago Christi* is that humanity, in all of its expressions, becomes incorporated into the family of God, as an ecclesial charismatic being fully participating in the triune life of God. Maximus the Confessor held that the relationship between God and humanity, even the cosmos, was participatory in nature (*metousia Theou*). The logoi of creation participate in the Logos of God. The hypostatic inherence (*enhypostasis*) of the human nature (the image of God) participates in the Logos and ultimately is fulfilled in the Logos becoming flesh. Human being is relational being, defined Christocentrically. The logos,[22] or God's wisdom, will, and purpose, of the *imago Dei* is Christ and subsequently our incorporation into his body as his children. Consequently, the image of God is realized through participating in divine *familitas* through Christ, a family that is home to all, exclusive of none. Thus, the image of God in Christ becomes the theological ground for the belonging of all persons disabled or abled. Likewise, in *theosis*, we share the same purpose.

THE RELATIONAL CONTEXT OF A MODIFIED RATIONAL-VOLITIONAL MODEL

If the *imago* is primarily participatory or relational, then what do we do with human faculties in persons who have mental disorders, as well as others? This is the problem that Reinders posed but did not fully address. We know that gifts, such as reason, contribute to the embodied consciousness of persons with depression. Yet we must stress that these relative, limited, and varying attributes, such as reason, freedom, and moral agency, in prelapsarian humanity are both ontologically similar and to a greater degree dissimilar to their divine archetype. Their dissimilarity in the ontological difference (*diastema*) between uncreated and created being does not disqualify them as instruments of the *imago*. Attributes are simply radically redefined, severely limited (dependence), and properly subordinated in their function. Human attributes, as a diversity of gifts, are not defined by their autonomous capacity to achieve, but by their weakness and limitation in dependent participation upon God. Decentering and relocating the attributes, such as reason and freedom, means recognizing and unveiling the illusory notion of autonomy and returning to the contingent and participatory nature of our existence. Our faculties and powers, as persons, are relative. They were created to serve our relationship with the divine. Human attributes and characteristics were designed to participate and find their perfection in relation with the divine as God's gift.

After examining Christ as the image of God, we reemphasize that we are not discarding traditional attributes from some human experience, like the rational, the volitional, the moral, or the functional.[23] We are subverting, inverting, redefining, and refocusing them based on the true standard in Christ. The change is from Greek notions to scriptural and christological ones. Christ is the standard. Further, his Sonship dictates the goal, relationship with the divine. The powers of the image service the theanthropic bond. The attributive faculties were not designed as instruments of human autonomy to attain power. Rather than titanic[24] capacities to attain herculean achievement, *imago* attributes and functions reflect the ontological difference of created beings and so are to be cultivated in utter dependence and virtue. In the case of reason, because of its limits and the noetic effect of sin, it is coupled specifically with humility (epistemic humility).[25] The creation of the attributes in the *imago*, such as the rational image, was not intended for autonomous human development and the achievement of reason, ability, and morality. They are divine capacities to be in relation with God.

This *telos*, before the fall, from the foundation of the world, was to be satisfied in Christ. He is the true image that models this call. In becoming human for the salvation of all of humanity, he identifies with what we esteem to be the lowest stations in society.[26] Christ covers the full expanse, the ontological difference (*diastema*) between God and humanity, not in its heights but in its depth and depression. He redeems from what we consider to be the bottom up, as we would perceive the bottom and its margins. To become human is to be human at its truest, that is, at its weakest, in its differences, and in its divine dissimilarity. Thus, the true icon of God subverts and inverts our graven image, the self-portrait, that we paint of our pure reason, our will to power, moral goodness, and Platonic polis. It deconstructs the Promethean temples constructed to house our tainted, bloodstained trophies of human conquest and vainglory. The suffering servant has come to cast us down from the high places and to identify with our lowliness. Claims of power, ability, righteousness, and wisdom are toppled in Christ. If the image of God is to be renewed, we must become like a child, as the Christ child. We must become like the sick who need a physician, like the incarcerated who need liberation, the leper who needs to be cleansed, and the lost who needs to be found. We are all of these persons, as we morph from dust to dust. He identifies with the lost, last, and least of these. In identifying with our brokenness, Christ also becomes an embodied prophetic sign judging our feeble façade of human wisdom, ability, and power, the fig leaves that attempt to cover our nakedness.

Now let us examine how the Christian tradition, drawing from Scripture, has deconstructed, relocated, and redefined attributes, such as reason and will. Ancient Eastern thinkers like St. Maximus acknowledged an Alexandrian anthropology in which image and likeness refer to mind and will. However, such properties were not an end in themselves but instrumental to a higher call. These aspects of the *imago* served a greater relational microcosmic (of the universe) function within the image of God—to be deified in Christ and mediate a cosmic *theosis*. The *skopos* of the image is a relational one, involving participation in his Sonship[27] and partaking of the divine nature. The divine intention of our participatory (*metousia*) *enhypostatic* existence in the Logos is to be conformed into his image, sonship/daughtership. The Logos is a procession of knowledge (wisdom, the way of God) embodied in the *imago*. Unfortunately, the theological history of the rational image and the nature and place of reason have been too often informed strictly by certain inherited philosophical traditions, usually Platonic or Aristotelian, or by the prevailing philosophy of the day, as opposed to the Scriptures.

The New Testament witness to the rational image in Christ (the mind of Christ) starkly contrasts with the picture offered by many philosophical traditions. The rational image (*logikon*) fulfilled in Christ is not the Logos of Heraclitus, the pure idea of Plato, the form of Aristotle, the rational seed of the Stoics, the *gnosis* of gnostic assent, the Cartesian *cogito*, the Leibnizian rational monad, the categories of Kant, or any other conceived rational structure of philosophy. Though it answers and exceeds them all. The Logos is ultimately defined in christological terms over against philosophical categories. The Logos, in procession, is declared from the Father and, in mission, sent for our salvation. In this sense, there is no *Deus revelatus* that brings salvation through the efforts of humanity, including the efforts and heavy lifting from the *logos* of philosophy.

At this point in referencing *Deus revelatus*, I want to pause to speak parenthetically on the *Deus absconditus*, the hiddenness of God, that Luther stressed. God intentionally does not reveal himself in human ability, reason, or power, but in the crucified One. Unlike Luther, we acknowledge the analogical structure (similarity and greater dissimilarity) of the Creator and creature relationship (*analogia entis*). The dissimilarity is exacerbated through the fall that separates us from God. Like Luther, though, we hold that God is hidden from us and inaccessible through our glorified human means. Angels with flaming swords guard the gates of paradise from our reentering upon banishment and exile. Fallen, we need to follow God's *oikonomia* of redemption. Yet, unlike Luther, we would not restrict the knowledge of God solely to the revelation of the crucified Christ, as in his version of the *theologia crucis*. Salvation history is replete with revelation pointing to the Mashiach. Yes, the content, core, and culmination of God's salvific revelation, we concur, is found at the cross. We also assert that owing to the *analogia entis* there is a similarity in the relational structure between Creator and creation conducive to revelation. That relation is structural to God's salvation history and preparatory for the gospel. God is never without a witness. Thus, the *Deus revelatus* in Christ is not the sole event of God's revelation, though it is the crescendo of God's light and bearer of salvation. This light is incipient in the logoi of creation, is obscured with the fall, but is gradually restored. The light shines through the law and the prophets, growing brighter and foreshadowing the coming Messiah. However, as Romans chapters 1–3 demonstrate, the revelation of God in creation and the law is suppressed through human unrighteousness and idolatry. In turn, this light exposes our darkness, providing us with the knowledge of sin (Rom. 3:20) and God's wrath (1:18). The result is that our self-justification is silenced and nullified (3:19), preparing us to receive the righteousness of God that only comes by faith in Christ (3:22).

Having made that epistemological distinction between Luther's more limited theology of the cross and what I am claiming, I reassert the nature and significance of the knowledge of God in the crucified One. The *enhypostatic* participation of the human logos in the Logos in Christ is the sole threshold to the knowledge of God's glory, which is revealed by the Spirit in Christ's suffering on the cross. Our noetic attainments are nullified by the Logos suffering. Christ came to embody our spiritual disfigurement and disorder and not human glory. Christ came also to embody our mental disorder as well by becoming fully human. The image of God in Christ is not based on or attained by performance of our faculties but is given as gift. The Logos became truly human that we might become like God through the gift of the sanctifying Spirit. The contrasts we find penned in Scripture that set the revelation of God apart from this world's philosophical traditions are striking.

The theology of Paul intentionally deconstructs *sarx*-driven reason. Paul sharply illustrates the dissimilarity between mere human reason and reason subject to the Spirit. In 1 Corinthians chapters 1 and 2, Paul contrasts the wisdom of God with the wisdom of the Greeks, the mind of Christ with the mind of the "natural man," and the nature of knowledge revealed by the Spirit with the knowledge given in philosophy. In chapter 2, verse 6, Paul declares, "We speak a message of wisdom to the mature, but not the wisdom of this age or of the rulers of this age, who are coming to nothing." Paul affirms the faculty of reason and the value of knowledge, but he redefines them. For the apostle, true knowledge is not speculative philosophy that is blind to the wisdom of God and rejects the power of salvation found in Christ. The speculative philosophy that ruled Paul's day and the scientific, technical, instrumental reason that rules our day echo the will to power for "the rulers of the age" (2:6). It is a knowledge that builds human pride (8:1) and blinds the eyes of the powers of this world from the true knowledge of God (1:21; 2:8-9). In Paul's day, the rulers he refers to executed Christ and persecuted his followers. The apostle judges the philosophy of this world as foolishness and worthless according to God's standard of knowledge (3:19-20). The wisdom of the world does not arrive at the knowledge of the existence of God (1:21) or at the knowledge of salvation in Christ (2:8). Throughout history the great, influential atheistic philosophies of Nietzsche, Heidegger, Sartre, and today's so-called new atheists and the influential political philosophies of Machiavelli, Hobbes, Rousseau, Marx, Bakunin, and others offer their systems and solutions but do not direct us to the saving wisdom of God found in a crucified King. For Paul, the philosophy of this world is not the wisdom of God.

Paul contrasts the fallen use of reason (exaltation) with the spiritual (proper) use of reason as exemplified by the mind of Christ (crucifixion).

The rational capacity of humanity (*logikoi*), properly defined, ordered, and redeemed, looks quite different from what our hubris values, prescribes, and has "normalized." The knowledge (the Son) and love of God (the Spirit) are God's gifts of himself to us, not self-fulfilled human capacities. The gospel inverts our values and, in this case, our sense of the rational-volitional. The knowledge of God, via an epistemology of the cross, is set over against any inflationary notion and display of human reason and will. The knowledge of God apprehended exclusively by the Spirit is both *semeion* (sign as demonstration of power) and *sophia* (wisdom) that the Jews and Gentiles seek (1 Cor. 1:22). Yet, in their true form, the treasure of wisdom and knowledge (Col. 2:3) and the demonstration of God's power (1 Cor. 1:24; 2:4) are concealed in Christ from the philosophers of the ages and embodied in the Lord of glory (1 Cor. 2:8), who comes as a suffering servant to die on a cross. The wise, the rich, and the powerful stumble over this rock of offense. Christ, the wisdom of God, surprises us as God's righteousness, holiness, sanctification, and redemption. The wisdom of God is the power of God revealed only by the Spirit in the One who suffered and was crucified. Divine wisdom or reason takes on "disfigurement" (Isa. 53) and "disorder" in respect to what we prize and value.[28] He identifies with human disability but is despised and rejected by those who have constructed their own image of ableism.

Clearly, human reason is redefined by the divine Logos made flesh. The logos of the *imago Dei* is defined most clearly in "the logos of the cross" (1 Cor. 1:18). The logos of the cross—rejection, suffering, and redemption— "crucifies" and converts reason to epistemic humility, through an epistemology of the cross, an epistemology of foolishness and weakness (1 Cor. 1:20-29). Kevin Vanhoozer claims a virtue epistemology, over against epistemic vice or noetic sin, in terms of an "epistemology of the cross" that deconstructs human ideologies and is an "outright rejection of the attempt to think God on the basis of reason alone."[29] Christ, the wisdom of God, is understood over and against our fallen use of reason.

Christ crucified is God's concealed and saving wisdom, revealed by the Spirit. Christ did not come to fulfill or crown the reason and wisdom of this world, but he came to destroy it (1 Cor. 1:19). To the eyes of human reason, this divine wisdom is hidden (2:7), rejected (2:8), and foolish (1:18-25) in light of its own standards. On the other hand, the wisdom of God is cherished by the weak, the ignoble, the foolish, the lowly, and the despised (1:26-29). In an epistemology of the cross, human reason and power and the faculties of aptitude and performance that are treasured and flaunted by human ableness are ousted, brought to nothing (2:6), and redefined (1:18; 2:2, 6, 10-16) by Christ through the "logos of the cross," which is Christ crucified. Rational faculties apart from God's illumination are declared impotent. They truly are without power to save and are rendered null (1:19; 2:6) in the light of God's true wisdom and power. Christ is God's true wisdom and power, which brings salvation to the lost. This is the purpose of the incarnation, to renew the image of God in us. The rational image of God is fulfilled in the mind of Christ. This mind is submitted to the Spirit and the wisdom of God and led into humble service and sacrifice for others. Christ crucified (God disfigured and disordered), not human attainment, is the wisdom and power animating the *imago*. For in the cross we see his suffering, glory, and salvation offered. We are called to participate through baptism in the cross, its death, burial, and resurrection, a participatory *theologia crucis*. We participate in the cross through the doorway of the sacraments. The power of the sacrament of baptism and the Eucharist reveals divine agency for salvation and sanctification to those who have agency, compromised agency, and nonempirical agency. Through the water and the bread and wine, God gifts himself as a gift to us, and we are made partakers of the divine nature, *theosis*.

Ultimately, it is Christ who is the measure of true wisdom and power (1 Cor. 1:24) and not human reason and its attending will to power. The logos of the cross appropriated freely through the sacraments is the power of God unto salvation. This radical conclusion is essential for a theological anthropology that should not gauge humanity and its value based on the performance of rational intelligence or other ability quotients measured by physical, cognitive, financial, social, or other standards. Paul's indictment is against the "natural" (without the Spirit)[30] use of reason. By nature, we are blind to God and God's plan.

We are now in a position to redefine the image and even our faculties, including reason, in terms of Christ crucified, who is the measure of God. Christ in identification and solidarity with the broken, biological hypostasis of embodied consciousness (humanity) is the true measure of humanity. And ultimately mental disorder and depression need to be evaluated in terms of our relationship with God in Christ as: *creation* (limited created being), *fallen* (disfigured and disordered creation), and the *new creation* (the renewed image). The three states of our relationship with God have historically informed three theological types of depression: *natural, consequential*, and *purgative*, which will be unpacked in the following three chapters. At this point, let us examine the structure of our relationship with God through Christ, as Creator and creation, and the ontological difference between the two.

Christ in his humanity identifies with the totality of our ontological difference. "What has not been assumed has not been healed" or redeemed, as Gregory the Theologian declared.[31] Further, even after the fall, Christ becomes sin as well (2 Cor. 5:21) that we be made righteous. Following the fall, the attributes of the *imago* are more or less marred, even spiritually disabled. Not that human nature changes ontologically; we remain human. The image of God, though spiritually disabled, remains good because God created it. However, it needs to be healed and saved by one who has not been marred by sin. Christ is hypostatically the true image because ontologically he is the archetypal Logos and the eternal Son. Thus, the *analogia entis*, or analogy of being, between created *adam* and uncreated being (God) is one of similitude and greater dissimilitude in being and attribution, but not an analogy of identity. The *diastema* of dissimilarity in the overall *analogia* is both ontological and hamartiological (effect of sin). A postlapsarian *analogia* results in further moral dissimilarity to divine likeness, departing from righteousness and true holiness. Following the fall, we may ask what has become of God's original intention of the image. Though it is impaired in *adam*, the image of God is revealed by God in Christ. Christ identifies with and subsumes all of *adam*, or created being, and the sin of *adam* (as the last Adam). He suffers sin's death that we may be joined to him, conformable to his death in order to partake of his resurrection. God becomes fully human and all that the condition entails, even spiritual disfigurement and disorder, that we may realize our full humanity and become like God. Even though Christ identifies with the poor and experiences marginalization as a Jew and a prophet, he does not necessarily possess every physical or intellectual impairment or every permutation of states within the human condition. However, he arguably suffered depression, perhaps from the garden of Gethsemane to Golgotha. In his person, he assumes all humanity, even all persons with psychiatric disabilities, representatively. In the Logos, the archetypal form of truth, goodness, and beauty in flesh, is the form of all forms, and the transcendental signifier[32] becoming human for all persons. The *analogia* between God and humanity does not fail but is concretized. In Christ, the *analogia entis*[33] is stretched to its limits and fulfilled in him.[34]

The conclusion is that the *imago* is defined by participation in the Son that persons may become new creations, sons and daughters of the most High God. The Son, in substance, is truly divine and is the true human image of God. The logos of the image is fulfilled in *theosis* through our *enhypostatic*[35] relation in Christ, where we become renewed in the image of God (righteousness and true holiness) as God's children. The precise nature of the relationship between the divine and human in the person of Christ is of course hammered out in the Chalcedonian formula (451 CE), which unites the two natures, divine and human, in one person Jesus Christ, truly God and truly human. Two distinct natures are joined in one hypostasis, "inconfusedly, unchangeably, inseparably, and indivisibly," not as two persons but "the Self-same Son and Only-begotten God, Word, Lord, Jesus Christ." The only begotten Son is one in being with the Father and the Holy Spirit, three distinct persons in one divine essence. The Father sent the eternally generated Son to become man that we might become like God, *imago Christi*.[36]

ANALOGIA ENTIS AND A RELATIONAL MODEL OF THE *IMAGO DEI*

The turn to a participatory or relational model of the *imago Dei* reflects a larger turn to relationality in other fields, such as postmodernism,[37] disability studies,[38] and theological anthropology. In terms of theology, Stanley Grenz traces the emergence of relationality and the relational *imago* with the Reformation. That period emphasized the loss of the structural notion of the image of God in terms of reason, will, and righteousness due to human depravity.[39] Human reason is fallen. The will is bound, and original righteousness has faltered and needs to be restored. Luther and Calvin stressed divine relationship and humanity's position before God. Human standing before God originally reflected the image of God but needs to be restored through right relations with God through Christ, who is our alien righteousness. Later, neo-Reformers Karl Barth (1886–1968) and Wolfhart Pannenberg (1928–2014) developed their own relational models based on the analogy between human constitutive relations and divine constitutive relations.[40] Barth's model, built around the "I-Thou encounter" of divine-human relationality, is ultimately shaped, to no surprise, by the revelation of the triune God through the incarnation. He rejects all philosophical anthropology.[41] Whereas Pannenberg, although upholding revelation, as Barth, also affirms human experience and anthropological insights that inform a theology from below.[42] Barth's *analogia relationis* is strictly grounded in his *analogia fidei*, rather than Erich Przywara's or Balthasar's *analogia entis* (analogy of being).[43] For Barth, relationality in the *imago* is based on God's self-revelation in the Lord Jesus Christ alone, no *tertium quid*. Barth could not accept revelation as fulfillment to a prior or general metaphysical construct that relates uncreated with created being, like the *analogia entis*.[44] Barth's refusal of any *praeparatio* or prolegomena becomes problematic even when examining the revelation of the incarnation. In order to recognize truly the humanity of Christ, it is vital to affirm in his hypostasis a truly human nature, created being. God chooses to work through creation. The context of creation needs to be affirmed as an acceptable means of facilitating revelation. The possibility of the incarnation and the prior *Heilsgeschichte* that leads up to it, beginning with the creation of *adam* and the *imago Dei*, are all an affirmation that God's revelation can be clothed in creation. We cannot disregard the context of creation, through which revelation, even the inspiration of Scripture, occurs. Revelation is communicated and unfolds contextually in space and time, in a world, through a worldview, and in the flesh of culture, even in a Jewish carpenter (John 1:14). Barth, at times, thought he could theologize on the revelation of God in Christ in a vacuum and remain immune to implicit philosophical assumptions or consequences of his claims. He manages this dilemma in spite of the fact that the Word is made human in human context, and that means cultural and historical context, which are not from above but from below.[45]

An analogy of being attempts to navigate between divinity and humanity that are not univocally related. The relational structure, both ontological and epistemological, between uncreated being and created being is not digital (exact or univocal) but analogical. Our understanding is cataphatic alongside an ever-increasing and infinite apophasis, conjunctive and ever disjunctive. Thus, the knowledge of God across analogical lines is understood as similitude (*analogia attributionis*) and even greater dissimilitude (*analogia proportionalitatis*) across infinity.[46] How does the analogy of being inform our discussion about the image of God? The analogy defines and informs the nature of the relationship between image and God. The *analogia* between uncreated being and created being begins in the *imago* with *adam* and is fulfilled and concretized in Christ.[47] Although the *analogia entis* seems to do much heavy philosophical and theological lifting, it is not an idol, rival, or salvific substitute for Christ, as is often portrayed by Barth and his supporters on this issue.[48] Contrarily, the *analogia* is the instrumental structure (ontological and epistemological) for receiving and understanding divine communication (knowledge of God) in the context of creation, beginning with the act of creation itself, which came into being by the eternal Logos (Word). Through the act of creation by the Word, the Word establishes the analogy between the Word and the logos (word) of creation. In creating all things by his Word, God presents creation as a gift and a revelation, which declare his glory[49] (Ps. 19:1-6). According to St. Maximus the Confessor, the Logos in creation prefigures the divine intention and the revelation of Christ to come, even a prolepsis of the incarnation,[50] the Word's cosmic incarnation.[51] Creation by the Word is a type of "incarnation" for Maximus in a figurative sense. Similarly, prior to the historical incarnation of Christ, God had revealed himself to his people, Israel, through the prophets, even abiding (the glory—*kabod*) with them in the tabernacle and the temple and through various theophanies. Further for Maximus, the Logos of Scripture is revelation that is prior to but also prefigures and points to Christ. To say that the Logos is not revealed analogically through creation and the Hebrew Scriptures but is only revealed in the incarnation is to deny God's revelation in the cosmos (Ps. 19; Rom. 1:19–20), in the law, the prophets, and the writings (Tanakh), and God's work in salvation history for his people. Regarding the necessary connection between revelation and the *analogia*, David Bentley Hart (1965–) boldly claims that "apart from the *analogia entis*, the very concept of revelation is a contradiction; only insofar as creaturely being is analogous to divine being, and proper to God's nature, can God show himself as God."[52] Contrarily, to Barth and other detractors, the *analogia entis*, and specifically the Logos revealed in creation, is not being held up against the incarnation as competing revelation or another means of salvation. There is no claim that the knowledge of God through the *analogia* is salvific; it is merely instrumental in the economy of preparation (*praeparatio*). Nevertheless, it is not that the incarnation is dependent on the preparatory revelation of the Logos in creation and in Scripture. Conversely, the logoi of creation and Scripture are proleptically dependent on the incarnation because the incarnation is the *skopos* (purpose) of the entire *economia* of the logoi beginning with creation.[53]

The Word became created, personal, human context through the *analogia*. God employed the context of creation to reveal his Word throughout salvation history (*Heilsgeschichte*) as *praeparatio evangelica*, a messianic hermeneutic, leading to Christ. The incarnation assumes the analogical framework in created being,[54] which is incipient in creation yet concretized and fulfilled in Christ alone. The Logos of creation is inseparably the Logos of salvation, from the *imago Dei* in *adam* to the *imago Dei* in Christ. Rephrasing the Athanasian idiom, Christ identifies with extremities of the ontological difference in created being that humanity may become like God. Further, the *analogia*, even with its faint similarities and greater dissimilarities, provides a reference to understand not only the connection between the invisible and the visible and faith and reason, but also theology. Theology then serves as a hinge to other disciplines (e.g., neurophilosophy), allowing for the full integrative work needed.

ZIZIOULAS AND RELATIONAL BEING

Much of our discussion on relationality thus far has drawn from Catholic sources on the *analogia* and from some patristic contributions, especially from Maximus the Confessor in the East, where the idea makes a significant ontological impact. Eastern Christian theology often stresses that personhood itself is construed as relational. As far as the analogy can be carried out, relations toward God and others define human personhood in the *imago Dei* as Bishop Zizioulas has noted, as "being-in-relation," which we began to uncover in the previous chapter.[55] Human being is defined by personhood. Personhood is not a mere attribute of human being but the very "hypostasis of the being."[56] Human being can be defined in its biological existence, and thus the human person may be called the *"hypostasis of biological existence,"* which is constituted by biological life that is uniquely differentiated as human.[57] Even the term for humanity, *adam*, includes male and female together. With the pneuma-breathed biological hypostasis of person, we affirm humanity in terms of its embodied conscious existence, which is not self-contained or autonomous but participates in the image of God for its very being.

Human life is not solitary in terms of person but is plural and in communion. With Zizioulas, the truth of the human person is not in substance or nature but as a "mode of existence," as derived debatably from the Cappadocians, and that mode is "being in communion," whereby a person locates their identity.[58] Further, personhood rests in being in communion with otherness not in the dissolution of difference but in the fellowship with it.[59] As the bishop affirms, "A human being left to himself cannot be a person."[60] Humanity is a differentiated unity of persons in communion that points to and directs the communal nature of our well-being. The self-determined, self-interested, inward-focused, autonomous individual defies divine intention. God created humanity as an icon of the divine to reflect holiness and love in communion. Personhood by nature reaches outside of itself in love to the other, *ekstasis*, that it may fulfill its purpose in God and creation.[61] True personhood is realized in love and service to God and creation. Relation and mutuality in love mark our common humanity and move the *imago* toward God in *theosis* as children of God.

Additionally, relation is structural to reality in terms of verbal and nonverbal interaction and communication between God and humanity, humanity with itself and with creation. Relation is a priori and conditional metaphysically and epistemologically to human being as a contingent and contextual being. Our relation and service to the other in love (ethics) precedes and trumps any ontology, as affirmed in Levinas' notion of "otherwise than being" and an "ethics of alterity" in which one transcends Heideggerian being and responds to the "other" (*il y a*—"there is"), by gazing into the face of the other and experiencing the pull and the gravity of the other, who in alterity refuses to be defined and colonized but instead imposes the command, "Thou shalt not kill."[62] The call of the other in God and neighbor is seen in the gaze and calls us to love and serve the other. Dependent on God and others, the love of God and love of the other mark the image of God in humanity and mark God's mission in us, a liturgy of love. As *Homo adorans* (humanity as worshiping beings), we are doxological creatures in relationship with our

God to love and serve. As *Homo extrenticus*, we are drawn to love outside of ourselves, and as *Homo socius* we extend that love to the other. Humanity is a relation of persons reflecting even the triune eternal, divine relation of persons as analogically the particular *hypostases* work within the general *ousia*.[63] For us as contingent beings and not subsistent relations within the divine nature, the analogy of our relations is rather an analogy of love. As God reached outside his divinity in the incarnation to assume our condition, we also are called in love to reach out the other in love. Our ministry with the world is to love one another as God has loved us.

THREE STATES OF THE RELATIONAL *IMAGO*: CREATION, FALL, NEW CREATION

In summary, we have identified a participatory (analogical) or relational *imago Dei*. The image is fulfilled in divine daughter/sonship *en Christo*, a process of *theosis*. We have characterized the image of God as identificational and soteriological. The identificational aspect highlights created being in its differentiation, dependence, disability, and weakness. Through the incarnation, Christ identifies with our humanity to the fullest extent. The soteriological aspect highlights that Christ identifies with fallen humanity. He heals and saves us in our brokenness through the love of the Spirit, which adopts us as God's children and transforms us in the *imago Christi*.

As we move from a relational anthropology to constructing a theology of depression, it is integral to further qualify the participatory image in its three relational states. *Creation* (natural), *fall* (consequential), and *new creation* (purgative) capture the movement and change of the relationship between God and humanity across salvation history. The relational anthropology that has been posited is relative to our relationship with God and the various states of that relationship: created state, fallen state, and newly created (redeemed) state. Thus, we are defining humanity theologically in its relationship with God. These three states that have been identified in terms of their soteriological correlations are somewhat similar to the states (four) identified by Peter Lombard in his *Sentences* that Christ assumes for the purpose of redemption.[64] It would be easy to move, like Lombard, to four states and cover the glorified image. But, in distinction from the controversy with disabilities,[65] I am asserting, contra some in disability studies, that mental disorders will be fully redeemed in the glorified state.[66] Thus, we will work with just three relational states and their related problems. These three relational states will be the basis from which to investigate historical sources for a theological typology of the etiology of mental disorders and depression that will be explored in the next three chapters.

CREATION: THE NATURAL OR EXISTENTIAL
RELATIONAL STATE

The image of God in creation, in its natural or existential condition, is contingent as opposed to necessary. God alone is necessary being. As Aquinas asserted in the revelation of God as I AM that I AM, the existence of God is necessary; and therefore, the existence is the same as his essence (*ipsum esse subsistens*). On the other hand, created contingent being is caused, participates in existence, and is becoming (has potentiality according to its essence). There is a difference between existence (*esse*—that something is) and essence (*essentia, quidditas*, quiddity—what that thing is). We exist as contingent, limited, and dependent beings participating in God's being and have no ground in ourselves. Contingency flies in the face of our modern notion of autonomy that defines human nature. Though we are dependent on and participate in divine being, our being is differentiated from God, as we noted in the *analogia entis*. Also, created being is further differentiated within itself. This differentiation is evident in the expansive and detailed taxonomic distinctions from domain to species. In terms of the image of God, Maximus the Confessor viewed the problem of the one and the many through the one Logos bringing the many logoi of creation together through humanity, the microcosm of the universe, and its *theosis*. The divisions brought together by humanity were the uncreated and created, heaven and earth, the intelligible and sensible, the universe and paradise, and male and female.[67] A redeemed humanity in Christ brings the many together in one.

As postmodernism has prophetically reminded us, the diastemic nature of created being reveals that *différance*[68] is not only ontological but epistemological and semantic. Context and shared meaning are defining. Of course, with postmodernism it would even deconstruct Maximian logocentrism, which is why I would see meaning as shared rather than infinitely deferred as Derrida would have it. For our purpose, the point taken is that difference and the narrative of the other are vital to a theological anthropology. Embracing difference provides equal access to the total human condition, specifically for those who experience disability and disorder. In this sense, we are further qualifying difference with limitation and thus subverting the notion that ability is normative.[69]

As contingent limited humans who live in a fallen world, we live on borrowed time tending toward death. Our frail form is shrouded with weakness, disability, and disorder as it relates to the image of God in Christ, such that no human is fully "able." Yet not all persons' adverse circumstances can be labeled or compared to (physical, intellectual, or psychiatric) disability. The angle taken here is that we are all spiritually broken before God. Ableist normativity is a construct, and an unattainable and false one at that. Perhaps lack of ability relative to the omnipotence of divine being is the norm for humanity. In spite of the social construct of limitation, onto-logically, limitation rather than ability seems to be the norm, though both are relative. Socially we unjustly value and measure human persons based on ability and performance and stigmatize those with less ability, augment-ing any existing so-called impairment.[70] Medical standardization of physi-cal and cognitive norms is needed for obvious practical purposes. But there is also a need for balance and to hear the voices of difference that should inform a social model of disability and public policy.[71]

Related to contingency and limitation are our inherent frailty and weak-ness. From dust we were created, and to dust we will return. We are clay jars, earthen vessels, as sacred writ reminds us. We are as the withering grass under the burning sun or as a vapor dissipating into the sky. We are also reminded on Ash Wednesday that we are unstable, temporal creatures bor-rowed from the ground. And on Good Friday we return to the ground. Our flesh is naturally susceptible to decadence, decay, and disorder, even depres-sion. Even the earth from which we are drawn, and all things, were cre-ated from *tohu* and *bohu*, concepts connected to *creatio ex nihilo*.[72] The *nihil*, or void, from which creation is brought into being can reflect the figurative divine kenosis needed to "make space" for nondivine reality (created being).[73] The thinking here is that the infinite God freely chose, not out of necessity, to limit himself and "step back" to create a universe that is not a pantheist extension of himself but is created from no preexistent material. Creation has its own reality and integrity, though fully dependent on God for its being. Yet it bears its *nihil* as DNA that distinguishes it from uncreated being. The shadow of nothingness, the existential void, looms over humankind as the seed of its ontological difference, even as it participates in God. The *nihil* also extends to human freedom, which is another marker of the image of God along with contingency and dependence. Because our essence is not synon-ymous and fully present with our existence, we must *become*. We must par-ticipate in our essence, what we are to become, by obeying God's will for us. Existentially, we precariously stand in freedom between the gravity of noth-ingness and becoming what we were created to be. And in truly choosing, we must be given freedom, freedom to obey or disobey. Freedom posits the possibility and potentiality to "create," outside of the will of God, an inverted *creatio ex nihilo*. This nothingness is a moral privation that unfolds from the disordered will of *adam*. It is within this existential tension of freedom in becoming where mental disruption occurs, moving us to leap in obedience or lapse. This mental disruption or existential anxiety is claimed by Søren Kierkegaard (1813–1855) to be the ground for the natural or existential etiology of mental disorder, even depression. Simply, mental disorders can occur in the natural order of things.

It is essential to realize that the relational state of the image of God is not stationary. The human person is not pure act but must act to become. The relational image in creation is incipient in its potency and not static but dynamic, moving toward its logos of *theosis*. Mournfully, *adam* moved from a natural state of freedom to the misuse of freedom and sin. The ontological chasm and the contingent nature of created being, which foster human freedom and its primal motion to become, an existential instability, agitate us to choose. Kierkegaard depicts the existential objectless anxiety that arises naturally from our finitude, indeterminate freedom, and the infinitude of possibilities in his *Concept of Anxiety*. Kierkegaard identified what I am calling a natural or existential type of angst that can lead to disorder. Later, Paul Tillich (1886–1965) developed the natural tension found in the ontological difference where nonbeing lurks at the boundaries of being, evoking the angst of nothingness. Like Kierkegaard, Tillich claims anxiety is structural to contingent being itself.

In fact, our encounter with the nothingness of existentialism, the void, the *nihil*, or the nauseating vacuum of nonbeing is not merely introspection into our groundless existence as contingent and ex nihilo. The atheistic existentialists, like Heidegger, Sartre, and others, who have pondered the *nihil* without the knowledge of God construe it as ontologically structural to reality and the self. There is no God, and existence is gratuitous. The *nihil* is the shadow cast by our thrownness into being in the world (Heidegger's *Dasein* or Kierkegaard's "dizziness of freedom").[74] For Sartre, it is the need to choose what we are to become and nihilate our nothingness[75] or for Derrida the absence of presence concealed by text.[76] Without the knowledge of God to explain their epiphany, the existentialist's description of the gaze into the void may appear as such. Behind the contingency of our existence, the indeterminacy of our freedom, and the void of our being is the God of eternity who has made all things from nothing. God's shadow is the gap or interval between all God is and all creation is not, an infinite ontological and even meontological[77] difference.

The encounter with the void, at the least, is a gaze at the nothingness of our contingent being. But it is more. It is a gaze at our *created* contingent being, which was brought out of nothingness by the loving will of God. When that love is opposed, the gaze is lost in the consequential estrangement from God. An eternal and infinite chasm of separation from the one who is our ground and love itself swallows us in the space of our own non-being.[78] Such an experience can be damning, but not necessarily. According to Kierkegaard, angst can function as a pedagogy of meaning and purpose. Such an experience can also be a dark night on the journey of ascent that may require abandonment (purgation) and a hunger that yields quest and epiphany. Ontologically, there is an infinite prelapsarian (prior to sin) gap between God and creation that allows for the potentiality of development and even expressions.

Thus far we have been discussing the downward gaze at that *diastema*, but there is also an upward transcendent gaze. God, as hyperessence (*hyperousia*), is ultimately beyond being and nonbeing. But even the gaze toward God in the apophatic unknowing is an expanse that inspires holy fear and awe. Our God is a consuming fire, and it is a terrible and fearful thing to fall into the hands of the living God, Scripture warns. The "back side" of God, as seen by Moses, can be seen and seen differently with different results by both believer and unbeliever. This gaze is not only present but also eschatological. For the unbeliever, it is an angst of death that envelops *Dasein*, the enslavement in time to the fear of death (Heb. 2:15). For the believer it can be the fear of God that is the beginning of wisdom that awakens our conscience and brings us closer to God "that we will have confidence on the Day of Judgment . . . there is no fear in love. But perfect love drives out fear, because fear has to do with punishment" (1 John 4:17-18, NIV).[79] The *diastema* of being, the analogical interval, the infinite chasm of ontological difference allow for the natural or existential tension. Human freedom emerges and can potentially bring disruption and even disorder into reality, thus a proposed etiology of depression.[80]

THE FALL: THE CONSEQUENTIAL (LAPSARIAN) RELATIONAL STATE

We noted that out of the structural difference in the *imago*, the potential for ontological motion (becoming) and its attending anxiety erupt out of existential instability. Structural fragility creates the natural grounds for the human will to either realize its logos or fall out of order with the divine purpose. Our primal parents chose the latter and misused the gift of freedom. They sought the impossible, an autonomous life grounded in the nothingness of its own being. The fall marks our second relational mode of the *imago*. The falls alienates us from God and consequentially opens the doors to a cacophony of "complicated wickedness."[81] The Christian tradition has vehemently debated the nature of the fall, its extent, and its impact on the *imago Dei*. The intention of this work is not to unpack the complex and lengthy arguments from various theological traditions surrounding the fall except that it has adversely impacted the image, either marring it or with extreme views obliterating it.

The union between God and *adam* is broken. The image is impaired. The will is curved onto itself (*incurvatus in se*), and human mediation of the cosmos is disordered. Further, the attributes and functions of the image of God that were designed for relational dependence on God to fulfill his will are now detached from their source. The image and its attributes implode with the speed of sin and death, and yet are inflated again with the deceptive vanity of human, satanic conceit, propelled by the inverted and perverted prophetic mission to be like God. Human reason is impaired and disordered as a consequence of sin, the so-called noetic effects of sin. Mental disruption and the possibility of greater imbalance, such as physical sickness and mental disorder, begin to surface. The original blessing of righteousness is marred. Human relations with the divine are broken, as alienation and darkness engulf our mournful human condition. Disorder, a departure from God's *shalom*, permeates our relationships with God, each other, and the cosmos. From an impaired *imago*, traditional theories trace the impaired and disordered mental and emotional states that potentially emerge consequentially as melancholia. So goes the classical view of depravity and disorder.

Lapsarian consequences of sin, alienation, and disorder historically define a second theological type of etiology, a consequential type. Consequential disorder is not referring to any defect in the nature of humanity in the image of God, nor to any other secular categories. This theological type claims that mental disorders can surface from the fall and its consequences upon the entire cosmos, including the physical and psychological state of human persons. The image of God is intact but fallen, broken, impaired, and disordered in terms of its relationship with God. Human attributes and functions that serve that relationship are likewise impacted. Because of the fall, the image of God becomes an instrument of sin and humanity an enemy of God. Violence becomes a priori for humanity in its relations toward God, the cosmos, and each other. The human condition is characterized by its alienation and estrangement from God and God's blessing, as well as estrangement from the cosmos and itself. The primal transgression is met with death as a gradual deterioration (morally, physically, and socially) of humanity, including the image of God, a physical terminus, and eternal condemnation. When disconnected from the source of life, entropy sets in. The image of God, as well as the cosmos, though good by nature, is impaired and disordered as a consequence. Pandora's box is open, releasing sin, sickness, and suffering universally and indiscriminately. The image of God is in need of a Savior who will fully identify and assume what it means to be human not only in our ontological difference of weakness and poverty but also in terms of human depravity (2 Cor. 5:21), disfigurement, and disorder.

Various streams within the great tradition, such as the desert fathers, have emphasized the nexus, directly or indirectly, between the consequence of the fall and sin with depression. Evagrius Ponticus (345–399 CE) developed the notion of acedia and its relations with sin and the demonic. We will develop and engage this consequential type of mental disorder in the next chapter by examining the work of Evagrius and the Swiss theologian Han Urs von Balthasar and their contribution to a consequential theory of mental disorder.

NEW CREATION: THE PURGATIVE (REDEEMED) RELATIONAL STATE

Finally, the third state of the relational image is the new creation in Christ. Christ assumed our humanity that we may assume the *imago Christi* and become like divinity. In becoming human, he became fully human to the true extent of ontological difference, even our melancholia. In terms of our social valuations, we deem the poor, the racially oppressed, the marginalized, persons with disabilities or sickness, the elderly, and those with mental disorders to be at the bottom of the ladder of success and lower on the chain of human being. We have, implicitly or explicitly at times, judged some as less valuable, even inhuman. These would include the unborn, those with Down syndrome, racial and ethnic minorities, refugees, asylum seekers, immigrants, migrants, and other marginalized groups of people. However, in the analogical difference between divine and human, difference expresses humanity in its diversity and truest sense, or what I am calling hyperhuman expressions. In weakness, we prophetically make evident to ourselves the true state of our humanity. Our creaturely dependence undermines ableist normative claims made by those who wield the semiotics and artifice of constructed power.

God, in true power, descended to assume humanity in all of its colors, shapes, customs, statuses, and conditions. In order to assume and identify with humanity at its fullest, he reaches the edges and margins, where limitations define our humanity and even constructed limitations that oppress our humanity. The Son of God has taken on the μορφὴν δούλου (form of a slave—Phil. 2:7), a suffering slave (Isa. 53:11), when he became human. Written in exile, the song in Isaiah 53 (the fourth Servant Song in Isaiah) tells of a servant (v. 2), also translated "slave," who did not don human beauty or majesty (v. 2). He was far from desirable (v. 2). He was rejected and despised by humanity because he identified with their suffering and pain (vv. 3-4) and was enveloped in grief and stricken with afflictions. Yet, through his wounded condition, he brought us *shalom* (soundness, well-being, order) and healing (v. 5). His impairment brought enablement. He fellowships with us in our melancholia, and through him we find peace and healing.

The Son of God did not come to showcase and tout human glory, which is immersed in its own reason, righteousness, and ability. His mission was to carry our cross of suffering, shame, disfigurement, and disorder. He identifies with our broken condition, even our melancholia, through a *theologia crucis*[82] (a staurology) rather than a *theologia gloria*. The cross is an emblem of our spiritual disfigurement. It is also the form and shape (cruciformity) of divine disfigurement (a disabled God)[83] becoming human and dying our death. Traditionally, we know the atonement provides for the forgiveness of our sins, our adoption into the family of God, and our ongoing sanctification and renewal in the *imago Christi*. As he took up our humanity, even our death on the cross, we likewise identify in baptism with his example and sacrifice. In baptism we put on his death, burial, and resurrection, the *via crucis* that leads from disfigurement to transfiguration, from (mental) disorder to reordering and renewing the image of God. Various traditions, monastic, mystical, and contemplative, have mapped out pathways of ascent to union with God. Many incorporate a purgative dimension of spiritual alienation and despondency, an *apatheia* that fosters deeper spiritual growth. A third theological type, the purgative type, will be explored in the tradition of the so-called dark night of the soul as empathic and at times didactic, and sanctifying.

PART III

ETIOLOGY OF MENTAL DISORDER
The Theological Types

5

Theological Type 1—The Natural

We have examined several models of the *imago Dei* and their impact on persons with disabilities. A relational model, one that does not define humanity based on ability, best suits our purposes. We expressed the relational image of God in terms of Jesus Christ, the *imago Christi*, specifically in terms of identification and salvation of humanity. God became human that humanity may become like the divine. Through the incarnation, Christ identifies with our difference and weakness that we may be adopted as sons and daughters and be transformed in his image, *theosis*. We further noted three defining states of the relational image of God: creation, fall, and new creation. These relational states of the human condition can be tied to three theological types that have historically been used to explain the etiology of mental disorder. Traditionally, these three types have shaped a theological taxonomy that has been commonly accepted as an account for mental disorders. They are the natural or existential type, the consequential type, and the purgative type. In this chapter, we will be critically examining the natural type of mental disorder through the lens of two existential thinkers, Søren Kierkegaard and Paul Tillich.

The three theological types are surely not new innovations and are thus qualified here as historical or classical. Yet, these types need to be scrutinized and not taken in their entirety as gospel. The classical typology merely represents traditional ways in which we have theologically categorized etiology for mental disorders. Yet they remain in need of analysis and critical examination of their assertions and the problems they present.

Each of these types can be illustrated through examples provided by major theological figures of the church, such as the Danish philosopher Søren Kierkegaard and the existential philosophical theologian Paul Tillich (type 1), the desert father Evagrius Ponticus and the Catholic theologian Hans Urs von Balthasar (type 2), and the Spanish mystic St. John of the Cross and the Dark Night of the Soul tradition (type 3).

The natural or existential type (type 1) is characterized by Søren Kierkegaard's work in *The Concept of Anxiety* and Paul Tillich's *The Courage to Be*. Existential philosophers in general have been long preoccupied with this category of angst. For Kierkegaard, anxiety is structural to human freedom. True freedom by nature knows no necessity. Nothing is determined. The Danish philosopher construes anxiety as structural to freedom because it presents possibility with no necessity toward any particular choice within the possible. Freedom offers choice with no need or determination to choose one way or the other, thus eliciting the dizzying motion of anxiety. In the face of vertigo, one is faced with a leap to choose. Freedom becomes the natural grounds from which anxiety emerges.

The second example of the natural type comes from Paul Tillich, who identifies anxiety as structurally existential to contingent being. Created being is contingent being. Hence, contingent being exists not by necessity, meaning it does not have to exist. Also, since created being exists and is contingent, it need not continue to exist. It has a beginning and an end. We can imagine a time when it was not. Contingency entails the fragility and variability of being that could be otherwise, fostering a fundamental instability and existential anxiety at the core of human existence. In *A Courage to Be*, Tillich's celebrated correlation method is an exercise in philosophical theology that correlates faith in God with the problem of the perennial threat of nonbeing, making it an adaptable philosophical framework for our theological typology.

I want to call attention to several of the typological examples that are cited in the next three chapters. Existentialists often address "anxiety" rather than "depression." While our study is working with mental disorder, it is primarily working with the complex of melancholia or depression. Clinically speaking, anxiety and depression are both affective disorders, often comorbid and thus inseparable. So in one sense such examples do not divert, weaken, or render less relevant our case, which is to analyze mental disorder in general and depression in particular. However, more poignantly, the varying iterations of mental disorder in these illustrations, including anxiety, function representatively and even symbolically of internal human disorder. The monumental work represented here by figures of such caliber, including Kierkegaard and Tillich, in the area of psychological disorder is uncommon and thus invaluable. Neglecting their contribution and effort would be a greater disservice merely because they exemplify a different species (anxiety rather than depression) than the common genus (of mental disorders). Simply, our work is better served to include rather than exclude such monumental treatments of anxiety.

KIERKEGAARD ON THE STRUCTURE OF FREEDOM: A NATURAL PRELAPSARIAN PHENOMENOLOGY OF ANXIETY

Kierkegaard offers us one of the more notable philosophical accounts of natural, prelapsarian angst in *The Concept of Anxiety*. This monograph deals specifically with existential anxiety from a phenomenological standpoint, as opposed to a modern clinical analysis. Yet, even so, Kierkegaard acknowledges that the existential type contains elements of anxiety disorder that can fully develop into the clinical type. In this sense, his work anticipates modern clinical analysis. Nonetheless, his concerns in writing *The Concept of Anxiety* are generally theological and more specifically phenomenological rather than clinical, probing the problem of freedom, the origin of sin, the transmission of sin, and his own experience with anxiety. His approach is neither merely theological, though he addresses the dogma of hereditary sin, nor scientific, or what we would call soft science.

Kierkegaard employs what he calls a "psychological" approach that is not psychological in the modern sense but more of a phenomenological approach, addressing the experience of consciousness within the horizon of the subjective. He deemed that science could not adequately explain anxiety or explain the qualitative leap that comes from anxiety because anxiety has no object of which to inquire.[1] Simply, one is not anxious because of this or that. Existential anxiety is objectless. There is no anxiety of something so that it may become the object of analysis or that a causal connection may be made. With anxiety, only infinite possibility without necessity lies before, so that a leap is required to move from infinity into actuality. Rollo May puts it this way: "It is the quality of the experience which makes it anxiety rather than a quantity."[2] Although he did not have the neuroscience of today available for his research, a contemporary Kierkegaard perhaps would likely hold an emergent property dualism that argues from the qualia or experience of consciousness to support his understanding of anxiety rather than a mere chemical explanation.

The Dane himself was afflicted with anxiety and depression throughout his life, as revealed in his journals.[3] In a May 12, 1839, entry he pens, "All existence from the smallest fly to the mysteries of the incarnation, makes me anxious."[4] Kierkegaard's method of *unum noris omnes* (if you know one, you know all), tantamount to the Socratic "know thyself" of finding truth in subjectivity, is present in *The Concept of Anxiety* as well as other works. He sought to better understand not only the philosophical problems at hand but also, through psychological introspection, his own struggle.

Kierkegaard was challenged by the open-ended nature of existential anxiety. Existential anxiety has nothing before it, no object but nothingness. Anxiety is not anxiety "of something." Angst is toward the tenuous nature of human existence itself, which can dissipate into nothingness at any time. Anxiety is nonderivative, causeless, and ontologically structural to human freedom itself.[5] Freedom presents possibility, and it is the freedom of possibility that breeds anxiety with its infinitude of options and no necessity or innate determination to choose one or the other. There are options in the structure of choice yet no necessity to choose any one in particular. Freedom presents an indeterminate either/or, as when a person stands at a precipice and looks down. She experiences both a fear of falling and a terrifying temptation to jump. There is total freedom to do either/or that generates an angst or dread. One is captured by the vertigo of the gaze into freedom, which is bound by no necessity to choose one or the other.[6]

Our original parents, states Kierkegaard, were confronted with the same dilemma of freedom in both the positive and negative commandments to eat freely from the tree of life but not to eat from the tree of the knowledge of good and evil lest they die. The impasse was exacerbated by the fact that references to good, evil, and death were without meaning to inexperienced humanity. According to Kierkegaard, Adam and Eve had the choice to obey or disobey God without full knowledge of the choices and their consequences.[7] God gave them freedom of choice without necessity or determination, and the freedom that was placed upon them agitated the anxiety of possibility, an anxiety that precedes the "qualitative leap" to either sin or obedience. Kierkegaard later in the same work also acknowledges an anxiety postlapse that enters in the world with sin and that accordingly increases every time an individual posits sin.[8] In the prelapsarian case, a qualitative leap is necessary because anxiety has no object to which to transition, which in such a case would be a quantitative transition.[9] In the postlapsarian case, anxiety exists on the back end as a consequence of sin. Thus, both sin and obedience enter into the world through a leap.

Kierkegaard posits anxiety as structural to the possibility of freedom (the possibility of possibility) and presupposes all volitional motion. Existential dread is part and parcel of the human predicament and cannot be avoided. Anxiety precedes all sin, and thus has attached itself to the whole human race, and, in part, it is descriptive of the human condition.

Kierkegaard proposes the function of this primal anxiety. He asserts that anxiety is the "dizziness of freedom," and that same anxiety is also the matrix that generates the type of anxiety that leads to temptation and the leap of disobedience or obedience. The instability of freedom and its ensuing anxiety fuel and set in motion the conditions for testing. Anxiety and temptation both precede sin and are its conditions. Anxiety creates the climate that precipitates temptation, with temptation precipitating the enticement toward the possibility of choice (choosing against God). Our anxious predicament draws a double-edged sword that inspires creativity out of the *tohu* and *bohu* of freedom. Ironically, anxiety is both the agitation of temptation and the provocation to righteousness. Anxiety serves as an inspiration and stimulation, a motion, to grow or fall, and it can operate pedagogically or draw one back to perdition. Anxiety peculiarly fuels our determination and development out of their primal stasis and into choice and becoming. Thus, anxiety can emerge naturally as it precedes the choices of our becoming, bringing us to a moral fork in the road with the potential for lapse and consequential disorder of the pathological type. On the other hand, existential anxiety also precedes the leap of faith toward God. Nonetheless, in all cases it has the potential to be didactic, a notion that is often controversial in disability communities.[10]

Thus, anxiety is not always a sickness unto death. Kierkegaard claims that it also can be pedagogical or educative. Anxiety teaches the profundity of freedom and choice, the necessity of reflection in choosing, and thanksgiving for the power of choice that enables actualization. Kierkegaard declares, "Whoever is educated by anxiety is educated by possibility, and only he who is educated by possibility is educated according to his infinitude."[11] Anxiety enlightens us to the infinite possibilities and choices to reflect upon, as well as our own heart and condition that must choose and be responsible. It calls us to reflect, to be responsible, to be proactive and to step toward God. Kierkegaard wisely notes that

> when such a person graduates from the school of possibility, and he knows better than a child knows his ABC's that he can demand absolutely nothing of life and that the terrible, perdition, and annihilation live next door to every man, and when he has thoroughly learned that every anxiety about which he was anxious came upon him in the next moment—he will give actuality another explanation, he will praise actuality, and even when it rests heavily upon him, he will remember that it nevertheless is far, far lighter than possibility was.[12]

Anxiety functions pedagogically because it calls us to consider the anxiety of the "infinite possible" that lightens the human burden in comparison to the "finite actual." Again Kierkegaard asserts, "Only he who passes through anxiety of the possible is educated to have no anxiety, not because he can escape the terrible things of life but because these always become weak by comparison with those of possibility."[13] Ultimately, then, the anxiety of possibility "hands him over to faith," for if "he misunderstands the anxiety, so that it does not lead him to faith but away from faith, then he is lost."[14] One learns the deceptive nature of all our finite ways in anxiety and is not terrified but purged and is able to move forward toward faith and toward God.[15] Anxiety functions as a "schoolmaster" that can lead us to God (Gal. 3:24).

Though imbued with agony, anxiety can be pedagogical. The medievalist C. S. Lewis similarly notes the didactic function of suffering: "But pain insists upon being attended to. God whispers to us in our pleasures, speaks in our conscience, but shouts in our pain: it is His megaphone to rouse a deaf world."[16] Like Kierkegaard, Lewis acknowledges that mental anguish can lead to one of two results, a leap either toward repentance and faith or toward "final and unrepented rebellion."[17] Even so, mild depression can awaken one on the journey to the challenges that lie ahead and the call to change. On other the hand, major depression untreated can lead one through the shadows and into the valley of death with no exit. Melancholia is both comic and tragic.[18] At this point, I leave in suspension the controversial claim of didactic suffering until the next chapter.

In summary, Kierkegaard's analysis leaves us with inferences from existential anxiety that can be both affirmed and questioned. First, the Dane notes the potential didactic function of anxiety. Connecting mild structural anxiety with pedagogy may not be as daunting and futile a task as connecting it with clinical depression. Mild amygdalic anxiety is necessary for reactive survivalist responses. However, it is not our place pastorally to claim for anyone the didactic purpose of their clinical condition. Such is a hermeneutical path that the individual alone must determine and travel. Kierkegaard seems to speak to a species of anxiety that relates more to something structural and innate to the human condition. Anxiety is structural to human possibility and cannot be avoided, but one works with it and adapts to it through the reflective choices made.

Kierkegaard's anxiety of possibility demands that one reflect on choice and its consequences, as well as consider the power of choice to actualize from the infinitude of possibility. Choice gives way to thanksgiving because one is grateful for the possibility of choice over the range of infinite possibilities, even the worst outcomes that are eliminated in actualization. For

Kierkegaard our choices become practices for cultivating virtue. One learns to be thankful and wise for what the anxiety of possibility brings in terms of realization. Anxiety instructs us to face freedom and choice with reflection, responsibility, and faith in God. On the other hand, if one misreads the intent of anxiety and does not leap forward in faith, one is swept in temptation into sin and is lost. In this sense anxiety is the precursor to sin, and so its function must be understood properly and serve to bring one to faith.

Second, the notion that anxiety is structural can be both affirmed in one sense and problematic in another. The assertion that anxiety is structural, meaning such a state is not to be stigmatized as a particular condition, can be equalizing and liberating from the standpoint of demarginalizing those with disabilities. Existential anxiety as structural to freedom and human development would be essential to human becoming and not initially a malady or a disability of any sort. Kierkegaard's view may even be consonant with an evolutionary view that construes such conditions as evocative for adaptation. Depression or anxiety, often construed as an evolutionary mechanism in its mild forms, may not be a disorder but "rather an adaptation for bargaining, conflict avoidance, problem-solving, disease avoidance, or other purposes."[19] Depressive symptoms shut down the person's mind and body, placing them in "safety mode," while it allows the person to focus and perform only the most essential functions for survival in a time of adversity. Again, it is worth mentioning that the distinction is often made in evolutionary psychology between mild depression and mild forms of other disorders and their evolutionary role and the severe and destructive effect of clinical depression and other pathological disorders.[20] Coping and adaptation or lack thereof is determinant in evaluating the type, magnitude, and consequences of melancholia.

SOME DIFFICULTIES WITH THE NATURAL TYPE

Invariably, a problematic outcome to structural anxiety rests in its consequences for postlapsarian humanity. Following the Adamic fall, Kierkegaard holds that structural anxiety is compounded and gives way to postlapsarian anxiety and becomes a consequence of original sin that is passed on to all humanity. Of course, the entire Augustinian construction leads to several problematic issues, such as the difficulty with participating in and/or inheriting (seminal or federal headship views) Adam's sin, guilt, and punishment, rather than merely inheriting a fallen world and a proclivity to sin, as in Eastern Christian thinking. Augustine's conclusion is based on a dubious Latin translation of Romans 5:12 (*eph ho*), which was similar to the Vulgate's translation rendering "because all have sinned" as "in whom all have sinned" in reference to the Adamic origin and transmission of sin and death.[21]

Although the notion of inherited sin has been eschewed by a common-sense appeal to injustice, theology is having profitable conversations with science over the possibility of the genetic transmission of sin. Recent attempts to explain the doctrine of original sin in terms of genetic science, natural selection, the inheritance of traits, and the freedom to alter genetic prescriptions through epigenetics have proven fruitful for the ongoing integration of theology and science.[22] Our concern is the connection between sin and sickness, such as mental disorder. From the perspective of genetic science, it is not implausible that one can inherit the genetic proclivity for any number of mental disorders through natural selection. This claim is speculated by biological science. It is also not a stretch to recognize the noetic effects of sin. Sin is a behavior rather than a substance.[23] The brain and the mind are involved in all behavior, and behavior impacts the mind and brain. Hence, there is a relationship between sinful behavior and the brain and mind that is dialectic, or working both ways. Science seeks to analyze this connection by searching the brain for the neural correlates for our behaviors, with causation being even thornier to ascertain. Nevertheless, it is not a stretch to claim that certain sins can manifest as mental disorder and vice versa, but the converse is also true.[24] Mental disorder is not necessarily tied to sinful behavior either. Careful research and precise conclusions need to be drawn when discerning between causation, correlation, connection, coincidence, and unrelation.

A more bewildering problem is any proposed connection between punishment and sickness, a formula that has long been associated with the teaching of the church. The fatal nexus of humanity to Adam in terms of sin and death is of vast significance and consequence to the entire *ordo salutis*,[25] but our immediate concern is that sickness and death are often linked consequentially to sin because of punishment. Thus, the common logic follows, as we personally inherit original sin, guilt, and death because of Adam's sin, so we also inherit sickness personally, directly or indirectly, as punishment for Adam's sin. Simply, sickness is a form of God's punishment. Yet the witness of Scripture is not univocal on the matter and not always so evident about the origin of sickness.[26] We merely have to cite the exceptions. First, the Genesis account of Adam's sin does not reference sickness as punishment for original disobedience. In the story of Job, we find that although he was "blameless and upright," God permitted both Job and his family to be plagued with sickness. In other words, Job was both righteous and sick, dispelling the notion that only the sinner receives sickness because of just punishment.

With the Deuteronomist, we first see the causal connection between disobedience and curse strongly pronounced, including disobedience and sickness (Deut. 28–30). But this thread does not run consistently throughout

Scripture, let alone as a binding, unbreakable law, as evidenced, for example, in the Psalms and in the Gospels, where the causal connection is ambiguous or denied. Throughout the Psalms there are petitions for healing of sickness both physical and mental, for example, in Psalm 6:2-3 (NIV)—"Have mercy upon me, O Lord; for I am faint; heal me, Lord, for my bones are in agony. My soul is in deep anguish. How long, Lord, how long?" Yet in this psalm it is not due to the psalmist's sin but from the evildoing of others; 6:7-9—"My eyes grow weak with sorrow, they fail because of all my foes. Away from me, all you who do evil, for the Lord has heard my weeping." However, there are occasions in the Psalms, for example Psalm 38, where it seems David understands that God is punishing him with sickness for his sin (vv. 1-4):

> Lord, do not rebuke me in your anger or discipline me in your wrath. Your arrows have pierced me, and your hand has come down on me. Because of your wrath there is no health in my body; there is no soundness in my bones because of my sin. My guilt has overwhelmed me like a burden too heavy to bear.

On the other hand, in Psalm 32 it seems to indicate that the psalmist is afflicted and in anguish not because of sinning but because of not confessing sin, an insight that modern talk therapy has uncovered time and again. Psalm 32:3 (NLT) reads, "When I refused to confess my sin, I was weak and miserable, and I groaned all day long."[27] The witness of Scripture is not univocal on the matter of sickness and etiology, and specifically the causal connection between sin and sickness.

In the Gospels, the narratives depict a variety of events in which Jesus heals a wide range of illnesses both physical and psychological.[28] Usually the narratives do not make us privy to the reasons for the illness. They just invite us to behold *semeia* of the kingdom of God manifesting through Christ, as he preaches, teaches, casts out demons, and heals sickness. Though there are instances where connections are made, which at times can further complicate the problem for other issues, the Gospel witness is not univocal or precise on etiology.[29] In various cases, as in Mark 9, Jesus heals a boy who is deaf and mute by casting out evil spirits from him. The implication is that the evil spirits caused the deaf and mute condition, not punishment from God. After Jesus casts out the unclean spirits, the boy is healed.[30]

A host of questions and problems arises from such a possible conclusion. Are evil spirits real, or are they constructs from a prescientific worldview? If they are constructs from a prescientific worldview, has a biomedical or disease model replaced it?[31] In what way? If demons are real, do they cause sickness? What type of sickness, physical, mental, or both? Are any or all sicknesses caused by demons? If a sickness is caused by a demon, how is it possible not to demonize the person as well? Each etiological conclusion in Scripture concerning sickness or disability has its own related set of problems and questions that need to be addressed. Yet possibly the greater problem is that where at times illness seems to be attributed to sin or the demonic, at other times it is neither. There is no consistent voice in terms of singular cause. In John 9:1-4, when the disciples ask Jesus whether a blind man's conditions stemmed from his sin or his parents' sin, Jesus replies that he was born in this condition so that "the power of God could be seen in him." Did God foreordain this man's condition? Was his condition due to natural causes that God has allowed and will use this situation to show his power and bring a greater good? But clearly the blindness was not due to judgment. Again, each conclusion has its own set of problems and questions. Yet in this case the cause is not due to sin or the demonic, and thus any absolute single conclusion concerning etiology that utilizes Scripture remains inconclusive. Also, for each distinctive scriptural claim of causation there remains a plethora of related problems to resolve. Simply, Scripture presents a variety of angles on etiological and causal questions related to illness that cannot be reduced to the simple formula that sickness equals judgment due to sin.[32]

One of the main apologetic arguments in Marcia Webb's work on depression is to disconnect mental disorders from selfishness, sickness, or demonic activity, either by causation or correlation. I have concluded that the full scriptural evidence makes it difficult to identify any one single cause or correlation or even a single rule of interpretation as to causation or correlation, or the denial of these, because it seems to give mixed (a variety of) readings.[33] However, I think it is just as difficult to rule out absolutely all causation or correlation based on scriptural grounds as well. There is often too much unevenhanded proof texting used to support a position. Webb rightly recognizes that all have sinned and hence sin precedes sickness but is not necessarily the cause of it.[34] On pastoral grounds, and because of the susceptibility of a scrupulous and overactive introspective conscience of the depressed, she advises not to make the sin-sickness correlation in treating mental disorders, which I concur at times can exacerbate the problem.[35] In terms of the connection with the demonic, again, the body of evidence interpreted as a whole is multivalent. Webb argues that many of the instances of healing and deliverance in the New Testament were related to physical illnesses that today can be medically treated and were not mental disorders,[36] though it seems the exorcism of the Gadarene demoniac is at least one exception that she does identify.[37]

Amos Yong also presents a counterexample to the notion that sickness is consequential to original sin. He notes that an intellectual disability, such as Down syndrome or at least trisomy, existed in pre–*Homo sapiens* hominids. For Yong, in this case, with an evolutionary model, disability preceded the fall and was not caused by it. Disability and disorder, in an evolutionary scheme, assist in providing the variation needed for adaptation. Yong sees the problem as rooted in our Western construal of original sin. To remedy, Yong suggests four modifications to the traditional notion of the fall. One, *sin* refers to willful acts of rebellion from self-aware free creatures against God, and the punishment of death is separation from God rather than physical death, which science tells us existed prior to humans, thus prior to a literal reading of the Genesis fall narrative. Two, the consequences of sin in terms of disability are tied not so much directly to an original sin as to the subsequent acts of violence committed against each other and the world, and how disability is more a social consequence of such acts. Three, all are impacted by the universality of sin, so humanity is not divided into two classes of the abled and the disabled. Four, solidarity with Adam in sin is exceeded by our solidarity in salvation with Christ. Further, in reexamining the nature of the fall, Yong establishes "four fences" concerning disability theology and God's providence. The will of God is neither arbitrary in causing disability nor unaware of disability as if it were an accident. God's sovereignty coexists with human freedom. They are not mutually exclusive. Also, God's will is not opposed to the laws of nature and works with them for good. Finally, God desires that all be saved. He does not intend two classes of people, such as the saved and the damned or the blessed and the cursed.[38]

Responding to Yong's four modifications or reemphases of the traditional doctrine of original sin, I would, without debate, concur with his third and fourth emphases. I think emphasis number two is in part correct. Following the fall, throughout human history, acts of violence have escalated and with technological advances have exacerbated the efficiency with which we commit violent acts. No one is untouched by human violence, including other humans and the rest of the natural world. And as Yong affirmed, those with disabilities and disorders often can suffer more violence from social consequences than from the impairments themselves. I also concur with Yong on this first emphasis that sin refers to a willful act of rebellion against God by free moral agents, and the punishment is death. Thus, Yong rightfully asserts that an evolutionary reading of science and Genesis would require a spiritual reading that identifies death as a separation from God rather than physical death. I also agree with Yong's four fences to provide boundaries and balance for a theology of disability and disorder in light of God's sovereignty and human freedom. However, it does not exclude the possibility that even though disability and disorder can serve an evolutionary function under a sovereign God, sickness, including mental disorder, can occur consequential to the fall, as much of the Christian tradition has affirmed.

In terms of intellectual disabilities, it can be argued that they may be pre-Adamic in terms of genetic variation and mutation in an evolutionary account of creation and even in postlapsarian terms not related to the fall. Nonetheless, mental disorders are not objectively, biologically, definitively diagnosed, as is, for example, Down syndrome.[39] Since genetics contributes somewhat to the predisposition to mental disorders, it is possible in an evolutionary account of creation that they existed prior in our prehominid ancestry. But they would be impossible to diagnose prior to the evolution of consciousness, since that is a condition for experiencing and reporting symptomology, which are essential to diagnosis. Subjectivity is transcendental to the experience of the disorder. It can also be debated, though it is not germane to our larger study, that prior to the development of civilization, external stressors were not advanced or acute enough to create an environment that would stimulate the type of adaptation that would require depression as a survival mechanism. Further, neurological development of areas that are impacted by mental disorders may not have been advanced enough to experience mental disorders as experienced by *Homo sapiens*.

Thus, for our purposes, I will locate the possibility of mental disorders (the natural type) with the first self-aware hominids and within a larger context of human brokenness and alienation from God, whether such alienation is due directly to individual sin (the consequential type 2), the condition of humanity (the consequential type 2), demonic activity (the consequential type 2), or the natural development of things (type 1). Singular causation is not the major focus of our study; healing and restoration in Christ are our concern. According to theological type 1, mental disorders can arise out of the general human condition of weakness, alienation, and brokenness and may be directly related to multiple factors that are often difficult to pin down. Yet, in all cases, Christ has come to identify with our weaknesses and transform us in the image of God.

Bishop Zizioulas helps us to see that humanity is a relation of persons, human and divine. We need each other and God to be truly human. Thus, the fall produces broken relations. Indeed, the fall impacts reason, freedom, volition, and the like, but primarily it is a break with God and others that impacts the *imago*. The image of God is broken in that relations between God and humanity are broken as well as with humanity and itself and the rest of creation. The gravity of sin pulls us away from God and our proper logos and draws us toward chaos and the disorder of a self-centered life. Like a dying star that no longer has the outward flow of energy that gives off heat and light and begins to implode under the gravity of its own mass, we begin to die on the inside detached from our source of energy and light. Healing is relational restoration of primordial and experienced alienation, even depression.

Scripture was not intended to be a science book. Genesis 3 does not attempt to explain scientifically the origin and process of biological death. The Genesis narrative gives a theological account of death in terms of separation from God, as Yong and others have distinguished. When Adam and Eve ate from the Tree of the Knowledge of Good and Evil, they did not die immediately. When God said, "In the day you shall eat of the fruit you shall surely die," he meant that at that moment of disobedience our primal parents were separated from God and their life source, and the death process would begin physically and spiritually, as a sickness unto death. A star gradually dies until, in at least one possible scenario, no light can escape, and it collapses under its own mass and gravitational pull into a black hole that implodes on itself and allows nothing to escape. The inward focus and insatiable drive of sin on the self yields a similar deadly dynamic.

Scripture affirms our depravity and radical alienation: "They are darkened in their understanding, alienated from the life of God because of the ignorance that is in them, due to their hardness of heart" (Eph. 4:18, ESV). "And you, who once were alienated and hostile in mind, doing evil deeds" (Col. 1:21, ESV). Our estrangement is indeed existential, as Heidegger, Sartre, Camus, Beckett, Ortega y Gasset, and other existentialists have notably portrayed. The human predicament is alien to itself and the world around it. Apart from God, human essence and meaning are absent, and all that is present is the absurdity of such absence and the necessity to choose in the face of the encroachment of death. Some of the existentialists' valid conclusions come from the false premise of a godless tabula rasa, as opposed to humanity's alienation from the divine. It is imperative to emphasize the theological nature of our alienation, which does involve existential concerns but considers those issues from the fissure of our relationship with the Holy One.

In addition, we need to also recognize that although Scripture does not formulate a univocal principle that either uniformly affirms or denies causation or correlation between sin and sickness either from divine judgment or from direct inherent consequences in sin itself, Scripture does at times make the connection, and so it cannot be ruled out. Many recognize that the polyphonic witness of the New Testament attributes sickness directly or indirectly to three primary causes, God, the devil, or natural causes, rather than to no cause. With any of the three causal agents depicted in Scripture, in the end, infirmity and death, it is posited, can serve as a divine instrument for judgment, pedagogy, or sanctification.[40] Still, for hermeneutical or theological reasons surrounding theodicy, one can take a nonliteral reading of incriminating scriptural texts in order to exonerate the divine and place the onus on evil, free will, or incorrect interpretation. These moves are not necessarily irresponsible theological moves. Some even opt for open theism as a response, which I am certainly not supporting.

The fact is that *melancholia*, the term, is not explicitly mentioned in the Scriptures, but the symptomology is prevalent throughout, as a case could be made that Job, Jacob, Saul, David, Solomon, Elijah, Naomi, Jonah, Jeremiah, and others, and possibly even Christ in the garden of Gethsemane, experienced melancholia, all for a variety of reasons cited. In all cases, though, as Hans Reinders has firmly indicated, "nature only produces variations in human bodies; it does not produce meanings."[41] We socioculturally, and even theologically, construct meanings of "defective," "deformed," or "dysfunctional" that have little to do with the natural process.[42] In this way, theology and other disciplines, without scriptural and/or moral warrant, have unjustly claimed the high ground and have been wielded as weapons of violence against the weak and marginalized. Yet, even against such violence, Christ has come with good news for the poor and weak and a kingdom that reverses the advances of such onslaughts.

TILLICH: THE STRUCTURE OF CONTINGENT BEING: A META-ONTOTHEOLOGICAL APPROACH TO MEONTOLOGICAL ANXIETY

While Kierkegaard initiates the conversation and is a precursor to the so-called age of anxiety, Paul Tillich addresses anxiety at the height of the age following World War II.[43] Kierkegaard asserts that his approach is a psychological one, though it is more a phenomenological one. On the other hand, Tillich's approach works out of philosophical theology.[44] His claims is to address anxiety as a universal existential phenomenon within the human condition. Although primarily philosophical, his work in existential anxiety was seminal to the development of empirical existential psychology.[45] Both Kierkegaard and Tillich are working within a creational framework of the ontological difference between the divine and this contingent world. While Kierkegaard's theory locates anxiety in freedom, Tillich's ontological analysis locates anxiety in the universal threat of nonbeing against contingent being that looms at the threshold of *Dasein* in space-time. Anxiety is structural to the contingency of being.[46]

Tillich's method is to probe existential issues through philosophical theology.[47] He utilizes a correlation method that employs theology apologetically to respond to existential issues and questions. For example: God is understood philosophically as the ground or power of being; faith is realized as ultimate concern; salvation is communicated as the new being in Christ. A major existential concern of Tillich's is the threat of nonbeing that crouches at the limits of the finitude and fragility of human being and all reality. Nonbeing lurks at the boundaries of being evoking the angst of nothingness, making anxiety structural to contingent being itself. In *The Courage to Be*, Tillich employees a virtue approach (courage) to the meontological problem.[48] He analyzes the variety of definitions and usages of "courage" in history and philosophy from Plato, the Stoics, Aquinas, Spinoza, and Nietzsche, and then he applies his own distilled meaning, "self-affirmation in-spite-of," to the problem of anxiety in the face of nonbeing, a perennial issue tackled by thinkers from Parmenides to Tillich's own time.[49]

Tillich offers the reader a general definition of anxiety and then later defines three specific iterations of the undifferentiated type of anxiety—death, meaninglessness, and condemnation. Of anxiety in general, he succinctly posits, "Anxiety is the state in which a being is aware of its possible nonbeing" and consciousness of the tenuous nature of one's own meaning and value system regarding the self and the world.[50] He further asserts, "Anxiety is the essential awareness of nonbeing. Existential in this statement means that it is not the abstract knowledge of nonbeing which produces anxiety but the awareness that nonbeing is a part of one's own being."[51] Like Kierkegaard, Tillich concludes that anxiety has no object. The notion of nonbeing elicits anxiety in one who is encompassed by finitude. Thus, anxiety is structural, ontological, or rather meontological (the study of nonbeing), with the meontological as a limit of contingent being. Open-ended existential anxiety leads to fear. Anxiety, which has no object, drives one to conceive of objects of fear.[52] For Tillich, "all objectless anxiety strives to become object-directed, fear concretizes, and attaches itself to an object."[53] Fear has an object, while anxiety does not.[54] And underlying "the element of anxiety in every fear" is the fear of death.[55] According to Tillich, "All anxiety is ultimately grounded in the individual's awareness of her impending mortality."[56] One becomes conscious of one's own wispy existence and tenuous constructs of meaning, which are incessantly under the threat of vanishing.[57]

According to Tillich, we negotiate these objects of fear that we may give anxiety a face in order to encounter it with *the courage to be*. As it stands, the facelessness and terror of nonbeing cannot be encountered for more than a flash. The "naked absolute" produces a "naked anxiety" that threatens to extinguish "every finite self-affirmation."[58] For Tillich, there are three fear-induced manifestations or particular types that attach themselves to the basic anxiety of nonbeing that threaten humanity's self-affirmation of being: the anxiety of death, the anxiety of meaninglessness, and the anxiety of condemnation.[59] The threat of our nonbeing evokes a basic existential anxiety through the fear of these particular expressions or objects.

These hypostases of anxiety are existential and not necessarily neurotic or clinical, though they may become such, as Kierkegaard realized. Clinical anxiety, or what Tillich calls "non-existential anxiety," is a state of existential anxiety that becomes pathological because one has failed to face the existential type with courage and self-affirmation in the ground of being (God).[60] Tillich understands this slip into the neurotic as an escape, a bad faith. He claims, "Neurosis is the way of avoiding nonbeing by avoiding being."[61] Basically, one fails to face anxiety by not taking it upon oneself in courage, and instead draws away from it through despair and escapes into neurosis with a weakened and unrealistic sense of self-affirmation.[62] Facing anxiety and finding a way forward in courage in this sense is consonant with evolutionary strategies that avoid pathology through adaptation and learning. For Tillich, existential threat is structural and a "part of the normal range of experience of the average person within a culture," though nonetheless an assault on the person's being and structure of constructed semiotics and semantics.[63]

Both Kierkegaard and Tillich recognize two levels of anxiety, the existential type and the inherent life-threatening danger of the pathological type, such as a mental disorder leading to suicide.[64] Tillich is aware that the medical field and the fields of philosophy and theology need an integrative approach in treating pathological anxiety. The former field does not recognize the ontological root of anxiety or the category of the ontological in general, and so understands all anxiety as neurotic. While the latter acknowledges the category of the ontological, it does not have the training to identify and treat the clinical type.[65]

THE COURAGE TO BE AS SELF-AFFIRMATION

Returning to existential anxiety, we need to unpack Tillich's understanding of courage in the face of nonbeing as self-affirmation (in-spite-of). Self-affirmation is not a call to rugged individualism but a call to stand on the ground of being as a part of all that is in spite of the threat of nonbeing. In calling for self-affirmation, Tillich does not seem to be asking for a call to self-centeredness or a self-reliance that involves an inflated overestimation of the self in order to counter the weight of nonbeing. Rather, it is an affirmation of being in the world. Self-affirmation is pronounced in a context of the world and the ground or power of being. He states, "But the self is self only because it has a world, a structured universe, to which it belongs and from which it is separated at the same time. Self and world are correlated and so are individualization and participation."[66] The self is relational and participatory (*methexis*—having with; for our purposes, "having being with"). What he calls an "identity of participation" is the courage to be a part of being.[67] Unlike in traditional virtue approaches, Tillich's call to courage is not a call to the practice of *phronesis* but a call to an affirmation grounded in the self and ultimately in the ground of self, a yes to self and its undifferentiated ground. As a side note, affirmation in this sense is consonant with CBT (cognitive behavioral theory/therapy) and similar methods as an effective form of positive reinforcement for the nonanxious self as it perceives a nonthreatening world.

Continuing with the relational nature of the self in his *Systematic Theology*, Tillich pens, "No individual exists without participation, and no personal being exists without communal being."[68] With Tillich's anthropology, there is inherence between self and world, and both inhere within the structure of being, as a "self-world polarity that is the basis for the subject-object structure of reason."[69] This version of participation is his solution to the problem of the particular (individualization) and the universal (totality, humanity, the universe), their dialectic, and their unity as they participate in being. Besides the inherent problems with the modernist subject-object reductive structure, Tillich affirms the relational and participatory nature of humanity and the created order itself. Thus, in self-affirming, one is world and being affirming, ultimately affirming the power or ground of being. God, as ground or power of being, is the source for courage and ultimate concern.[70]

TILLICH'S META-ONTOTHEOLOGY

In self-affirming, we are acknowledging that we stand on the ground of being, which is God, and thus affirm the divine that undergirds all things. Tillich's notion of the divine is a complex matter and is not the object of our inquiry or critique here. However, it is noteworthy that his notion of the divine does not fall under the traditional ontotheological construct in terms of what he calls theological theism; that is, he cites Anselm, Scotus, and other Scholastics. If God is the greatest and highest being of traditional theism (ontotheology), then that God is still a part of creation and not the origin of being and thus not the wholly other, according to Tillich. As the ground of being, God is transcendent of essence and existence and prior to being and wholly other than being and semiotics, "the God above God."[71] Tillich's approach attempts to be a meta-ontotheological one in that it seeks to go beyond the God of being to find the God above and outside of being or ground of being. For Tillich, God is both *Grund* and *Ungrund* (ground and "unground," or groundlessness). The attempt to transcend and overcome ontotheology, as a method for moving forward theologically, was influenced by Heidegger, who sought not to name or to say anything of God.[72] Tillich, likewise, sought to transcend the nameable God of being. Courage or absolute faith finds its ultimate source in the "God above God," the God above the God of theism, who is traditionally expressed in terms of being, existence, essence, and semiotics (signs and symbols of God). However, like Heidegger's (early or latter), Tillich's God is accessible only through the subjective experience of "being there" (*Dasein*) or poetic language and further takes us from classical creedal notions of God that claim to be derived from revelation, which in turns actually communicates, in human terms, something of the very nature of God. The phenomenological tradition of Heidegger and Tillich is an attempt at existential correspondence between the divine and *Dasein* or, later, poetic language. The attempt by Tillich is to offer a nontraditional and deflated theology of revelation or divine communication over against the traditional philosophy and theology that Heidegger so rigorously denounced.

SOME PROBLEMS WITH TILLICH'S APPROACH

In summarizing Tillich on anxiety and courage, we recognize that he locates and identifies anxiety as structural to being owing to its contingency, which allows for the possibility and threat of nonbeing. The threat comes in the form of the anxiety of meaninglessness, death, and condemnation and is to be faced with our self-affirming, dependent stance in the divine ground of being that undergirds all things.

> Courage is the self-affirmation of being despite the fact of nonbeing. It is the act of the individual self in taking the anxiety of nonbeing upon itself by affirming itself either as part of an embracing whole or in its individual selfhood. Courage always includes a risk, it is always threatened by nonbeing, whether the risk of losing oneself and becoming a thing within the whole of things or of losing one's world in an empty self-relatedness. Courage needs the power of being, a power transcending the non-being which is experienced in the anxiety of fate and death, which is present in the anxiety of emptiness and meaninglessness, which is effective in the anxiety of guilt and condemnation. The courage which takes this threefold anxiety into itself must be rooted in a power of being that is greater than the power of oneself and the power of one's world.[73]

One note to emphasize is the ontological (within the ontological difference) nature of anxiety for Tillich. Anxiety is structural or natural and cannot be removed or cured. Like Kierkegaard, he affirms that anxiety is universal and a natural phenomenon. Tillich assures, "The basic anxiety, the anxiety of a finite being about the threat of nonbeing, cannot be eliminated. It belongs to existence itself."[74] Courage, though the ultimate response to anxiety, "does not remove anxiety." Since anxiety is existential, it cannot be removed. Courage is self-affirmation—namely, in spite of nonbeing.[75] Anxiety presents humanity with a continual call to face the threat and move forward or to turn and draw back, a continual ultimatum of life or death.

Unlike Kierkegaard, Tillich does not initially link "condemnation anxiety," a type of existential anxiety, with the notion of sin (postlapsarian anxiety for Kierkegaard) and is therefore free from the problems that are indigenous to an Augustinian hamartiology. However, he does connect guilt-anxiety to falling short of one's own standard, though not necessarily God's standard and thus sin.[76] Existential anxiety is simply viewed as universal to the human condition and not a transgression. Natural anxiety does not marginalize or create a second class of people but looms over every person at the boundary of their being. In this way all being, including our own, is marginalized or finds anxiety at our own margins. Everyone is called to face and overcome existential anxiety with courage. Although Tillich summons the virtue of courage to overcome anxiety, he does not use vice or sin language to describe fear or bad faith. For Tillich, "he who is not capable of a powerful self-affirmation in spite of the anxiety of non-being is forced into a weak, reduced self-affirmation."[77]

From the standpoint of traditional Christian theism, the obvious arguments are not necessarily leveled against Tillich's etiology of anxiety but against the remedy proposed. Tillich prescribes that one must transcend traditional theism and find "absolute faith" and mystical union with the "God above God."[78] Tillich's indictment is that the God of theism can be named and located historically and culturally, and understood semiotically, which not only limits the infinite God but also places God as a being among others and not as being itself.[79] As a being among many, God is reduced to and caught up in "the subject-object structure of reality," in which God and humanity are tyrannically objectified and controlled by each other.[80] Tillich believes this issue is the root of modern atheism, which revolts against such control of the divine and control of reality. Nietzsche prescribed that this "God" had to be killed. He also held that it was the root of existentialist despair. Hence, Tillich deems that traditional theism has instigated the age of anxiety and must be transcended if anxiety is to be overcome. Absolute faith must rest in the God who is outside and above the God of traditional theism, as mentioned above.

The problem with this construal or even any mystical construal of God or a religious experience is that it transcends semiotics. Thus, it transcends language, referents, and meaning. Unless joined with cataphatic revelation or cosmological inferences, there remains no access for critical analysis. One is trapped in an impasse of agnosticism. Mysticism throws us right into an epistemological crisis and potentially into nihilism, since the mystic does not know whether she has been absorbed into the void, the *nihil*, being itself, the divine, or self-deception. The claim that mysticism brings absolute certainty ironically invites absolute agnosticism. There is no way of knowing, meta-knowing, or communicating whether or what has enveloped the mystic. Even in traditional apophatic theism, the cloud of unknowing still shrouds something, the cataphatic. Our knowledge of God is analogical. We find both continuity and a greater discontinuity of language and being when we comparatively think of God on our own terms. With Tillich's God above semiotics, or any mediation, there is no real knowledge or certainty to evaluate. In the end, this uncertainty may become the source of our anxiety, the *nihil*.[81]

Epistemological and theological problems aside, we can affirm the anthropological claims in both Kierkegaard and Tillich that highlight the structural frailty in human nature. The indeterminate and contingent nature of human being naturally lends itself to the possibility of disorder. That is not to undermine the declaration in Genesis regarding creation "that it was very good." The connotation of "good" in this context means it is as God wanted or intended it to be. The structural type of disorder acknowledges that creation is finite, contingent, and limited, but also in a nascent state that is intended for development, and part of the challenge of its development is rooted in its own finitude and its need to depend on the divine. Truly, in God we live and move and have our being. Ontologically, we are not autonomous or self-sufficient but, in our frailty, depend and participate in divine being for existence but also in divine will for our becoming and our *telos*, which is to be sanctified by the Spirit in the *imago Christi*. In the incarnation, Christ came to identify with our nature, our sin, and even our disorder to bring us healing and redemption.

6

Theological Type 2—The Consequential

In this chapter we will continue to examine the etiology of mental disorders through a theological typology that has been characteristic of the Christian tradition's reading and interpretation of psychological distress. The premise of the consequential theological type is that, owing to the fall, either directly or indirectly, persons can suffer from mental disorders. The direct or indirect transmission of mental disorders, and sickness in general, is primarily tied to a cosmos that is radically out of order with God and is inundated with traumatic and stressful circumstances that can contribute adversely to mental health. Traditionally, other factors such as sin (committed and committed against us) and demonic activity have been directly or indirectly attributed to mental disorder. Simply, the fall has seismic consequences that impact through a variety of means all of life, including mental health. We will examine the consequential type of mental disorder through the lenses of the desert father Evagrius Ponticus (345–399 CE) and the modern Swiss Catholic theologian Hans Urs von Balthasar (1905–1988).

Evagrius and Balthasar are two among many Christian thinkers who have typified the consequential type of theologically informed etiologies. The desert ascetic Evagrius Ponticus studied and wrote extensively on the condition and sin of acedia and concludes that it originates from demonic activity and instrumentally manifests in human cognition (*logismoi*). Evagrius prescribes that acedia is combated through *apatheia*, ascetic practices, and scriptural affirmations, among other remedies. The desert father devised a sophisticated, state-of-the-art diagnostic and treatment plan that anticipates both modern cognitive behavioral therapy and charismatic spiritual warfare. We will also assess the work of Hans Urs von Balthasar, who identifies both the natural type (1) and the consequential type (2) of mental disorder. We will draw primarily from his work *The Christian and Anxiety*, which in part is a response to Søren Kierkegaard's *Concept of Anxiety*.

EVAGRIUS PONTICUS: ACEDIA AND THE DEMONIC

Evagrius Ponticus (345–399 CE) was a third-generation anchorite and desert father who was taught by Macarius the Great, who was acquainted with Antony of Egypt.[1] Evagrius, an ascetic, anchorite monk, was born in Pontus in present-day Turkey to an aristocratic family who had likely entrusted him to Gregory of Nazianzus for his education.[2] Little is known about his early life, but it is apparent from his writings that he received a comprehensive and in-depth education.[3] Evagrius was trained in the classics, including Greek philosophy, and later inherited the oral tradition of the early desert monasticism of Antony of Egypt. He was ordained a reader by Basil the Great and later ordained a deacon by Gregory of Nazianzus.[4] After the Second Ecumenical Council in 381, Gregory left his position, and in 382 Evagrius journeyed to Jerusalem to become a monk in the monastery of Rufinus and Melania the Elder.[5] In 383 he took on the anchorite life and set out for the desert in Nitira and then in Kellia, both in Egypt. He died there in 399.[6]

Evagrius' ascetic struggles in the desert are documented in his own prolific writings, in the writings of his student Palladius, and through the teachings of his most renowned student, John Cassian, who promulgated the tradition of Evagrius and the desert fathers to the West. Because of his Origenist influence, Evagrius was criticized in his own day and throughout church history, mainly because of Origen's teachings, which were condemned in the Second Council of Constantinople in 553.[7] Despite his Origenist affiliation and even gnostic tendencies, Evagrius was extremely influential in the West through Cassian and in the East through Maximus the Confessor, St. Symeon the New Theologian, and those who followed them. Out of his lived, monastic experience in the isolation of the desert and within the four walls of his cell, Evagrius developed his practical theology of "spiritual warfare," which involved identifying the core demons and sins that sought to overthrow the faith of every monk. One primary area of focus was his work with acedia (mental sloth or apathy), translated by Raposa as "boredom," by Bunge as "despondency," and by Feld as "sadness."[8]

Evagrius began to catalog his confrontations with temptations and the demonic in around 375 CE. He compiled a general list of eight evil thoughts or temptations (*logismoi*) that were basic categories under which all other evil thoughts could be located. A few centuries later under Pope Gregory the Great, these eight evil thoughts would be reduced to seven and later become the proverbial seven deadly sins. Evagrius enumerates:

> There are eight basic categories of thought in which are included every thought. First is that of gluttony, then impurity, avarice, sadness, anger, acedia, vainglory, and last of all pride. It is not in our power to determine whether we are disturbed by these thoughts but it is up to us to decide if they are to linger within us or not and whether or not they are to stir up our passions.[9]

The project of Evagrius was to offer spiritual wisdom to young monks to help them identify and resist such *logismoi*, which ultimately he discerned came from demons, and attain a passionless state, *apatheia*, toward such thoughts as one grows in the knowledge of God through contemplation and prayer.[10] For Evagrius, discerning and interpreting the *logismoi* were key to this endeavor. The evil thoughts house the passions (*pathe*), and both the thoughts and passions are inflicted upon the isolated and battle-fatigued soul by the demonic.[11] Evagrius candidly diagnoses that "the etiology of all passionate thoughts is demonic."[12] Early Judeo and Christian worldviews, and even folk religion globally, have always constructed sophisticated demonologies out of their spirit beliefs in order to give an account of the complex existence and interaction of evil in the lives of everyday people, especially in areas of causality that were outside of human understanding and control.[13] For Evagrius and the early monastic tradition, the desert, the archetypal site of temptation, was the arena in which evil, the demonic, was encountered. The desert was the domain of liminality that provided the grueling environment that could foster the needed spiritual transfiguration. Acedia would surely add to that environment.

The desert is traditionally a place of spiritual retreat and abandonment where one may not be distracted by worldly allures, and where one can offer full attention and consecration to God. The flip side is that the desert fosters isolation and even the inertia that settles in from being sealed off and imprisoned in an anchorite's cell. Such loneliness is a breeding ground for boredom, despondency, depression, and mental struggle or spiritual warfare. The Scriptures depict the desert as the place where prophets and ascetics are forged through trial, tribulation, and temptation. Moses leading God's people, Elijah fleeing from Jezebel, John the Baptist receiving God's call, and even Christ's temptation were all on the battlefield of the desert. The called of God are brought to the wilderness to be tempted by passion-fueled thoughts that could lead them away from God's purpose and assignment. Resistance in the face of such an onslaught would prove one worthy of the call and prepare one to advance for future assignments and even future trials and struggles.

Acedia, like all *logismoi*, acts as demonic arrows shot at the mind of the monk in the day of evil in an attempt to render him powerless in a slumber of sloth or to even abandon his habit. Acedia, a sadness and slackness of the soul, functions like a thorn in the anchorite's side as he attempts to carry out his devotion and discipline but is thwarted by despondency:

> Despondency:
> breezy love,
> trampers of steps,
> hater of love of work,
> fight against solitude,
> thunderstorm of psalmody,
> aversion to prayer,
> slackening of asceticism,
> ill-timed slumber,
> sleep, tossing and turning,
> burden of solitude,
> hatred of the cell,
> adversary of ascetical efforts,
> counter-attack against endurance,
> impediment to reflection,
> ignorance of the Scriptures,
> companion of sadness,
> daily rhythm of hunger.[14]

Gabriel Bunge, in his work *Despondency*, elaborates on Evagrius' symptomatology of the acedia-laden monk: restlessness, doubt, worry, psychosomatic illness, aimless busyness, prayerlessness, and doubt of call are among the manifestations of despondency that assail the victim.[15] It does not take much effort to imagine how the isolated, incarcerated, inert, and monotonous life of an ascetic hermit could lend itself to depression and despondency. Such conditions of an anchorite are the very ones that a modern therapist would warn a client to avoid, such as lonely, cloistered, and sedentary conditions, as well as monotonous routines. Remedies such as social interaction, conversation, enjoying the outdoors, diversions, and trying something novel are often prescribed, but these are diametrically opposed to the ascetic life. The monk has no escape or any such modern diversions to offset the ennui. Bunge describes it as an "inner restlessness" that strikes directly at the discipline and rule of the anchorite to remain within the four walls of his cell day in and out and accomplish the tasks and routines at hand.[16] The attention of the monk becomes edgy and erratic, and out of tedium he is jerked from one impulse to the next, never settled and completing nothing. Underneath the uneasiness and apprehension ultimately lies the impulse to abandon one's habits and vocation, giving way to speculation that one's station in life may be the very cause of the plaguing condition. The monk impulsively begins to doubt the call that brought him to this point.

For Evagrius, these *logismoi*, like acedia, are demonically incited in the mind and emotions of a person in the form of passionate thoughts. It has been noted that Evagrius anticipates discoveries in cognitive science and cognitive behavioral theory that identify depressive feelings as a product of cognitive distortions about self, the world, and the future (Beck's cognitive triad).[17] However, the *logismoi* are not merely cognitive distortions or irrational inferences about reality as identified by CBT, though they are at least that. For Evagrius the irrational thoughts are also demonic, and if received and acted upon can lead one into sin and perdition, hence deadly sins.

CRITICAL ENGAGEMENT OF THE EVAGRIAN TYPE

If acedia is incited by demonic beings, what are we to make of Evagrius' conclusion? Neoplatonism frequently influenced early Christian worldviews, even to the extent of varying degrees of syncretism. Both Christian and Neoplatonic worldviews of Evagrius' day would comprehend reality as both invisible and visible, immaterial and material. The mind forms thought in the invisible realm, while the visible, phenomenal realm is apprehended by the senses of the body, the world of the intelligible and the sensual, respectively. Epistemologically, one ascends from the visible to the invisible to contemplate and attain the knowledge of God or the One in Neoplatonism in which the One is apprehended by pure intellect. In Christian thought, contemplation (*theoria*) involves knowing God (*theologia*) devoid of sensual stimulation and images specifically through the practice of asceticism and prayer. In both Christian and Neoplatonic worldviews there are intermediate beings: angels and demons in Christian thought and a cosmic god or gods of lesser emanations than the One in Neoplatonism. It was not a stretch for Evagrius to hold that evil intermediate beings sought to impede ascending and uniting with Christ by tempting the thought life.

Evagrian anthropology defines humanity as rational (*logikon*), gifted with reason (logos) that is the image of God and gives humanity *capex Dei* (God capacity).[18] A human being also has irrational and emotive powers (*thumos*; *epithumia*) that make us animal-like or irrational (*alogon*).[19] These irrational powers (alogical)—namely, desire and anger—blind the mind and obscure and deceive thoughts as they form *logismoi*.[20] Although Evagrius locates the origin of these thoughts in the demonic, the person is not rendered powerless of choice. Each has the free will to receive and act on these thoughts or to resist them and think on those thoughts that are virtuous.

Evil is not created by God, nor is it a thing itself, but it is a privation or absence of good, as was commonly held by desert theologians. The human person and all its capacities and powers, including free will, are intended for good if used properly for the intended end, whereas evil is a misuse of the good that God purposes, a misappropriation of the powers that God bestows for a good and right end. Thus, evil is demonic but enters into the world and the human sphere by our own permission. The remedy for Evagrius is then a keen, scrutinizing self-awareness that discerns and unmasks the subtlety and intricacy of spirits and thoughts as well as their strategies and redirects thoughts upward through prayer in faith, hope, and love.[21]

Feld's reading of Evagrius' strategy is not dissimilar to the modern strategy of cognitive behavioral therapy or integrated usages of CBT, as mentioned above.[22] CBT, which is based on research and empirical evidence, is one of the most widely used and effective forms of therapy for most mental disorders. CBT claims to equip clients with the resources to identify, evaluate, and change distorted automatic thoughts that are causal to emotional oppression and self-defeating and destructive behavior. The major premise in CBT is that thinking is the most empirically based influence on feelings and behavior, and that a change in thought patterns will result in change in one's emotional and behavioral life. CBT is an autodidactic, problem-solution, learning model of short-term treatment that enables clients to test empirically the reality and rationality of their own thoughts and to modify thought patterns to be more adaptive, mindful, realistic, and hope filled.

Feld notes a threefold pattern in Evagrius similar to CBT strategy that begins with observation of one's own thought life, followed by an analysis of such thought and identification of its content and the demon behind it, and finally an unmasking of the demon and its deceitful nature.[23] CBT of course does not locate the origin of thoughts in the demonic, but it does seek to identify distorted thinking as the cause of depressed feelings and behaviors. Following this threefold strategy, the monk would enter into contemplation and prayer to order rightly his thoughts. Self-awareness—namely, cognitive awareness of *logismoi* and cognitive restructuring through discernment and prayer—could make for an "Evagrian version" of CBT. With CBT and other forms of therapy, a client is guided, analyzed, or counseled by a therapist who works through various strategies and methods to assist in solving various problems. Notwithstanding the success of the Evagrian method or modern CBT, critics abound. The "triumph of the therapeutic" has seen the the priesthood and the healing charisms of the church replaced by the modern-day Western therapist with "life, liberty and the pursuit of happiness," that being the salvation offered by the gospel according to the American dream.[24] Improvement in mental health conditions is to be applauded, though standards based on unrealistic premises may be detrimental in the long run. In fact, there is increasing research and literature that counters the claims of CBT's effectiveness and asserts contrarily a decline in its ability to treat symptoms long term.[25]

In the monastic tradition, primarily in the East, monks and nuns were often trained under the tutelage of a spiritual father or mother. Spiritual parenting was a significant gift and had a significant role in the development of sons and daughters in Christ within monasticism. A spiritual mother or father became such because they were first spiritual daughters or sons of a master who came alongside a novice training and nurturing them in the wisdom of the Christian life. The long tradition of spiritual mothers and fathers extends back before the church to the Hebrew Bible with Jethro and Moses, Moses and Joshua, Elijah and Elisha (and the school of the prophets), Jeremiah and Baruch, and, in the New Testament, Christ and his disciples, Barnabas and Paul, Paul and Timothy, and so forth. The spiritual parent specializes in the instruction, counsel, and formation of the disciple, and Evagrius served in this capacity for Palladius and others.

The anchorites were forbidden by their mentors to engage in needless chatter or improper soul baring (*parrhesia*), and later monastic rules included vows of silence.[26] The solitary conditions of the monk were much too conducive to foster depressive states. So-called talk therapy, incorporated in CBT, psychodynamics, and other therapies, has proven to be effective. The sacrament of confession and heart-to-heart sharing were needed and practiced in the fourth century as well and provided a means to combat the tendency to repress and stay isolated. Externalizing what may be internally troubling or even toxic in healthy and supportive contexts and ways can be cathartic and a means of release from hindrances and emotional impasses. Spiritual parents could serve as surrogate therapists of the soul and minister an empathic ear and wise counsel out of their own experiences of struggle and victory. In counseling, a therapist equips the person to discern cognitive distortions that impact emotions and behavior. Further, the therapist equips the person to restructure their ideation with reality and hope-based thinking, often through affirmations and other techniques. Evagrius as a spiritual father directed his sons to employ *antirrhetikos*, or Scripture-based counterstatements, to combat the demonically incited *logismoi* and to redirect thinking away from sin and toward God.[27]

Aimless and endless rumination is a common symptom of depression. The stream of consciousness and inner monologue of automatic thoughts seem to run rampant, internally voicing scripts of helplessness, hopelessness, and worthlessness in depressive states. Counteraffirmation from Scripture would serve as the "sword of the Lord," which would break the endless chain of despairing rumination and invite the mind into a liberating dialogue with God.[28] The integration of cognitive restructuring with Christian belief formation for discipleship has been found to be beneficial not only for those with mental disorders but also for those in recovery and those simply on the pathway of Christian discipleship.[29]

The human person is not a solitary individual but a relational being in community with God and others. Mental health and disorders, contrary to the modern paradigm, are not individualistic issues. Sociocultural, economic, philosophical, theological, and other factors contribute to the making up of our identity and to the constructs of mental health and mental disorders. Future systemic change and systemic support need to increase nurturing wholeness to create healthy communities. Both church and society have offered much in this respect but have so much further to go in terms of erasing stereotypes and stigmas and combating through education our notion of rugged rational individualism.[30]

While the Evagrian method anticipates and, in many ways, is consistent with modern therapeutic practices, it operates out of a radically different worldview and thus arrives at different conclusions when interpreting ultimate causality of phenomena like acedia. Some are problematic. Modern cognitive behavioral theory locates depressive feelings and behaviors in distorted cognition, which in turn has neural correlates. On the other hand, Evagrian methodology locates acedia ultimately in the demonic with tempted and distorted cognition as the mediating or penultimate cause and not the ultimate cause. Some of these conclusions create further questions that can be problematic and would need to be engaged in other studies.[31] Is a spirit worldview, one that holds a place for the existence and activity of angels, demons, spiritual powers, gods, and God, prescientific and precritical? Is such a worldview merely a projection from a prescientific mind that seeks to explain causation, phenomena, events, or issues without the proper ratio-empirical equipment?

THE REALITY OF SPIRIT AND EMERGENCE

Most modern astrophysicists, like Stephen Hawking, strongly affirm the universe as finite, unbounded, and a closed, self-sufficient, self-explaining system, which means that the universe contains its own explanation (causal closure) and is its own reason for being and acting, apart from any reliance on divine agency or something external to the universe.[32] The universe is causally closed. The notion of a causally closed universe creates problems accounting for divine agency and action or any kind of spirit agency and action.[33] As a response, some have continued to hold a firm bifurcation between faith and reason and theology and science that allows them to maintain traditional classical Christian notions about the nature and action of God and God's interaction with the universe. In what is more of a dualist model of reality (God and creation), God's nature is more of a fixed "substance" than a process that is impassable but allows for interaction with an ex nihilo creation directly through revelation or indirectly through natural law. This model dialogues and interacts with the sciences; however, revelation is held over science, governing and guiding it, while science is subservient and confirms revelation. On the other hand, other theologians have attempted to be more conversant with science, allowing the sciences to take the lead and provide direction for theology. Some interdisciplinary theologians, such as Philip Clayton and Robert J. Russell, have sought to integrate modern science with process theology through the framework of emergence.[34]

Emergence is an interdisciplinary framework that attempts to explain the activity and interaction of systems, mechanisms, substances, properties, and actions within and between the various levels of fields that comprise the study of the universe, from the microphysical upward to the macrophysical, to the chemical, biological, psychological, sociological, and onward. The attraction to emergence is its explanatory power in that it eludes the extremes of reduction on one end and dualism on the other. Although emergence identifies the universe as physical, containing many nonphysical systems and properties, it captures the relationship between levels without reducing any level to the level below it, such as saying that all mental activity is merely and solely brain chemistry (reductionistic physicalism)[35] or that because one states that all mental activity is merely brain chemistry then mental activity truly does not exist (eliminative materialism).[36] Additionally, emergence understands the supervenience of each level on the level beneath it in a nonreductive manner, giving room for new properties and laws without resorting to any type of nonphysical substance, some version of Cartesian substance dualism.[37]

As theologians have incorporated the theory of emergence, there has increasingly been a movement toward open panentheistic emergent models to best explain the God-universe relationship.[38] "Open" refers to the nature of God as passible and limited in his consequent nature. Yet many embrace the dipolar nature of the divine in process theology and hold to an impassible and eternal God in his antecedent ontological nature.[39] The dipolar nature of God is joined with the panentheistic idea that "all is in God," as analogically the mind dwells in the body (body-mind combination), so God dwells in the world (God-universe combination).[40] Such models claim to account for God's activity in the world without breaking, intervening in, or superseding the physical laws of the universe.[41] Open panentheistic emergent models seek to account for God in naturalistic terms that cooperate with the physical laws of the universe. However, panentheists, such as Philip Clayton, also argue for the openness of human consciousness (consciousness as an emergent property of the brain) to other agencies, including human, divine, and spirit.[42] Of course classical renewalist[43] perspectives have always claimed divine-human and spirit world–human interaction.[44] Nonetheless, charismatic renewalists usually hold to a classical dualistic spirit-matter worldview and often have scientific integration as a lower priority and so are technically less engaged. However, there are exceptions, and they tend to run along the lines of integrating a Pentecostal spirit worldview with open panentheistic emergent lines, for example, the work of Amos Yong.[45]

Hypothetically, assuming for the sake of argument, because it is debatable, difficult, and virtually impossible to prove scientifically, that spirit is an emergent property that can interact and influence human consciousness, then possibly human consciousness can be open to demonic activity as well as divine activity. This hypothesis would open the door to more questions to consider. Do demons exist? Do demons have ontic or merely metaphorical status? Or are they fallen angels who tempt humans? Do demons cause, influence, or feed off mental disorder? How does one know? To what degree can the demonic influence mental disorder? How does one know what is of demonic origin, personal-volitional origin, or divine origin? Do demons act with God's permission, on their own, or both, and is their action connected with one's personal sin and/or so-called generational sin?[46] How do all of these questions bear on theodicy? These questions are highly speculative, theological, and pastoral and extremely significant and even problematic. The most difficult questions related to Evagrian acedia center on demonstrating the existence of the demonic, demonstrating that the demonic is connected to sin and causal to mental disorder, and diagnosing demonization without demonizing persons, which seems like a tall order and again highly problematic. Prior, we had addressed some of these questions in part, but they require their own study apart from this work to tackle fully the concerns and implications that are involved in claims of the demonic.[47] Thus, the Evagrian consequential model, which connects acedia and depression to the consequences of sin and ultimately the demonic, needs to address further questions and problems as a part of a different study.

BALTHASAR—NATURAL TYPE: THE STRUCTURE OF TEMPTATION (1); AND CONSEQUENTIAL TYPE: CONSEQUENCE OF SIN AND SALVATION (2)

Hans Urs von Balthasar addresses in theological terms both the natural and consequential types of anxiety. Balthasar, the twentieth-century *nouvelle theologie* Swiss Catholic, in his short work *The Christian and Anxiety* identifies anxiety as structural to temptation and consequential to the fall and Christ's work of salvation. Balthasar's text, as opposed to the other two treatises examined in chapter 5, works strictly out of theological categories. This is not to say that Balthasar's work does not have philosophical appeal. Balthasar engages the world philosophically in most of his works, especially through the transcendentals, and finds their fulfillment theologically in the triune God. *The Christian and Anxiety* is no exception. Balthasar offers a deeply penetrating philosophical analysis of the subject but concludes his study theologically in the "light of Christ and the Trinity."[48]

Balthasar begins *The Christian and Anxiety* with a brief critique of Kierkegaard's *The Concept of Anxiety*. His fundamental problem with the work is that, in his estimation, Kierkegaard deals with a point of Christian dogma from merely a psychological perspective, and so his monograph lacks theological examination. In fact, "God and Christ are rarely mentioned explicitly in this work, which was in fact meant to be a theological work."[49] His condemnation is against Kierkegaard's use of "psychoanalysis and existential philosophy," which Balthasar sees as a reflection of "the finite mind horrified by its own limitlessness." Instead, the piece should have been a "serious theology of anxiety" drawn from the fountain of revelation, the Word of God.[50] Balthasar does not restrain his sentiments in his critique.

Balthasar condemns Kierkegaard's relegation of anxiety to something structural to humanity and not something structural to humanity's relationship with God. His basic argument against Kierkegaard is that the Dane makes the case for anxiety as something interior to humanity, ontological, and structural to freedom, as opposed to relating anxiety directly to the presence or absence of God in relationship with humanity. In other words, Kierkegaard detaches fundamental anxiety from any connection to humanity's relationship with God or separation from God. Balthasar's argument contra Kierkegaard's is, "The mind is made anxious, not by the void of nothingness in its own interior dimension, but by the void that yawns wherever the nearness and concreteness of God have withdrawn into a distant estrangement and have yielded their place to 'someone over there,' to an abstract relation to an 'other.'"[51] Anxiety is structural to temptation rather than to freedom, and it necessarily functions to test faithfulness to God amid God's apparent hiddenness.

Adam was not tempted "based on a 'creaturely anxiety' about being able to fall," "but God had to leave open to man the space that made it possible for man to move away. God could not spare man the experience of being tempted by what God had excluded and forbidden, which precisely by being forbidden acquires its power over man."[52] God grants the space for temptation in that once "this space had been entered, anxiety is the order of the day."[53] Thus, "nothingness" is the immediate basis for anxiety, but not from a nothingness of humanity's finitude in the fact of infinite possibility, per Kierkegaard, but rather from the space needed for tempting and testing allowed by God. Thus, Balthasar would agree with Kierkegaard that prelapsarian anxiety is structural, but not structural to freedom but structural to temptation by divine design. God's protection is suspended by God temporally to allow for temptation and testing, and such an "absence" or space that allows for temptation births anxiety in the human mind as it faces the test of obedience or disobedience to God's will.

Once the space of temptation is opened, "the space can no longer be closed, and anxiety can no longer be banished. From now on anxiety is intrinsic to the mind on the basis of the gaping void that incubates temptation, but this immanence of anxiety within humanity has a transcendent prerequisite: alienation from God."[54] Anxiety is innate to humanity, Balthasar concurs with Kierkegaard, but a closer reliance on the scriptural account rather than on the limitation of philosophical ontology reveals clearly that anxiety is derived from temptation, not the "void of nothingness" that characterizes the possibility of freedom. Instead, for Balthasar, anxiety is initially related to one's relationship with God and not to the ontological structure of human being or freedom. Following the fall, the anxiety of temptation is compounded into the anxiety of sin, as a consequence. Balthasar seeks theological ground for his notion of anxiety, yet he does not directly address Kierkegaard's concern, as well as Tillich's and ours as well, for the *nihil* stemming from ontological difference. Though Balthasar clearly held to the analogical structure of the divine-creation relationship, he does not address it, which begs the question, leaving it inappropriately unanswered.

As Balthasar contends that humanity cannot be gripped by a "neutral" anxiety that rests in human freedom unrelated to the divine, so he also holds the same for anxiety related to sin. There is no neutral ground of philosophical introspection to stand on in the midst of the Lutheran dialectic between the anxiety of sin and the anxiety of the cross. Here, Balthasar believes both Kierkegaard and Luther missed the mark. The both-and of *simul iustus et peccator* becomes an "in-between," a place of neutrality or a theological stalemate. Balthasar views the "in-between" dialectic as truly a "neither-nor," which he claims is an impossibility while one is truly in Christ.[55] One is either in Christ or not in Christ. Balthasar's participatory understanding of the cross and salvation will not permit for the type of dialectic that trapped Kierkegaard. We do not merely stand in a legal, forensic state before God but are also virtually joined in union with the crucified One and risen together through participation.

Balthasar will not tolerate an either/or of being in Christ, which seems to be the position from which Kierkegaard posits freedom and the leap of faith. In this valley of decision, the Dane is neutralized and paralyzed by the "rupture between the finite and the infinite that it [the finite mind] finds within itself, with its own unfathomable freedom."[56] Such is the "anxiety of one faced with the abyss of his own mind," and hence Kierkegaard's departure from dogmatics into psychology, a field in which "dialectical anxiety is at home."[57] The Swiss theologian's participation in the cross and salvation is a step out of the dialectic with salvation in front and anxiety and sin left behind.[58]

While for Balthasar, Kierkegaard's notion of anxiety does not take into account humanity's relationship with God prior to its relationship with freedom, the Swiss theologian's own identification of anxiety rests solely in relationship to God, rooted in revelation rather than psychology, making it a more a theology of anxiety in his estimation. Although he is eager to correct what he construes as a nontheological notion of structural anxiety in Kierkegaard, Balthasar still proposes a "neutral anxiety" or general anxiety "as a fundamental given of human existence" common to day-to-day human life in this world that falls upon the just and the unjust.[59] He is never clear as to when it originates, but it seems to follow the fall as a consequence and leads to sin-anxiety or salvation-anxiety. Balthasar hints, "Now, however, we must complete the thought and note that this neutrality is immediately displaced, down to the very root of existence, by the difference between this turning toward and this turning away . . . the contrast that divides the anxiety of the wicked from the behavior and attitude of the good."[60]

Before the fall, anxiety arises in the interval of temptation and testing where God allows for such space. Following the fall, anxiety seems to be accepted as naturally part of the human condition. At one point, he compares this general anxiety with that claimed for the "age of anxiety." Balthasar distinguishes between the iteration of anxiety that has been epidemic in the so-called modern age of anxiety, due to the "mechanized world where colossal machinery inexorably swallows up the frail human body and mind only to refashion it into a cog in the machinery," and the general phenomenon of the malady, which has been common since the beginning.[61] The latter is generic, universal, and natural to humanity, while the former is a peculiar, individual manifestation of the latter that is specific to the spirit of the age. Balthasar seeks to bring the modern iteration into perspective and remove it from the status of something ontological unto itself and transtemporal, per Kierkegaard, and relocate it to a hypostasis of the neurosis found in this peculiar age. Hence, in demystifying so-called existential anxiety, he deflates its value as structural and universal and makes it idiosyncratic of modernity.

In this sense, Balthasar's position on general anxiety, though not stated as such, is similar to a physiological perspective that understands the phenomenon as part of the human condition that can be constructive or destructive. However, at one point he makes the reaching conclusion that the modern neurotic type of anxiety is relegated to this age alone and was not a manifestation in the "earlier, humane world," an inference without ground and highly unlikely to be the case.[62] Of course, each manifestation of the species is unique to its context and conditions and so is unrepeatable in that specific sense, but it is apparent that mental disorders occurred in the premodern world, though they may have manifested differently in different contexts. The historiography of the phenomenon and its descriptions attest to the occurrence of the species since the beginning of recorded time, though the variety of species, subspecies, and manifestations of anxiety are not always the same and may vary causally and descriptively across time and culture.[63]

Following, Balthasar moves from general or natural anxiety to anxiety that is related to sin and punishment, anxiety as consequential. This move brings us to a consequential etiology (type 2), stemming from the consequences of sin, or conviction of sin. Balthasar identifies both a "sin-anxiety" that comes from sin and the anticipation of death and wrath and a "salvation-anxiety" that works by grace to lead one to repentance and salvation.[64] Balthasar has no problem clearly connecting anxiety and sin, a move that certain progressive theologies today may find troubling. Balthasar understands our common sin as a two-sided coin of autonomy and atheism, a "despairing dialectic between the identification of itself with God and the denial of God, only to arrive in the end, at a chaotic failure to distinguish between the two."[65] Modernity has never been kind to any type of "sin preaching," especially any type that connects sin with judgment and punishment, and somewhat right-fully so. Sinners in the hands of an angry church have not fared well in the past. So we are leery about sin preaching and stone casting, although Scrip-ture at times seems to make the connection between sin and its consequential impact on our mental states.[66] Nonetheless, Balthasar seeks to remain faithful to the scriptural witness holding to the notion that sin-anxiety, or anxiety caused by sin and guilt, brings tribulation and torment as the wicked seek to evade the light of the all-seeing God and God's judgment.[67] The sin-laden soul swallowed up by the dread of the terror of the Lord and incarcerated in hopelessness learns that anxiety is also a call that can lead to freedom by turning to God for salvation, or what he terms salvation-anxiety.[68] He cites the conditional passages of blessing and cursing in Deuteronomy 28–30 as the ground for this salvation-anxiety. Deuteronomistic thinking promises systematic disorder and ruin in every facet of life for the disobedient but promises systematic order and fruitfulness in every facet of life for the obedi-ent. This same anxiety that comes to the one deserving wrath can also come to lead one to turn to God and further lead the faithful to be tested on the journey to greater faithfulness.[69] Balthasar is matter-of-fact.

However, we have already considered some of the problems with this line of thinking when examining Kierkegaard. Biblical figures, such as Job, Christ, or Paul, shoot down the common kneejerk connection between sin and sickness or affliction. They were not afflicted because of their unrigh-teousness and God's judgment. They were righteous and yet still suffered infirmities. Reinders summarizes the problem well when considering many have sinned the same sin but only some suffer certain consequences like mel-ancholia: "If it were true that God sends disabling conditions upon some but not on others without there being a clear moral difference between them, this would mean that in distributing good and evil, the divine will works about as randomly as chance and fortune. This would render the very notion of a divine will meaningless."[70] Deuteronomistic themes, inconsistent in them-selves, are also simply not found consistently throughout Scripture. Nonethe-less, it seems in Balthasar that anxiety is a prophetic instrument of God that is utilized to test the untested, to call the fallen back to righteousness, and to lead the faithful unto blessing and glory.[71]

He then turns to the New Testament and illustrates how "the anxiety of the good" operates on the soul when confronted with Christ and leads to salvation-anxiety. The anxiety of the good, as Balthasar calls it, is the revela-tion of the goodness of God to convict contrite hearts, leading to repentance and salvation. In one instance, Balthasar cites that anxiety of the good occurs with the disciples who beheld the Christ phantom hovering over the deep sea:

Zechariah (Luke 1:12); with Mary overshadowed by the Spirit (Luke 1:29), a relieved Joseph (Matt 1:20); Peter under the burden of guilt (Luke 5:8-9); the disciples on Mount Tabor (Matt 17:6); the women at the tomb (Luke 24:22); the astonished Paul on the road to Damascus (Acts 9:60); and John the Revelator, who fell as dead before the Son of Man (Rev. 1:17).[72] These expressions point to the incarnate One who carries the "anxiety of the Redeemer" that marks the distinction between the anxiety of the old and the anxiety of the new.[73] Anxiety that comes from the law producing condemnation, and anxiety from the goodness of God in Christ that leads to repentance and redemption.

In the "anxiety of the Redeemer," the Son of Man has come to overcome our anxiety and fear by taking it upon sin himself, and victory is found in a resolute decision to participate in his death and resurrection.[74] All that the "Old and New Covenants know of anxiety is here gathered together and infinitely surpassed, because the person is the infinite God himself."[75] In the anxiety of the Redeemer abides the vicarious suffering of the Son of Man for the impure and the unrighteous and their anxiety that anticipates the judgment seat.[76] In his infinite love for the world, the Redeemer took on himself the absolute anxiety of the human race, "which undergirds and surpasses every other anxiety and thus becomes the standard and tribunal for all," and "the absolute measure of the abyss and of every other abysmal experience," and vanquished it on the cross in the abandonment of the Son by the Father.[77] Christ has conquered the principality of anxiety through his weakness, and the faithful from their weakness participate in the victory that begins at the cross. The love of God compelled Christ to suffer the anxiety of this world one time for all. For Balthasar, owing to the power of the cross, a Christian has no permission to be overtaken by sin-anxiety following such a victory, because Christ no longer permits it.[78] The child of God has "anxiety-free access to God in faith, hope, and love," whereby nothing shall separate them from God.[79]

Ideally, we can concur with Balthasar that Christ has made a way for the faithful to overcome sin and anxiety. However, in practice it is unrealistic to think that members of the body of Christ will never experience anxiety related to the consequences of sin. More so, rest assured the general anxiety that is universal to human life will continue to linger. Regardless to what degree a tradition within Christianity holds to an accelerated view of sanctification or realized view of eschatological salvation, absolute sinless perfection has never been the overall teaching of the church. Balthasar is not making a claim for such a teaching either. He is merely proclaiming that Christ has made a way for Christians to be victorious over sin and anxiety as they walk with Christ. Even after conversion, Christians remain in this world and are embodied in passions and so are susceptible to temptation. Even Christ was tempted. Pauline theology makes space for the postconversion struggle between the flesh and the spirit in terms of the *sarx* and carnality (issues surrounding *sarx* and *pneuma* in Romans, Galatians, and 1 Corinthians).

A theological etiology of mental disorder needs to be comprehensive, acknowledging the natural or structural factors that make mental disorder possible, as well as recognizing that sin and the fall can have an impact on mental states as well. The uncertain relation between a hypothetical demonic and mental disorder, as well as the consequential connection between sin and melancholia, would need to be fully addressed elsewhere in an in-depth work that is faithful to the scriptural witness, specifically the witness to salvation in Christ, as well as the latest research afforded by the sciences. In considering sin and its relation to mental health, we are again reminded that theologically and socioculturally we make meaning of natural phenomena.[80] Often, the meaning we attribute to natural phenomena or even to biblical notions of sin has more to do with our social or political posturing and the power we seek than to the divine will.[81] Any meaning that regards our fellow sisters and brothers as defective or disqualified and thus less than human is clearly our (de)vice and not from the mind of God, who made all things good and humanity in his image.

7

Theological Type 3—The Purgative

We return to one of our key themes, the Athanasian idiom, "For the Son of God became man so that we might become God." The goal of the incarnation is our sanctification, or what the Eastern Church referred to as deification, or *theosis*. The third relational state of the image of God in Christ is the new creation, and the third theological expression of mental disorder is the *purgative* type. In terms of humanity, new creation means the children of God regenerated and transfigured by the Spirit in the image of Christ. We stated above that the purpose of the relational *imago Christi* revealed in the incarnation is identificational (with our weakness) and soteriological (sonship/*familitas* and *theosis*). A theological anthropology stemming from new creation informs a theology of mental disorder in a unique way. The notion that suffering is a part of our spiritual growth is as old as Job and exemplified in Christ, who "learned obedience from the things he suffered" (Heb. 5:8). It is also an equally age-old problem in theodicy that questions either the goodness or the omnipotence of God for allowing evil or at least pain in our lives. Much of a New Testament theology of sanctification depicts the ongoing internal struggle between the spirit and the flesh (e.g., Rom. 6–8; Gal. 3–6; Col. 3). One is able to grow in holiness and Christlikeness by yielding to the sanctifying work of the Spirit and resisting sin and temptation (Rom. 8:13; Gal. 5:16). First Peter 4:1 captures best the concept of purgation as sanctification from sin: "Whoever has suffered in the flesh has ceased from sin." What does purgation look like, and what is its psychological impact in terms of mental health? Also, when is mental anguish no longer purgative or sanctifying, and when is it pathological and dangerous?

ST. JOHN OF THE CROSS: THE DARK NIGHT OF THE SOUL

The third theological type of melancholia is the purgative type, and it is best typified in the work of St. John of the Cross (1542–1591), or what is commonly known as "the dark night of the soul" after the poem and commentary *The Dark Night* by St. John of the Cross. There appear to be three general usages of the term: the one of St. John of the Cross, another a popular idiomatic use, and one that represents a "dark night tradition" encompassing the dark night phenomena prior and up to St. John of the Cross and following St. John.

The first usage stems from the poem "The Dark Night" and the larger commentary on the poem, both written by St. John of the Cross in the late six-teenth century. The title *Dark Night of the Soul* refers to the seeker's privation of sense and spiritual perception, which results from divine purgation and purifi-cation on the ascent to God. The novice embarks on a journey of contemplative prayer that involves three stages: purgation, illumination, and mystical union with God. Through the course of the sojourn, the ascetic experiences varied forms and degrees of spiritual darkness and abandonment that are instrumen-tal in purging the soul of trust in its own capacities and intellectual constructs to apprehend and follow God. The first night is the purifying of the senses, while the second night is the purifying of the soul or spirit. The seeming divine abandonment and ensuing spiritual darkness, along with the accompanying pain and suffering, are what constitute the "dark night" (DN).

The second usage of the DN is the popular undifferentiated[1] use of the phrase to serve as a catchall for any general period of darkness and suffer-ing religious or otherwise,[2] for example, "the president went through a dark night of the soul when he lost the election." In this case the term and its understanding are not used critically and are loosely employed for mass con-sumption as a device for comprehending setbacks in the self-actualization process within the self-help genre. Not being strictly tied to religious experi-ence, the popular usage does not necessarily entail connection with St. John of the Cross and the systematic and strategic contemplative analysis through the usual three-step pattern of mystical union.

The third usage of the DN is related to what may be called the "tradition" of the DN. The tradition builds off of the classic work and pattern of St. John of the Cross but recognizes that abandonment by God for the purpose of purification may take on a variety of patterns or forms that may include but also vary from the one laid down by St. John of the Cross.[3] An example of applying the DN tradition as a theoretical framework for interpreting other types of spiritual anguish is the case of Mother Teresa of Calcutta. Some have interpreted the recent revelations of the life of Mother Teresa and her longtime undisclosed struggle with spiritual aridity as the DN.[4] With the case of Mother Teresa, her struggle may not have taken the exact pattern prescribed by St. John, but it nonetheless is understood as a type of the DN and thus is part of the DN tradition.

Clearly, both the first and third usages are evidently tied to a distinct pattern of Christian ascetic theology and the Christian journey of holiness, as opposed to the second usage, which is not necessarily connected to Christianity, religion, or any systematic or rigorous pattern. It is also significant to note that although the DN narrative often comes from the Catholic tradition, such melancholia is not relegated to strictly that tradition. Julius Rubin documents a similar phenomenon within Protestantism that he simply calls *religious melancholy*, drawing from Burton's *Anatomy*, where it is first identified. Rubin's work traces religious melancholy from the Protestant Reformation to Puritanism, the two Great Awakenings, Wesleyan-Arminian perfectionism, and modern-day evangelicalism. He posits that Luther's *Anfechtung*, Calvin's anxiety, Cowper's depression, Finney's mourners' bench, Noyes' suicide, and similar conversion pathologies are products of the excesses of sinners or saints pursuing conversion or final salvation within the ecclesial cultural of revivalism. Distinctive of this pursuit is a radical awareness of sin, guilt, separation from God, and eternal damnation that seems to find no remedy or solace even through spiritual disciplines.[5] The purgative type developed in this chapter will explore the usage in St. John of the Cross and in the larger tradition of the DN and is closely related to this notion of religious melancholy.

ST. JOHN OF THE CROSS: THE DARK NIGHT OF THE SOUL AND DEPRESSION

St. John of the Cross was a major figure in the Catholic Reformation along with figures such as his mentor, Teresa of Avila, Ignatius Loyola, and Francis de Sales. He is mostly known as a Carmelite friar who worked reform within that movement and as a Spanish mystic who wrote two commentaries, *Ascent of Mount Carmel* and the sequel *The Dark Night*, which expounded on an untitled poem of eight stanzas often referred to also as "The Dark Night." In these works, St. John builds on the traditional threefold path of Christian mysticism: purgation, illumination, and union. Purgation consists of the standard privation of desire from the sensible and intelligible realms and the accompanying sensual and spiritual aridity that follow the privation. The DN is both active and passive and consists of two nights of abandonment: the dark night of the senses and the dark night of the soul or spirit. On these two dark nights, by the grace of God, one mortifies the desire of the senses, and the soul and is purged and purified from every obstacle that prevents one from climbing the ladder of ascent to God.

The DN's relation to the purgative type of depression is that the DN tradition describes phenomena that can be construed as melancholia or similar to it. The purgative type can identify depression in two ways, as either a component of an overall divine strategy of sanctification for the godly or a collateral phenomenon that accompanies such a strategy. Several seminal questions arise from either assertion that can guide our analysis and interaction with the purgative type of depression. Is there a distinction between the DN and what we call depression? How can we make that distinction and why? Does God employ the DN or suffering pedagogically, and can suffering be salutary? If so, what are some of the problems with this methodology?

First, is there a distinction between the DN and what we call depression? St. John anticipates this problem and couches the question within a larger question. One can rephrase it this way. How does one know whether the origin of the aridity and spiritual privation is from the DN or from "sins and imperfections," "weakness and lukewarmness," or a "bad humour or indisposition of the body," such as depression?[6] St. John gives neophytes three signs that will enable them to make the distinction and identify the DN. First, following the purging of the sensual desires, seekers will find "no pleasure or consolation in the things of God" or "anything created."[7] St. John concludes that if this aridity were due to "sins or imperfection," then the soul would still enjoy the pleasures of the world, which, in the aridity of the DN, the soul does not.[8] However, he notes that such a lack of enjoyment and emptiness toward heavenly or earthly pleasure may also proceed from a "melancholy humour" as well as the DN.[9] Thus, a second sign is needed.

In the dark night persons may be focused on God with all of their being and still feel backslidden and far from God because the enjoyment and sweetness of sense and spirit has ceased. The arid soul incessantly and carefully pursues God but misperceives itself and believes that it is not in pursuit of God and that it does not serve God. Conversely, in a lukewarm state this dynamic will never be the case. St. John points out that the lukewarm do not carefully follow after God and are quite indifferent to their spiritual state when not following God.[10] In the case of depression, St. John acknowledges that the state can be comorbid with aridity and even augment its affect.[11] However, one can distinguish between the two in terms of the drive to serve God, which remains in the arid state.[12] The pervasive gloom of depression strips one of any desire for pursuing either worldly or divine pleasure. Aridity will likewise strip the soul of both sensual pleasure for the world and the divine. Nonetheless, even in this arid condition, the believer in the DN will yet be willing and strong in spirit to continue to seek God. The difference between depression and aridity is that the former will inhibit the seeker from following after God, while the latter will not ultimately impede one from seeking after the divine and will maintain a purgative effect.[13] Further, in the former condition, the depressed will be remiss of any negligence in pursuing God, while God will supply the one under aridity with the strength of spirit needed to sustain the journey toward union with God.[14]

The third and final sign of the DN is when the soul can "no longer meditate or reflect in the imaginative sphere of sense" on the divine.[15] Such cognitive exercises are no longer accessible by divine permission. In order to purge the senses and the mind of false constructs, God ceases to communicate through the medium of outward or inward senses but exclusively "by pure spirit" and an "act of simple contemplation, to which neither the exterior or interior senses of the lower part of the soul can attain."[16] The third sign indicates the DN, because with "sins and imperfections," "weakness and lukewarmness," or a "bad humour or indisposition of the body" this level of divine communication is never attained. For St. John of the Cross, ultimately, these three signs indicate the conditions of one experiencing the DN. However, having all three signs merely denotes that one is experiencing the DN, but it does not indicate that one does not have depression as well as the DN. They simply are distinct.

The Spanish friar acknowledged that depression may be comorbid with the DN and may exacerbate it as well. The three signs merely indicate that depression and the DN are not synonymous, though they may coexist and share symptoms. Thus, since some symptomology is shared between the DN and depression, we may identify the DN as a "theological melancholia." However, for St. John the two are not synonymous, as the DN originates with God for the *telos* of sanctification, while depression, St. John seems to suggest, is more related etiologically to the body (natural) and in the end deprives one of both sensual and spiritual pleasure. Likewise, as mentioned above, St. John identifies three signs that mark the DN as discrete from depression.

FURTHER INSIGHTS ON THE DISTINCTION BETWEEN THE DARK NIGHT AND DEPRESSION

Kevin Culligan, a psychotherapist from the Order of Discalced Carmelites, comes to similar conclusions concerning the DN in his essay "The Dark Night and Depression."[17] Culligan differentiates the DN from depression based on certain accompanying signs, specifically sustained prayer in pursuit of God, which is present in the former and lacking in the latter.[18] Culligan explains the Christian life of prayer, through St. John's template, as a three-stage journey to union with God.[19] The three stages are discursive meditation (beginner), contemplative prayer (proficient), and union with God (perfect). These three stages of course correspond to the classic triad of purgation, illumination, and union. In the first two stages, which correspond to the two DNs, there are significant losses or deprivation that obstruct the seeker from praying in the discursive and contemplative modes. In the first night, the DN of the senses, "persons lose sensory satisfaction" in prayer.[20] Beginners are unable to practice discursive meditation no matter how much they exert their external senses, minds, or imagination.[21] Further, "they no longer derive emotional satisfaction from their spiritual journey."[22] However, in spite of such impediments, the beginner presses forward and will not relinquish her prayer life, which marks her from the depressed, who remain inert and lethargic toward the exercise.

In the second stage of contemplative prayer during the DN of the spirit, the "proficient" are stripped of all idols and false images and constructs of God and are left abandoned. Following, they are enlightened to their own interior emptiness and disorder to the point that they feel as if they do not know God anymore.[23] The divesting of false constructs and false security elicits excruciating spiritual pain that further assists purgation and allows for the light of God's purifying self-communication to pierce the darkness and ultimately ascend to the apex, union with God.[24]

Culligan, like St. John of the Cross, distinguishes the DN from clinical depression on the grounds of symptomology. Both involve loss of pleasure in worldly and divine things. Yet the DN does not yield "the dysphoric mood,[25] the psychomotor retardation, the loss of energy, or the loss of interest or pleasure in hobbies and enjoyable activities, including sex, that one typically sees in clinical depression." With the DN there is indeed a profound sense of incompletion and emptiness but never "morbid statements of abnormal guilt, self-loathing, worthlessness, and suicidal ideation that accompany serious depressive episodes."[26] Overall, Culligan, the psychotherapist, explains that "depressed persons typically looked depressed, sound depressed, and make you depressed," while he seldom feels burdened when listening to persons describe "the dryness of the dark night."[27]

Along with St. John, Culligan claims that the DN and depression can be comorbid, and he treats each separately and distinctly. As a spiritual guide he gives proper spiritual direction for the DN, and as a therapist he recommends treating clinical depression therapeutically. However, neither St. John nor Culligan addresses how one phenomenon may cause or exacerbate the other. Following analysis of the DN, we can answer our directing questions. Is there a distinction between the DN and what we call depression? The DN, though a "theological melancholia," is distinct from clinical depression. How can we make that distinction and why? We make this distinction based on differing etiology and symptomology. The DN seems to come from the divine, while depression in a sanctified person has natural causes, whether biological, psychological, and/or social. The symptomology of the DN allows for continued pursuit of God even under aridity, while depression does not. We also make this distinction, along with Culligan, in order to maintain distinct treatment: spiritual direction for the DN and therapy, medication, proper diet, sleep, exercise, and other treatments when needed for clinical depression.

Psychiatrist and spiritual director Gerald May concurs with the distinction made between the DN and depression. Like Culligan, May notes that the classic symptoms of depression and the overall glum impression made by the depressed are either absent or clearly less pronounced in the DN.[28] On the positive end, "the person's sense of humor, general effectiveness, and compassion for others are not usually impaired in the dark night as they are in depression."[29] May also concurs that the DN and depression are frequently comorbid, often leading to or aggravating the other.[30] The two are not mutually exclusive. They can involve the instigating of the other and thus need to be given proper attention. In any case, we hear wisdom in May's strategy that "it makes more sense simply to identify depression where it exists and to treat it appropriately, regardless of whether it is associated with a dark-night experience."[31] Further, "the presence of the dark night should not cause any hesitation about treating depression."[32] Culligan calls it "a collaborative approach" entailing spiritual and psychiatric treatment.[33] Consequently, although technically the DN and depression are not synonymous, there is no need for mere taxonomy's sake to treat these as unrelated phenomena. As May[34] and others[35] have stressed, religious persons often erroneously conclude that being a believer on a spiritual journey precludes the possibility of clinical depression and thus a need for therapy or medication. Misconceptions entail the notions that the sanctified are beyond depression, treatment of symptoms is a sign of spiritual weakness, or psychiatric treatment can obstruct spiritual progress.[36]

Psychiatrist Glòria Durà-Vilà and colleagues, in a 2010 article entitled "The Dark Night of the Soul: Causes and Resolution of Emotional Distress among Contemplative Nuns," document and analyze their work in an ethnographic study of a group of ten Augustinian nuns in the Spanish Monastery of Santa Monica.[37] Symptoms that otherwise might have been categorized and interpreted as depressive were reframed by the nuns through the DN framework and reinterpreted as both existential (our type 1) and purgative (our type 3) and a vital part of their spiritual growth. A DN hermeneutic that fostered a meaning-making approach to existential anguish and spiritual aridity assisted the sisters to cope and grow through what could have been a detrimental experience. Similar to our previous interlocutors, Durà-Vilà et al. also differentiate between the DN, which is salutary and sanctifying, and clinical depression, which is pathological. They also identify distinct treatments for each, spiritual direction and psychiatry, respectively.[38] In the case of the DN, existential and spiritual resources of critical reflection, meaning construction from suffering, illumination, and progress in formation empowered the participants to overcome their struggle and find peace.

Philosopher Anastasia Scrutton critiqued the Durà-Vilà et al. study, taking issue with the alleged bifurcation made between the DN and depression and any divine salutary interpretation of either. First, she believed that the two manifestations cannot be so easily delineated. Second, any view of divinely authored suffering that is salutary is highly problematic for reasons related to the problem of evil and theodicy. As a response, Scrutton ultimately identifies three current theologies of depression. They are spiritual illness (SI), spiritual health (SH), and potentially transformative (PT).[39] SI interprets mental disorder as stemming from sin, the demonic, and/or divine judgment (our type 2). SH understands depression as a sign and even an instrument used by God to make believers holy, similar to the DN (our type 3). PT holds that "depression (along with many other instances of suffering) is inherently bad and undesirable, but can become the occasion for the person's spiritual growth (e.g., compassion, insight, appreciation of beauty)."[40] PT is similar to but not quite our type 1, Kierkegaard's pedagogical anxiety. Ultimately, Scrutton wants to eliminate all types but the PT type.

The first two types, SI and SH, for Scrutton, are popular Christian theologies of depression that she deems problematic. Her main focus in the article, though, is on SH. Based on her evaluation, Scrutton contends that SH should be replaced by PT.[41] Scrutton evaluates the notion of SH on two criteria. The first criterion is the "therapeutic value of a belief," "that it can help sufferers to make sense of their experiences, and to find aspects of them transforming."[42] The "meaning-giving" dimension of SH "brings meaning and value to experiences in a way that purely biomedical approaches cannot."[43] Although Scrutton affirms the therapeutic value of belief, she wants to be careful to guard against the often related notions that suffering is from God, is positive, or should be romanticized.[44] This is the second criterion, that the "belief is realistic or true to experience." She contends that positive or romantic notions of suffering are not realistic or true to the insider who is experiencing suffering but come from the outsider and should be eliminated from a theology of depression.[45] Yet we also acknowledge that not all persons with mental disorders can be characterized as suffering.

In her estimation, the suffering of depression is always negative, is not from God but natural in origin, and is not to be idealized, though God can bring good out of it.[46] Scrutton perceives that SH contains an effective meaning-giving dimension. Persons who believe that their plight of darkness and anguish is part of a greater divine mission are more likely to find meaning in the journey that will carry them through.[47] However, in that very sense of triumphalism, SH is susceptible to romanticizing suffering, expressly giving it divine origin or sanction, thus opening the door to the problem of evil and the aporia of theodicy issues that surround such a problem. Furthermore, the SH/DN candidates who construe their despondent state as divine providence may be less apt to receive treatment for depressive symptoms or even desire to terminate the DN, which would involve aborting the divine mission.[48]

In light of these criteria, Scrutton proposes the PT theology of depression to replace the SH/DN model and an SI model (depression as spiritual illness stemming from sin, the demonic, and/or divine judgment). The PT type maintains the effective meaning-making dimension, as well as bypassing the problem of evil and ensuing theodicy solutions. This model holds that depression and accompanied suffering are not divine in origin but natural phenomena and are inherently evil and not good. Thus, suffering, which is not derived or permitted by God and is inherently evil, is not to be idealized.[49] Nonetheless, God is able to bring good out of evil, and depression can become potentially transformative and salutary.[50]

Ultimately, Scrutton would have both types, SI and SH/DN, classified as potentially transformative for several reasons. Those experiencing depressive episodes under SH/DN need to be treated psychiatrically and not have symptoms dismissed as a divinely authorized component of the DN. The former can also have transformation outside of a religious hermeneutic. Scrutton perceives that both SI and SH/DN can contain depression and suffering, which are natural in origin and negative in experience and thus are not attributed to the divine, but can be (PT) transformative depending on the sufferer's response to therapeutic and meaning-making beliefs, which do not necessarily have to be connected to God or a religion. This move allows Scrutton to eliminate the question of evil and theodicy in depression, and also make a transformative experience available to the nonreligious.[51] However, in response, both Culligan and May, who separate the DN from clinical depression yet recognize their comorbidity, would also, like Scrutton, see the need to treat the depression psychiatrically. Thus, those with pathological depression under any of these typologies receive treatment without having to conflate the types in the manner of Scrutton. We can still allow the types to be separate and maintain their integrity. The other contentions related to suffering and theology will be examined in the next two sections.

THE PURGATIVE TYPE AND SUFFERING

The DN, as a purgative type of theological melancholia, and clinical depression are distinct manifestations and are treated distinctly. Yet their comorbidity requires acute, informed sensitivity in making and treating the distinctions properly. We now move to our final questions: Does God employ suffering pedagogically, and can it be salutary? If so, what are some of the problems with this methodology? St. John's, Culligan's, and May's analyses of the DN declare a resounding affirmation, while Scrutton has apologetically eliminated that option. Clearly, the instrumental use of abandonment and purgation collaterally resulting in spiritual suffering for the purpose of utter dependence and union with God is the driving motif and *telos* of the DN. St. John and the others mentioned unequivocally value the pedagogical and purgative value of spiritual darkness.

Culligan concurs as he interprets both the DN and depression in terms of loss. Loss in both cases does not represent "signs of dysfunction" but rather "reminders that we do not find our ultimate fulfillment in this world."[52] Bonding in relationships of all types, personally, materially, and emotionally, is essential to becoming fully human. And yet our attachment to the things of this world is penultimate and cannot fulfill our deepest longings, which are for God and so demand a "letting go."[53] Culligan claims that loss, represented in the spiritual metaphor of darkness, is more of a blessing than a curse, because "the losses of life, with all of their pain and suffering, are continual reminders of this reality."[54] Darkness "teaches us that no spiritual feeling, no self-concept, no image of God, no human relationship, no worldly achievement is worth more than God."[55]

May has not only spiritually directed and therapeutically treated persons in the DN, but he has also passed through the valley of the shadow of death himself.[56] May documents his own spiritual experience through cancer and other ailments and concludes that the DN was a gift from God that taught him many lessons, including the illusion of control, letting go of the illusion, and the meaning given in not being in control and the unknowing.[57] May acknowledges that finite expectations and contingencies, among other factors, allow for suffering to be normative and a challenge to be overcome, even serving pedagogically along the way not as an end in itself but as a vehicle to greater understanding and even peace with God.

Some type or degree of suffering is unavoidable and expected both in a fallen world where evil afflicts the unjust and just alike and in a world of ever-changing environments and contexts that require stress and tension to cultivate adaptation and thus survival. Consequently, suffering that is adaptive, transformative, and even redemptive would seem almost required in some cases in order to perpetuate. However, suffering does not necessitate that it must come directly or indirectly from God. It can be natural. Yet suffering of natural origin can potentially function transformatively under the providence of God as persons seek to respond in a way that can be mathetic and edifying.[58] On the other hand, Scrutton, in opposition to the DN tradition, refuses to locate suffering in the active or permissive will of God and views it and mental disorder as evils to be faced. For Scrutton, God is not responsible for evil but provides the means for human efforts to combat it. She contests that suffering, however, is not to be idealized from an etic perspective, further burdening those who suffer. Suffering, as romanticized, exemplified, objectified, and even commodified, for the benefit of the outsider (the etic), is to be avoided at all costs, and this is Scrutton's dispute with idealized interpretations of suffering. Suffering in itself is not redemptive but has the potential to redeem inherent in and depending on the person's response.[59] Thus, the therapeutic value of beliefs and the meaning-making component of PT are essential. However, Scrutton realizes that not all suffering may be PT, and this is a significant distinction to make. Not all suffering is "soul making." In the case of the Holocaust, for example, suffering is a horrendous evil that only serves to dehumanize and is not soul making but more so "soul destroying" (my word).[60]

We can infer that suffering may have natural and/or evil causation that can impel adaptation and even spiritual growth. However, to eliminate entirely the divine from the DN or to eliminate the divine providentially or redemptively from either the structural type 1 or the consequential type 2 seems to go against the nature, extent, and *telos* of scriptural salvation.

SOME THEOLOGICAL CONCLUSIONS

With the purgative type of theological depression, as canonized in the DN tradition, we have the classic understanding of spiritual darkness as an essential apophatic instrument of the divine employed to purify the sensual and spiritual passions of seekers and to lead them to rely solely on the hand of God for guidance into mystical union with the divine. An encounter with the numinous, a *mysterium tremendum*, purges even one's sense of self as distinct from the divine, a "self-depreciation"[61] (Gal. 2:20). The purgative tradition extends from the Hebrew Bible, with Job, Moses, David, and Jeremiah, to the New Testament, with Christ in the garden of Gethsemane and Paul with his thorn in the flesh, to the church age, including Antony of Egypt, Evagrius Ponticus, and Teresa Avila up to today with Mother Teresa of Calcutta. The DN tradition has rightfully distinguished between theological melancholia, or purgative spiritual darkness, and pathological melancholia, or clinical depression based on distinct etiology and treatment. In terms of comorbidity, treatment needs to be proper to the type: spiritual direction for the DN and psychiatric for clinical depression. In both cases, suffering can be transformative. Depending on one's theology proper and soteriology, God's agency is directly causal to the DN and/or its collateral suffering as in a Calvinistic system; or as in a Wesleyan-Arminian system, God's agency works with human free agency and suffering is understood collaterally as a consequence of human freedom and the fall.

However, conflating the two or three types into an undifferentiated PT, as in Scrutton, can be problematic as it lacks any theological impetus. Scrutton holds that all mental distress that is spiritual, pathological, and/or transformative in terms of etiology and treatment is the same. If all types have the same natural, atheological etiology and the same treatment, psychiatric if needed, and a general set of therapeutic, meaning-making beliefs,[62] then any recourse to transcendent divine agency is needless. John Swinton's response to Scrutton's article makes precisely this point. Swinton contends, "Has the atheological approach of the PT model that Scrutton seems to prefer numbed us to the fact that God's direct involvement in the spiritual illness (SI) and the spiritual health (SH) models may not be epiphenomenal or quite so easily disposed of?"[63] He concurs with Scrutton that at times certain SH models "can hurt people and that an emphasis on depression as an SI is a negative interpretation that serves to further stigmatize people experiencing depression."[64] However, are various aberrant forms of SH enough to exclude the theological for an undifferentiated brand of "therapeutic deism?"[65] John Swinton's response is that "stripped of its transcendent dimensions this model begins to look suspiciously like a form of spiritually oriented self-actualization wherein a person can overcome the pathological dimensions of depression and come to a place where they see and interpret it as a transformative experience."[66]

Any version of therapeutic deism (also moral therapeutic deism) fails to account for the fallen nature of humanity (type 2—consequential type), and most of all for the salvific purpose of God in Christ that responds to the consequences of the fall (type 3—purgative type), and thus is limited in its redemptive value and power. An atheological PT may provide some support to the overall therapeutic process on the psychiatric end of treatment in a similar, but maybe lesser, way to how mindfulness or cognitive behavioral therapy lends to a therapeutic and meaning-making approach. However, the ultimate cause of depression is unknown, and several contributing factors, such as genetics, physical health, biochemistry, abuse or trauma, environment, stress, and life circumstances, are significant, but we have also learned that there are spiritual factors as well. A robust Christian theology of depression must interact with the relevant key loci of the field, such as the Trinity, Christology, the incarnation, soteriology, and their interdisciplinary implications on mental health and wholeness. The following chapter will begin that task.

PART IV

A TRINITARIAN THEOLOGY OF MELANCHOLIA

8

The Melancholic God

Does God Get Depressed?

We made the move early on that a theological anthropology must be rooted in the image of God. Relationality is a central feature of that image. The image does not reflect autonomy but participation (in God). Specifically, Jesus Christ defines the image of God with the goal of transformation in his image. Through the incarnation, Christ takes on our human condition in order to redeem us. One aspect of our condition is suffering. If Christ assumes our humanity, he also assumes our weakness and suffering, which includes our melancholia. But can we then say that God suffers—or that God can be depressed, even? A related question is whether it is possible or necessary for God to suffer as God (in his divine nature) in order to vindicate human suffering. From here, we must consider how Christ, as divine mediator, properly takes on and simultaneously addresses our melancholia.

INCARNATION AND KENOSIS

We have been working with two guiding principles from the early Christian tradition. The first comes from Athanasius, "God became man so that we may become God." The second comes from Gregory of Nazianzus, "What has not been assumed has not been healed." Both theological idioms speak to divine identification with human nature and salvation. God becomes human to mediate *theosis* to his creation. As we apply the notions of the image of God and incarnation to a theology of depression, there are two components to our application. One is identification, and the other is salvation. As divine mediator, Christ identifies with our full humanity, even our mental disorders, so that we may be transformed into his image. Identifying with humanity is instrumental to salvation for humanity. We have claimed that the *imago Christi* is the goal of sanctification; specifically, it refers to becoming Christlike, sons and daughters of God. We are brought into the *familitas* of God and participate in the transfiguring love of God, which is shared perichoretically by the Father, Son, and Holy Spirit. Christ assumes all three relational states—creation, fall, and new creation, yet in a unique way as the Son of God and Savior. Through the incarnation, he becomes created being and is united as divinity to human nature in one person.

He identifies with our predicament to take away the sins of the world and restores our relationship with God. As a human person, he is tempted, resists sin (Heb. 4:15), and is made an offering for our sins (2 Cor. 5:21). He assumes and dies our death on the cross and descends into hell and on the third day rises again. In rising, he does not need to become a new creation. His rising is not for him. The resurrection is for us. As the "resurrection and the life," he raises us as a new creation in Christ. As Christ was baptized into our humanity as a sin offering in death, burial, descent, and resurrection, so we are identified with his humanity and image. We fellowship with his sufferings and conform to his death in order to partake of his resurrection. Romans 6 discloses the stark reality of our baptism and identification with Christ. When Christ died, we died. When Christ was buried, we were buried. When Christ resurrected, we arose from the dead with him.[1] The incarnation, culminating with the cross, used here as shorthand for Christ's death, burial, descent, resurrection, and ascension, is the means by which God identifies with our humanity and sin and heals and saves us from despondency and death. Thus, he identifies with each of the three relational states in order to redeem and fully sanctify us in his image.

When Christ assumes our full humanity, it includes even our condition of melancholia. In that way does God in Christ identify with our mental disorders? And how does identification work toward healing and sanctification? What does healing look like for those in Christ who are depressed? How does Christ reorder our spiritual disorder and transfigure our moral disfigurement through the cross? In attempting to answer some of these questions, let us move to the motive of the incarnation, divine love, and whether such love necessitates a kenosis.

Moved by relentless love, God identified with our humanity that he might redeem us. In Philippians 2:7, Paul is specific. The human form Christ took on was the form of a slave. What does assuming human nature involve, specifically in terms of taking on the form of a suffering slave, as Scripture depicts? Did he literally empty himself of his divinity in order to become human? Or did he become human, and in doing so, figuratively become "nothing" because he did not hold onto divine privilege but descended to come as a slave? The theologically operative term in this discussion is *kenosis*. Here we are referring to the significance of the so-called kenotic hymn in Philippians 2:5-11 and that passage's relation to the incarnation as suffering servant. The theological interpretation of 2:7 refers to the free choice of the second person of the Trinity to humble himself and take on human nature in the *forma servi* (form of a servant). Through this act of undying sacrificial love, he identifies with our humanity that he may save it. The noun *kenosis* is not found in Scripture but is derived from its verbal form in Philippians 2:7. The verb in question is ἐκένωσεν (*ekenōsen*) from the root κενόω (*kenoō*) "to empty out" or "to be emptied." A traditional and soft definition of kenosis that does not involve a divesting of divine properties is given by Gordon Fee as "some form of self-limitation of divine prerogatives on the part of the earthly Jesus."[2] Fee exegetes the usage of the term in this passage as modal and metaphorical rather than literal.[3] Fee assesses the christological data in Philippians and related data concerning Christ's human nature found in the book of Hebrews, Paul, and the Gospels. He concludes that Christ is depicted as exercising full humanity and at times choosing "to limit certain divine prerogatives" without ever divesting himself of divinity or emptying himself of being truly God.[4] The addition of the human nature with the divine Logos in the person of Christ allows for full human attributes and their functioning to occur alongside divine properties in the person of Christ. And further, because of the communication of those human attributes in the one person, we can claim that the divine experiences humanity and suffering. The divine freely chooses to suffer rather than not to suffer (a limitation) when choosing to become human in the incarnation.[5]

Fee conveys the traditional view of kenosis with a modern sensibility. Still, over the past few centuries there has been a growing movement away from the traditional view of kenosis toward kenosis as divestment of divine attributes. The contemporary move toward kenotic Christology began in seventeenth-century Lutheranism, reflecting on Luther's theology of the cross. Modern kenoticism flourished in the nineteenth and early twentieth centuries first in Germany and then in England. Gottfried Thomasius (1802–1875) laid out his groundbreaking, seminal text on kenotic theory, *Christi Person und Werk*. In the text, he critically sifts through Chalcedonian terms like "true deity, true humanity, and the real unity of Christ's person" to understand the hypostatic union.[6] His conclusion is that the Logos divests itself of the divine mode of being, which he posits as nonessential, in order to fully assume a human nature (*assumtio humani*).[7] He goes on to define "essential" by distinguishing it from attributes that he deems accidental. Further he bifurcates attributes that are immanent (love, holiness, truth, self-determination) from those that are relative (omniscience, omnipotence, omnipresence).[8] Thus, divine nature is divested of the accidental and relative attributes. Thomasius' became the model upon which others kenotic theories are built and even radically altered. Such proponents include Hugh R. Mackintosh (1870–1936), Charles Gore (1853–1932), P. T. Forsyth (1848–1921), Hans Urs von Balthasar (1910–1988), Jürgen Moltmann (1926–), and Thomas Altizer (1927–2018), among others.[9] Altizer and Balthasar represent some of the more radical reworkings of kenosis. In order to identify truly with humanity, Altizer calls for the "death of God" in Hegelian fashion, whereby God with the incarnation commits suicide by emptying himself of his transcendence into the immanent unfolding of the world process, culminating in the death of Christ and thus the radical deification of secularity.[10] Balthasar's kenosis is revealed in the incarnation and culminates in Christ's descent into hell. Balthasar grounds kenosis in the immanent Trinity. He identifies it as a superkenosis.[11] The Father's love is eternally emptied into the Son and similarly echoed with the Spirit and in the act of creation and the incarnation. Balthasar's kenosis, drawn from 1 Peter 3:19 and a later version of the Apostles Creed, drastically requires the Son of God to identify in solidarity with condemned humanity in order to save humanity by descending to the depths of hell, suffering, and assuming their punishment.[12]

Kenosis as a theological mechanism has been applied to a variety of loci. We see kenosis, with differing foci and strategies, appropriated to the Trinity, creation, Christology, and, in most cases, the incarnation (ontologically or functionally). Christology kenotically understood is "the Incarnation in terms of the Logos 'giving up' or 'laying aside' or 'divesting itself of' or 'emptying itself of' certain properties that normally belong to divinity."[13] These properties are deemed temporal to the incarnation. Contemporary kenotic Christologies attempt to account for the Logos' assumption of full humanity in one person in light of historical criticism of the gospel and modern science. Theories attempt to respond to problems revolving around the true humanity of Christ. They usually involve historical[14] critical[15] issues that bear on the nature, extent, and accuracy of Christ's knowledge.[16] How does one hold in tension in one person, impassibility and passibility, eternality and temporality, uncreated and created, life and death, omniscience and ignorance, omnipotence and weakness, omnipresence and physical location, among other seeming antinomies? Contemporary theories of kenosis attempt to answer that question.

Kenoticists claim that the traditional construal of the incarnation, as laid out at Chalcedon, holds incompatible properties (divine and human) in one person. Proponents claim that kenosis involves the Word freely choosing to lay aside divine attributes that they deem nonessential or contingent to divinity, like omniscience, omnipotence, and omnipresence, in order to be in union with human nature.[17] The notion is that Christ renounced, laid aside, self-limited, or willfully chose not to exercise certain divine attributes. These properties are then designated nonessential or accidental to divinity, in order to fully assume a human nature and function as a human as portrayed in Scripture. By definition, can there be any accidents in God? Various kenotic theories that have had radical bearing on the incarnation in terms of either reworking or replacing the Chalcedonian definition have sought to accommodate the full humanity[18] of Christ in light of his divinity.[19]

Our purpose is not to critique existing kenotic theories and defend the traditional definition, which would take a volume itself. At this juncture, we are theologically employing the notion of kenosis referenced in the Philippian hymn to understand how through the incarnation Christ took on the form of a slave in order to assume the depths of the human condition, including disorder and depression. We affirm unabashedly that the Logos assumed the human predicament. Yet, in becoming human, the Logos does not stop being fully divine, nor does it change his ontological nature. Neither are the two natures fused together to form one nature (monophysitism). Nor is there a *tertium quid*, two separate natures and the person of Christ.

The divine nature cannot be divested of divine attributes and remain divine. We only have to refer to Anselm's definition, not necessarily the argument, that states *aliquid quo nihil maius cogitari possit*, God is a "being than which no greater can be conceived." Many so-called contingent or nonessential attributes, such as omniscience and omnipotence, are necessary to a notion of a being than which no greater can be conceived. It would seem that we could think of a being higher than a nonomnipotent kenotic God, or a kenotic God who is omnipotent and chooses not to divest of it.[20] Similarly, the other omni-attributes would follow. The nature of "omni-" would seem to preclude any relative or accidental status. Further, the doctrine of divine simplicity would signify that there is no real distinction between the identity and attributes of God. Divestment of omni-attributes would seem to involve divestment of the divine nature and thus divinity.[21]

COMMUNICATIO IDIOMATUM

We affirm that the Son of God assumed a human nature, but not at the expense of the divine nature. The logic of Chalcedon and virtually the entirety of patristic interpretation understand the incarnation as an addition (of a human nature) rather than a subtraction or divestment (of a divine nature). Whether one looks at the patristic *communicatio idiomatum* as the communication of powers from nature to another nature or the medieval *communicatio*, in which both natures are communicated to the one person, neither view claims a change of divinity.[22] The key to a *communicatio* is the "union" (*unio hypostatica sive personalis*) within Chalcedonian boundaries of the two natures, not the emptying or merging of one nature into another, the divine into the human or the human into the divine. The ontological difference and infinite analogical interval of dissimilarity between uncreated and created being makes such a conflation unfeasible.

Modern kenotic theory, originally coming out of Lutheranism, may be an ill-fated attempt to compensate for a hyper-divinized human nature of Christ, which is a result of sharing attributes across natures. A Lutheran *communicatio*, which distinguishes four genera of *communicatio*, often allows for a sharing of properties across the two natures. Sharing not merely assigns them to the one person but ascribes properties of the divine nature to the human and the human to the divine nature.[23] The distribution occurs from divine to human nature (*genus maiestaticum*, a genus of majesty) and from human to divine nature (*genus kenoticum* or *tapeinoticum*, ταπεινωσις, a genus of humility). Thus, one nature is ascribed to possessing the property of the other, in violation of Chalcedonian terms and boundaries.[24]

The *communicatio idiomatum* genus of majesty, often discussed in sacramental theology in the sixteenth century, may have opened the door in the nineteenth century to a kenotic response to such a move. The traditional doctrine of the *communicatio idiomatum* was an attempt to resolve these problems without denying or divesting of either the divine or human natures. The doctrine, in one form, claims that because of the hypostatic union of the divine and human natures in one person, the properties or attributes of the divine nature (the Logos) can be ascribed to the one person Jesus Christ, and the properties of the human nature (of Christ) can be ascribed to the one person Jesus Christ (*genus idiomaticum*). What is predicated of the Logos is predicated of the person Jesus Christ. And what is predicated of his human nature can be predicated of the person Jesus Christ. However, that which is of the divine nature cannot be ascribed to human nature and the converse. There is no communication or sharing of *idiomata* between the two natures, just in the person. Neither can one ascribe the properties of one nature to the other nature (*genus apotelesmoticum*). For example, the Logos is not the soul, reason, or body of Christ, as in Apollinarianism. The two true, full natures must be kept distinct and not conflated into one nature in the one person (monophysitism). Also, the attributes of each nature must not be confused between the two natures.

In the crucifixion, Christ died. While we can then say that "God died," it was not the Logos that ceased, but rather the human nature of Christ that died. Further, owing to the hypostatic union and the communication of attributes, the human death of the man Jesus is ascribed to the person Jesus Christ, the God-man. Hence, God was crucified. God died for us *in* Jesus Christ. The attributes of both natures are shared in the one person. The attributes of both natures are the attributes of the one person. Both the divine attributes (e.g., omnipotence and omniscience) and the human attributes (e.g., growing in wisdom, suffering, limitation of knowledge) can be ascribed to the one person. The person Jesus Christ, in obeying the will of the Father, acts according to both natures and the *idiomata* proper to each respective nature without confusing, changing, dividing, or separating the natures.

There is no need for a kenosis as divine divestment. Full humanity can be experienced in the *theandric* person, Jesus Christ, without resorting to stripping away divinity. In the Gospels, Christ acts humanly from his human nature and divinely from his divine nature. We can draw this conclusion because the two natures exist and are vital within one concrete person. There is no irreconcilable dualism or polar opposition that needs to reduce or deny one nature or the other.[25] In Christ, we are speaking of a new person, not of humanity and divinity or their respective agencies in separate terms but of a union in one person. The analogy of difference is made concrete. Any kenotic qualifiers within the Trinity, creation, or incarnation need to abide within the orthodox definitions. God is one in being and three distinct persons neither confounding the persons nor dividing the essence. The second person of the Trinity, the divine Logos, descends into the womb of Mary and is incarnate in the one person Jesus Christ. He possesses a fully divine nature and a fully human nature united in one person (*unio hypostatica sive personalis*) with the attributes of each distinct nature shared in one person.

THE QUESTION OF DIVINE IMPASSIBILITY AND SUFFERING

Historical critical issues surrounding the knowledge and ability of Christ led kenoticists to accommodate and sacrifice what they deem to be nonessential, archaic, or incompatible notions and attributes of the divine. This entailed the omniattributes discussed above, as well as the concepts of divine impassibility, immutability, and simplicity.[26] Our response to the question of kenosis leads us to the larger question of divine impassibility/passibility, and specifically how it relates to suffering and the suffering of mental disorders, such as depression. Although many claim that disability does not necessitate suffering,[27] which is true, I am making the claim that mental disorder is frequently accompanied by suffering. If we are to address how theology defines, informs, and ministers to depression, then we must identify how God relates to suffering and mental disorder. The notion is that if God cannot feel and know experientially what we are going through when we suffer, then he cannot understand, relate to, take on, and heal our psychic wounds and grief. As is often stated, love that does not feel or suffer is not real love. Suffering takes on ultimate meaning and is endurable if we know that God suffers along with us.

Thus, as with the problem presented by kenosis, we need to address the larger theological category of divine impassibility/passibility and mental disorder. Divine (im)passibility or *apatheia* is a multifaceted problem whose due argumentation demands space beyond our study.[28] For our purposes we will briefly explore the following: the view of the Christian tradition on divine (im)passibility, recent problems with the doctrine, arguments against impassibility, arguments for it, and finally conclusions on (im)passibility as we move toward a theology of depression.[29]

THE CLASSICAL UNDERSTANDING OF DIVINE IMPASSIBILITY

The doctrines of divine impassibility and incarnate passibility through Christ's human nature have long been the normative stance of the vast majority of the church up until the past two centuries. A list of notable figures holding the traditional, or classical, view reads like a who's who in historical Christian theology: Justin Martyr, Clement I of Rome, Ignatius, Aristides, Theophilus of Antioch, Athenagoras, Irenaeus, Clement of Alexandria, Tertullian, Novatian, Origen, Athanasius, the Cappadocian fathers, Augustine, Cyril of Alexandria, Leo the Great, Anselm, Aquinas, Calvin, and Arminius, among others.[30] The view of impassibility was also upheld in the Chalcedonian definition, the Fourth Lateran Council, the Thirty-Nine Articles of the Anglican Church, and the Westminster Confession, among other documents.

The Christian tradition has for the most part, until the past two centuries, affirmed that God is *apathes*; he does not experience suffering.[31] Traditionally, the issues surrounding divine impassibility are related to and often a consequent of the concepts of God's simplicity and immutability. There is an ontological difference between uncreated and created being. Contrary to created being, God does not have parts and does not change. The medieval Scholastic theologian Thomas Aquinas (1225–1274), who best exemplifies this position, grounds divine impassibility on immutability and ultimately divine simplicity. For Aquinas, drawing from Augustine, Anselm, and others in the tradition, divine simplicity[32] is foundational to all subsequent analysis of God's attributes.[33]

With created being, Aquinas, like Boethius, makes a distinction between "that a thing is" and "what a thing is"—*diversum est esse et id quod est*. Created being does not have existence in itself nor its essence in its existence, but its *actus essendi* (act of being) is caused by God, who actuates its potentiality, its essence. Contingent being does not have existence in itself nor contain the reason of its being in its essence. Contingent being does not essentially exist but exists by virtue of participating in *esse* (existence). And the various essences within contingent beings participate in their respective acts of existence. Participation limits and defines their respective acts of existence relative to their nature. For example, as a human individual, I am a contingent being. My existence is not necessary, meaning it does not have to be, nor is it self-caused or self-generating. My human nature in itself does not necessitate that I have to exist. There was a time when I was not, and there will be a time when I will not be. My being is contingent upon God's being, which is necessary. I do not possess aseity, meaning I cannot account for myself or exist in and of myself. But I am dependent on divine being, which alone accounts for and exists in itself. I am not self-generated, nor do I possess my own raison d'être, but God causes my existence.[34] In terms of my essence, who or what I am participates in *esse* (existence) and is in potentiality realized through the act of existing.[35] I am a being that must become what I am. As a being that "becomes," I am a composite of existence and essence and also potency and act. In order to become I move, as body and soul, from potency to act and experience change. I am mutable and, further, passible as I experience change through what I feel and suffer, as I am acted upon externally or act upon myself.

On the other hand, with God, there is no difference between God's *esse* (existence) and God's *essentia* (essence). God is *actus purus* without potential. He has no need to actualize his essence, nor is he in the process of becoming.[36] God's existence is God's essence.[37] Divine being is necessary and not contingent because God is subsistent being itself (*ipsum esse subsistens*). God is identical to his existence, nature, and his attributes. Thus, God is not partite and bound within the parameters of existence and essence, act and potency, substance and accidents, or form and matter compositions. Since God's existence is his essence, there is no real distinction within the divine nature.[38] God and God's nature are the same. Otherwise stated, God is God's nature, including the attributes or properties of that nature. God's identity and attributes are convertible with each other, and the divine attributes themselves are convertible with each other. The simplicity of the divine nature cannot allow for change in its essence. Hence, God is immutable.[39]

With an essence that is fully actualized, pure act, God does not become, and God does not become something that God is not. The divine nature is not an essence with potential, meaning that there is no potency to become and hence change. Containing no potency, the divine nature has no need to self-actualize but is pure act. Thus, for Aquinas "it is evident that it is impossible for God to be in any way changeable."[40] Divine simplicity grounds the attribute of immutability from which follows impassibility.[41] As existence in itself (*ipsum esse*) and pure act (*actus purus*), God has no potency, thus no motion to change. God cannot act in a way that brings change to the divine, nor can God be acted upon in a manner that would allow for change, such as suffering. In this manner, God is uniquely distinct from created being. Any attempts at anthropomorphizing, conflating the divine nature (monophysitism), or devising a univocal exchange between uncreated and created being, are a confusion of the ontological difference and a metaphysical and logical impossibility. God exists in God's self (*aseity*), but creation does not exist in itself. It participates in existence as an act of God. Also, as pure act of perfect love,[42] or love fully and completely actualized, God does not need to be awakened, informed, inspired, moved, or changed by human experience in order to love more completely, effectively, or salvifically.[43] Further, God cannot be impacted, like human persons, by evil, sin, or loss within the created, temporal order that occasions suffering, lest God be deprived of perfection, power, and goodness. Divine existence is neither contingent nor corporeal and is not subject to its conditions. As humans, we suffer because we are embodied and part of the created order and its predicaments.

As we have noted, the Christian tradition has acknowledged in the hypostasis, Jesus Christ, God takes on the human condition and all of its contingency, including suffering and death. He assumes our feeble state through his human nature, not his divine nature. Christ is also tempted in every point of sin as we are tempted but found sinless. When Scripture says prophetically that Christ is acquainted with grief and sorrow and learns obedience through suffering, it refers specifically to his human nature. Yet, suffering is ascribed to the person (hypostasis) of Jesus Christ. The person of Christ also holds the divine nature. Thus, these scriptural descriptors around passibility can further be ascribed to divinity—thus, God suffers. In this sense the impassible is passible. The transcendent God is said to suffer and even die in Christ, but through his humanity. God does not (and cannot) suffer in the divine nature on our behalf. In terms of suffering and empathy, what is needed is univocal and communicable by nature. God as an ontological outsider (an etic perspective) cannot grasp our weakness and frailty from an emic perspective as an insider. There is no univocal translation between the divine nature and the human nature to transmit human suffering. God can only truly suffer for us as one of us, not only because it is the only logical possibility as divine

being, but also because it is the solely true empathic way. Ontological dispar-
ity prevents true univocal empathy. In this way, God *knows* human suffering
by means of human suffering, that is, by suffering as a human. It is not for
divine need, of which God has none, that God became human, but for our
need to be forgiven and redeemed. God has no ontological lack because he is
distinct from the created order. There is no divine need to be de-divinized,
redeemed, or completed, as with Moltmann or with Jenson, by becoming
fully passible to actualize his destiny.[44]

Although the majority position regarding suffering has been divine
impassibility, there has been variation within that position and additionally
other recognized models. A common taxonomy is *strong* or *extreme impassi-*
bility, *weak* or *qualified impassibility*, *strong* or *extreme passibility*, and *weak* or
qualified passibility.[45] We can easily plot these on a continuum in our mind.
The qualified positions have been the majority positions, with qualified
impassibility dominating much of church history and qualified passibility
dominating the past two centuries. The development[46] of the doctrine in
terms of a qualified impassibility becomes the normative position from Irenaeus,[47] Tertullian,[48] Origen,[49] Gregory Thaumaturgus,[50] Lactantius,[51] Athanasius,[52] the Cappadocian fathers,[53] Augustine,[54] Cyril of Alexandria,[55] to Leo
the Great,[56] culminating with Chalcedon.[57]

Early patristic development of impassibility sought to preserve *apatheia*,
while maintaining the balance between the following: uncreated and created
being, transcendence and immanence, divine otherness and divine relations
with creation, divine dissimilarity and similarity of analogical language in
Scripture concerning (im)passibility, and divine impassibility and divine
passibility in the hypostasis through Christ's human nature.[58] The doctrine
eventually develops into the orthodox definition, in which the two natures
are distinct but joined together united in one subject (*unio hypostatica sive*
personalis). And the attributes of both natures are ascribed to the one person
Jesus Christ. Cyril of Alexandria describes the two natures in one person "not
as referring to two persons or two hypostases divided from one another and
completely diverging into distinct and separate spheres. For there is only one
Son, the Word who was made man for our sake. I would say that everything
refers to him, words and deeds, both those that befit deity, as well as those
which are human."[59]

In the one person are predicated the properties of the divine and the
human natures. The properties or attributes of the divine nature (the Logos)
can be ascribed to the one person Jesus Christ. And the properties of the
human nature (of Christ) can be ascribed to the one person Jesus Christ. Leo
the Great (400–461 CE) in his *Tome to Flavian* asserts, "The union of the two

natures which meet together in Christ made no confusion of their properties in the union: but the properties of the two natures continue unimpaired and entire even in the union."[60] He continues:

> For as the God is not changed by compassion, so the man is not consumed by dignity. For each nature in union with, the other performs the actions which are proper to it. The Word those which are proper to the Word, the flesh those which are proper to the flesh. The one is resplendent with miracles, the other succumbs to injuries. And as the Word recedes not from equality with the Father's glory, so the flesh parts not with the nature of our race. For (and it must be said again and again), one and the same person is truly the Son of God, and truly the Son of man.[61]

Further, the two natures are not merged in monophysitism but are united in the hypostasis, where the *communicatio idiomatum* actually occurs. However, the communication of attribution does not directly exchange properties between natures. We can predicate suffering and death to the divine. Yes, "One of the Trinity was crucified."[62] God does indeed suffer, but it occurs through the human nature of Jesus Christ. Yet, ultimately the divine nature is impassible, Cyril of Alexandria noted, because God is (*asomaton*) without a body, incorporeal.[63] God can only suffer as human in the person of Christ through the human nature.

MODERN PERSPECTIVES ON (IM)PASSIBILITY

The Chalcedonian position had been normative for fourteen centuries following its declaration, as exemplified by prominent figures such as Anselm, Aquinas, Calvin, Arminius, and others (with the notable exception of Martin Luther).[64] However, over the past two centuries, following on the work of Hegel and then the nineteenth-century kenoticist movement within Lutheranism, there has been a transition from the metaphysical concern of impassibility to the more existential considerations of human travesty that impact theodicy. The developments led to the modern theological responses of passibilism.[65] Two world wars, the unspeakable horrors of the Shoah,[66] and other mindless attempts at genocide[67] have caused the masses and even scholars to question God. Does God have any empathy for our plight? Does he feel the pain we feel from these horrendous happenings? Many modern theologians retorted that a God who could not or would not suffer and even die with us could not love and would not be worthy of worship.[68]

The passibilist empathic argument is summarized by German Reformed theologian Jürgen Moltmann (1926–) in *The Crucified God*: "A God who cannot suffer is poorer than any man. For a God who is incapable of suffering is a being who cannot be involved. Suffering and injustice do not affect him. And because he is so completely insensitive, he cannot be affected or shaken by anything. He cannot weep, for he has no tears. But the one who cannot suffer cannot love either. So he is also a loveless being. Aristotle's God cannot love."[69]

Moltmann's attack is leveled against Plato and Aristotle and their influence on the Western tradition of Christian theism. Moltmann's argument and the arguments of many of the other proponents of the passibilist argument depend on the so-called Hellenization hypothesis of Adolf Harnack and others. The claim is that patristic and medieval constructs of God slavishly and uncritically borrowed from Greek philosophy, especially Plato and Aristotle.[70]

Moltmann's vision of the "crucified God" is representative of the modern perspective. Moltmann radically responded to the problem of evil and Chalcedonian impassibility with a demanding apologetic of *theopatheia* (the passible or suffering God). Moltmann relates a story that comes from Elie Wiesel, a Holocaust survivor as a youth from Auschwitz and Buchenwald. The words of Wiesel echo and fuel Moltmann's drastic reaction to an indifferent God. In his book *Night*, Wiesel recounts:

> The SS hanged two Jewish men and a youth in front of the whole camp. The men died quickly, but the death throes of the youth lasted for half an hour. "Where is God? Where is he?" someone asked behind me. As the youth still hung in torment in the noose after a long time, I heard the man call again, "Where is God now?" And I heard a voice in myself answer: "Where is he? He is here. He is hanging there on the gallows."[71]

For Moltmann and others who embrace divine pathos,[72] the suffering of God is the only appropriate Christian response to the modern atrocities of human suffering. He retrieves Luther's theology of the cross as the hub of his theology, and the crucifixion of God is the touchstone. In Moltmann's Trinitarian *theologia crucis*, the true nature of God as love is revealed and known through the event of his death on the cross. The crucified God stands over against traditional Christian theism and a retreat to the theodicy of atheism.[73] God demonstrates and vindicates his love by taking on the human condition in all of its excruciating suffering, even death. He experiences death's anguish and separation down to the core of the triune relations of the persons. Moltmann proclaims, "The content of the doctrine of the Trinity is the real cross of Christ himself. The form of the crucified Christ is the Trinity."[74] The Trinity, as the history of God, subsumes and overcomes the history of our godforsakenness.[75] The dereliction at the cross results in the Fatherlessness of the

Son and the Sonlessness of the Father, the ultimate surrendering and giving of love.[76] The Son of God is given up and rejected by the Father and dies, and the Father eternally grieves his loss, while the love of the Spirit overcomes the forsakenness of humankind.[77] The cross diffracts and fragments the Trinity.

From the classical position, there are many points to contend with Moltmann. The most severe blows must be dealt to his demand for the death of God in order to justify God in the eyes of suffering humanity and to redeem humanity as well. God is seemingly required to prove himself worthy of his position of divine Lord and Savior by assuming (through the Son) in his own divine nature our broken human condition. In this case, the purpose of the incarnation is not unilateral toward creation, which is to become human to save humanity. The incarnation is needed for creation *and* God. For Moltmann, the incarnation is divinely self-directed and self-developmental. God needs to become human to justify and save himself. The Son must experience our pain, shame, and death in his divine nature in order to justify his divinity. However, contra Moltmann, an incarnation that is divinely directed, involving death to the divine nature, nullifies its intent and goal, which is to justify and deify human nature rather than to "complete" the divine nature. In this case, if the divine nature overwhelms and suppresses the human nature within the person of Christ in order to fulfill the purpose of the atonement, not only is the incarnation null, void, and unnecessary, but also the whole notion of divine mediation likewise is nullified. There becomes no need for an intercessor between sinful humanity and a holy God. Further, taking on the hypostasis and corporeality in order to suffer becomes instrumental to God's self-centered use of the human condition. The incarnation becomes a means to God's own end. And humanity becomes a means to God's own end. A divinely effected incarnation seems wrongheaded, as human suffering becomes a means to actualize and justify God's own divinity, hardly a loving, sacrificial act.

The plot thickens. Further, the Son undergoes rejection from the Father, while the Father experiences grief and loss over the death of the Son—a "God against God" scenario, as Bruce Marshall puts it.[78] Marshall also rightfully finds it problematic that Moltmann allows death to bear on the structure of God's own being through the divine nature.[79] The entire drama occurs within the divine nature, separating and alienating the divine persons, and thus dismantling and reconfiguring the eternal Trinity. The abandonment and separation occurring between Father and Son disrupt and separate the persons to the point they dissolve the intra-triune relations and annihilate the Trinity, which is clearly problematic. Not only does the Father's rejection of the eternal Son separate the second and third persons and dismantle the

Trinity, but the divine nature takes over the hypostasis in Monophysitism. The cross as an event in which the Trinity is reconstituted in history now becomes a type of theopanism,[80] or an inverted or immanent cosmic deification through God's kenosis in the world process. Moltmann, and others who claim that divine impassibility is a slavish borrowing from Greek paganism, has exceeded that claim with his own anthropomorphic echo of Greek mythological tragedy in this scenario of theocide.

Moltmann is also adamant that this event of divine and human justification through the revelation of God's kenotic love is exclusively revealed at the cross. The cross becomes a God- and Savior-making event, over against the classical view of divine being in three persons as an eternal immutable reality. I concur with Moltmann that "the inner criterion of whether or not Christian theology is *Christian* lies in the crucified Christ."[81] I concur that the "Christian faith stands and falls with the knowledge of the crucified Christ, that is, with the knowledge of God *in* the crucified Christ . . . the 'crucified God.'"[82] The trajectory of salvation history indeed reaches its pinnacle with the apex of love and redemption at the cross where the fullness and mystery of the ages in Christ is revealed. Contrarily, Moltmann extends the impact of the cross beyond its traditional soteriological function to inflated epistemological proportions. Over against any prior analogical, preparatory revelation of God in creation, true knowledge of God is restricted to the revelation of the cross. The cross becomes the limit and sum of the revelation of God, an epistemologically totalizing notion.[83] Even further, for Moltmann, the economy of the cross alone must strictly define the doctrine of the Trinity.[84] Moltmann, appropriating Luther, puts it this way: "Christ the crucified alone is 'man's true theology and knowledge of God.'"[85] Thus, all that God was and is and is to come must be revealed in the cross event. Unfortunately, the result of collapsing and exhausting the immanent Trinity in the economic is a historical, anthropological, and meontological reduction of the divine.[86]

With Moltmann's crucified God, the cross event must manifest a univocal correspondence between the divine nature and persons. The full limited, depraved, and judged human condition in all of its permutations must be assumed by the divine nature in order to justify both God as Savior and humanity as saved. In order to assume the full and total experience of human depravity and suffering ("all the depths and abysses of human history" which become God's history),[87] Moltmann is hypothetically requiring the divine to partake of every combination of transgression and demonization known to human experience, which seems inconceivable and a theological impossibility. Such an undertaking becomes a prerequisite for the identity of the second person of the Trinity in Moltmann's scheme. If such an enterprise is the preposterous condition of justification for God and humanity, then we are abandoned to a reductio ad absurdum of infinite proportions.[88] Bruce Marshall reminds us that the church fathers realized that the identity of the divine persons is necessary and cannot depend on anything temporal or contingent.[89]

There are several problems here to enumerate. Dominican theologian Gilles Emery echoes our concerns and asserts additional ones. He cites erroneous dialectical tensions in the divine, the "historicization of God," the epistemological primacy of the cross, radical kenotic redemption, "infernal torments inflicted upon Christ," a "functional interpretation of trinitarian language," and an eradication of the persons of the Trinity as gravely troubling when considering passibility.[90] Needless to say, there is an irreconcilable christological conflict between the classical view and the contemporary view of divine impassibility. Moltmann's view has been one of the more espoused and influential perspectives on the subject.

We also find varying analyses and arguments as well from Barth (voluntary divine passibility),[91] Balthasar (Trinitarian superkenosis, kenosis of the Son and descent into hell),[92] and Jenson[93] (divine actualization in the world process), among others. These proposals incorporate arguments from the Hellenization of early Christianity,[94] an argument from divine pathos in scriptural language,[95] and/or some version of theodicy[96] that further features one or more of the following strategies: (1) divine actualization to overcome evil, (2) divine empathy as therapeutic or salvific, (3) divine suffering authenticating love, or (4) divine self-punishment absorbing human evil and damnation used to exonerate God and bring salvation to humanity.[97] We have examined and initially responded to all four arguments.

CONCLUSIONS ON (IM)PASSIBILITY

In this work, I have not argued specifically against any of the theodicy strategies listed above, except divine becoming. In fact, I affirm the core meaning that they seek to convey. The intent is the Logos empathizing, suffering, substituting for, and overcoming our sin and death for our salvation. God's unchanging love, which by definition is a self-sacrificing *donum*, is causal to the salvific mission carried out through the incarnation. However, I am making the claim of *theopatheia* within a Chalcedonian hermeneutic that understands that the incarnation assumes all pathos that has been mentioned above in the person of Christ. However, the herculean undertaking is through his human nature, as univocally necessary—God as human for humanity. Human suffering can only be truly understood when one suffers as a human.[98] Ultimately, neither nature, divine nor human, in itself suffered, since natures do not suffer but permit the person to act or suffer.[99] Persons act, not natures.

The person of Jesus Christ suffered for us without the need for the divine nature to become human nature or for the divine nature to suffer. The ontological difference in terms of nature cannot be overcome. The divine nature cannot be transformed into the human nature with either nature remaining. The difference is only met in Christ the mediator through the two-nature and one-person hypostasis.[100] However, we are reminded that impassible does not mean dispassionate, inert, or indifferent.[101] Weinandy makes the argument for an impassible God who is not only able to suffer for us as a human but experiences a wide range of passion. This God is not inactive and static but in full action according to intra-trinitarian relations within the perfection of divine attributes, including God's unconditional love.[102] Human suffering can only receive experiential empathy from like human suffering, not from an etic or foreign nature, specifically since suffering is ultimately registered somatically.[103] The invisible God does not have a body. On the other hand, the type of love needed to embrace and overcome the scope of sin, brokenness, and suffering in this world needs to be superior in every sense to that which is empirically available in this world. Such a love must transcend the outermost limits of human love, empathy, and pathos. Love must be conditionally unaffected or moved by evil. Since God's divine love is pure act, it is unconditional or without conditions and is unalterable and immutable, unlike conditional human love, and meets that need. God's compassion is a function of God's love, untouched by sin, evil, or the love of concupiscence.[104] The incarnation meets both criteria in love and suffering. In this sense, God in Christ loves divinely by suffering humanly. As Rob Lister states it, "God remains the conqueror and not the victim of sin and evil."[105]

Lister, who holds to an impassibility in which God is "voluntarily impassioned," makes it clear that "God's love is a characteristic of divine stability. It is this ontology of perfectly pitched intra-Trinitarian love, as opposed to metaphysical dispassion/disinterest, that is the basis of God's intrinsic invulnerability to involuntary affective manipulation."[106] Another intriguing voluntarist proposal that allows for a qualified passible impassibility comes from Anastasia Scrutton. She retrieves the subtle distinction made by Augustine and Aquinas between passions (*passiones*) and affections (*affectiones*). The two are conflated in modern thinking but distinct in ancient and medieval understanding. Her reading of the two theologians qualifies "passions" as involuntary, unreasonable, and part of the sensitive (sensory) appetite, while "affections" are voluntary and rational and part of the intellectual appetite.[107] Thus, emotion is essential to God's wisdom and providence and can be predicated of the divine as a rational property, similarly to current cognitive theories. Hence, one can predicate affection of God, such as love, joy, and righteous wrath, stemming from the rational and volitional properties of the divine intellectual appetite.

Even with Scrutton's distinction, which would locate affections in the divine intellect, such pathos could not involve a contradiction with the other operations of the divine attributes or a change in the divine nature. God's pathos is a pure complete act of eternal perfect love, operating in tandem, integration, and unity with the other divine properties, notably God's sovereign and providential wisdom, which manifests the *oikonomia* of God. The love of God is the pure, perfect light of the divine nature that passes through the intra-trinitarian relations. In passing, it refracts in creation and in the human heart, expressing all of the colors of the Spirit's fruits of joy, peace, and goodness.[108] Similarly, God's just wrath is perfectly tempered, rightly ordered, analogically[109] and anthropomorphically revealed in Scripture, and perfectly accommodated to finite and limited creation. His wrath is fitting with his love to work salvation in all things. The wide range of time-bound and circumstance-limited natural human emotions, not consequential to sin, that spring from the capacity of the *imago* ultimately reflect the divine nature. Our emotions were crafted and intended from the divine exemplar and analogue, the eternal perfect and holy love of God. Yet divine love is perfect love. It knows none of the fluctuation, waning, weakening, abating, conditionality, and other imperfections and failings of created corporeal being. Lister reemphasizes, "This intra-Trinitarian love is perfectly willed; it never wanes, and it never needs to be bolstered from without."[110] Thus, God's perfect love revealed through Christ our Mediator and Reconciler is the divine antidote to the cruel contingency of melancholia, which we have identified as a relational disorder. In Christ, we find relational redemption as our advocate, healer, and friend in each state of melancholia: natural, consequential, and purgative.

GOD AND DEPRESSION

We have addressed much concerning kenosis and divine (im)passibility, although we have not exhausted the topic. Many questions remain unanswered in this study, since they are outside of our scope and intent. We undertook the study of divine passibility to ascertain whether God can suffer depression. In the person of Jesus Christ, we can answer that question in the affirmative. Christ our Mediator took on our mental disorders that we might find peace and salvation in his name. We are reminded from chapter 4 that depression is a relational disorder. God became relationally one with humanity to redeem our relationship with him from creation to fall to new creation. Further, we can conclude that in terms of our three relational states, the divine nature cannot be transformed into created being; it cannot become sinful; it cannot grow in holiness. Only through the human nature can God suffer and relate to mental disorder and depression. Our ultimate concern in addressing divine suffering is to ascertain whether God in Christ addresses, empathizes, experiences, or even heals depression or mental disorder. Does God heal the depressed? When considering the three types of depression and their relational states, we can affirm that Christ addresses, empathizes, experiences, and even heals or overcomes suffering through resurrection, eschatologically now and not yet. Our fellowship in his suffering yields participation in his resurrection and a new creation. He participates in our suffering that we may participate in his victory, eschatologically realized.

Taking on a full human nature, the Logos assumes the ontological difference of created being and faces all of the challenges and vicissitudes of the flesh, including existential anxiety. The angst that emerges from the dilemma within freedom (Kierkegaard) and within temptation (Balthasar) is before Christ at all points. We see this highlighted in the desert and in the garden of Gethsemane. Although he steps into the vertigo of infinite possibility but maintains faith on every occasion, he nonetheless comes face to face with agony, dread, and even depression. At Gethsemane and Golgotha, he faces his own dark night of the soul (type 3) when confronted with the cup of bitter sorrow. His human will, like ours, would prefer to avoid the agony of death that lies ahead. Yet he does not choose self-preservation, as we would, but denies himself, accepts the will of the Father, and fulfills the *missio* as a true Son. Although Christ is without sin and does not directly experience the second type of depression from the consequence of depravity, he does become a sin offering. He bears the burden and consequence of our temptation and sin, including depression. He faces depression as our representative, and, as a result of the temptation, he faces it in his own humanity.

From Gethsemane to the dereliction at Golgotha as Christ faces the crushing weight of the sin of the world on his soul, he despondently cries out, "My soul is overwhelmed with sorrow to the point of death" (Mark 14:34, NIV), and later, "My God my God why have you forsaken me?" (Mark 15:34, NIV). He who learned holy obedience as a suffering servant was baptized in our grief, sorrow, and depression, taking the sins of the world as the sacrificial Lamb of God. Christ faces not only natural creaturely angst but also the anguish that results from taking on our sin and agony. Our maladies are his that by his wounds we may be healed, ἰάομαι, a word often used in the New Testament for physical and spiritual healing. What the first Adam, as representative, and his progeny have done to the race through sin, the last Adam has undone at the cross. As our divine mediator and vicarious substitute, he freely assumes the conditions of melancholia and absorbs them in his sacrifice. From the brutal cross of disfigurement, he returns to dust to reclaim us from the fiery depths unto resurrection, a transfiguration. The resurrection is the source and *telos* of our healing (*soteria*) as we begin on the trajectory of realization that we are wholly a new creation, spirit, soul, and body.

Yet, for us as participants in the new creation, there is a tension. Our full realization of a new creation is now and not yet. We have the earnest of our inheritance through the sanctifying love of the Spirit. His indwelling presence is a deposit on the kingdom as well as an assurance of what is to come. In this sense healing is not synonymous with curing, until death finally dies in the second death (Rev. 20:14). We are not promised that we will escape suffering for our faith. Yet the Spirit comforts us through it. The servant is not greater than the Master. We each have a cross of sacrifice to carry daily. By that cross, we partake of his sufferings and draw from the healing power of his resurrection. We participate in Christ. Likewise, he identifies with us in all relational states, including our various melancholias. We will explore in the next chapter how he is our advocate, healer, and friend.

9

Toward a Trinitarian Theology of Depression

ON THEOLOGY, SALVATION, AND CRITICAL
DISABILITY STUDIES

In the preface I referenced how religion, and specifically Christianity, in "ministering to" persons with disabilities, including mental disorders, has often failed to "do no harm." We have often misspoken on behalf of God, and worse, been guilty of malpractice through both ignorance and sins of omission and commission. Far too many people with disabilities and their families have been victims of negative and painful experiences from the religious community. Gaventa comments, "Both the medical and social models were and remain leery of religious and spiritual interpretations of disability, in large part, I believe because of the experience of judgment and exclusion that many people with disabilities and their families faced in their churches, synagogues, and mosques and other places in which the religious attitude about cause and treatment impacted cultural beliefs and traditions."[1] Nonetheless, Gaventa also goes on to mention "the growing research into the connections between spirituality and health in the past fifty years" and the positive impact that spirituality and its institutions and practices have had on the arenas of disability and mental disorders.[2] Though often the last institution of society to do so, the church is attempting to redeem itself in its ministry with persons with disabilities and disorders.

Yet, in spite of self-corrective measures, religion is still condemned by some in disability studies for what they deem to be structural problems that are entrenched in the very nature of religion and at the root of what religions like Christianity attempt to do, which is to proclaim and minister salvation. Christianity, by its very evangelistic nature, can easily be construed as ableist and oppressive. Fiona Kumari Campbell, a leading critical disability studies scholar, fervently contends, "A chief feature of an ableist viewpoint is a belief that impairment (irrespective of 'type') is inherently negative and should the opportunity present itself, be ameliorated, cured or indeed eliminated. What remain unspeakable are readings of the disabled body presenting life with impairment as an animating, affirmative modality of subjectivity. Instead of ontological embrace, the processes of ableism like those of racism induce an internalisation which devalues disablement."[3] In critical disability studies there is a suspicion against all attempts at amelioration, curing, or removing a disability or disorder. Such attempts imply that we are claiming that one has a defect or is inherently defective, which reifies and strengthens the regime of ablenormativity. As mentioned above, owing to much harm and malpractice inside and outside of religion, such suspicion, to some degree, has been warranted.

Christianity and our theological work at present are proclaiming healing, restoration, and salvation in Christ and may be construed as oppressive or reinforcing ableism. Although the church, using all ethically sound means available, is called to be an advocate and work for justice alongside persons with disabilities, the salvation the church offers in Christ can include these but categorically also transcends any medical or social "ameliorating, curing, or eliminating" of a disability or disorder. The Christian faith has traditionally declared that we are all made in the image of God, and that image is good. Scripture and Christian tradition also recognize that we all have fallen short of God's and our own best expectations. Yet even a broken humanity and world are not inherently defective and are still considered good by God and redeemable. The universal and leveling nature of our weakness and sinfulness does not divide humanity up into binaries of ability and disability, especially morally speaking. We are all human and exist in the analogical interval between created and uncreated being. Further, we have all made choices that have separated us from God and are in need of restoration. The salvation that is needed is not prescriptible by or in any human terms but is initiated and fulfilled by God alone. Christ did not come to ameliorate a fixable or mendable condition. Something of a more radical order is required. His mission was to birth an entirely new creation—a new heaven and a new earth. In all of our differences and relative abilities that are affirmed by God, we all, regardless, must be born again because of sin. God's death on our behalf is an indictment against and hardly a capitulation to the cult of normativity or the pathologies of ableism/nondisablement.

The new creation is as subversive to the binaries and regimes of our power constructs as any radical critical theory can get. Paul declares, "All have sinned and fallen short of the glory of God." But because of God's saving grace, "there is no longer Jew or Gentile, slave or free, male or female. For you are all one in Christ Jesus" (Gal. 3:28, NLT). Paul does not literally mean that these distinctions no longer exist. They existed in the apostle's day when he penned these letters. A literal reading is not warranted here. These distinctions were not dissolved, though clearly the transformation of the gospel initiated redemptive trajectories that were injected into society with its proclamation and expectation to leaven the lump of society over space and time. In these texts, Paul is highlighting our solidarity of unrighteousness in Adam and the solidarity of our righteousness in Christ. Surely there are poignant differences in our semiotic constructed realities, but there is unity in our common human need for the love of God. We are all disabled by sin and death, which are the sole limits and boundaries established in the call for salvation. We are all disabled before death, which is not to minimize the problem of ableism or the plight of those with disabilities. Clearly, we realize that our spiritual "disability" or adverse, "disabling" circumstances like unemployment, poverty, or divorce are not the same as (physical, intellectual, psychiatric) disabilities. Simply, sin and death set the theological limit and boundary for our common need for salvation and not human ability or disability. Hence, our theological anthropology is not based on ableist amelioration but on deification as a work of the Spirit of God alone. This designation of moral disability in no way removes, dilutes, or replaces the need to work justice with those who experience disability and disorder. Such work is the consequence of our redemption. Healing and salvation were normative for the ministry of Christ and the disciples in the Gospels and are for the church today. Our claim is that melancholia can be a redemptive experience.

Even critical disability and crip[4] theorist Robert McRuer recognized, in a qualified sense, our universal disability and the impossibility of attaining ableist normativity when he claimed that "everyone is virtually disabled, both in the sense that able-bodied norms are 'intrinsically impossible to embody' fully and in the sense that able-bodied status is always temporary, disability being the one identity category that all people will embody if they live long enough."[5] The entropy of death works on us all. Researcher Nitsan Almog also cites the same McRuer statement to summarize her study of university students with and without visual impairments. The study examined academic pursuits and social barriers from the students' perspective. At the end of the study, the students and the researcher concluded "that the boundaries between disability and able-bodiness are extremely fragile."[6] The impossibility of the pure category of ableist normativity allows for us all to be located on a broader register of disability. Likewise, in terms of righteousness, sin, and death, Christian theology is making a similar case that none are righteous, and all are in need of redeeming love.

While some critical disability theories rigidly condemn any attempts to ameliorate or heal and interpret such gestures as power plays to strengthen existing ableness normativity and marginalizing of persons with disabilities, theologically, we do not want to perpetuate or be an accomplice to oppression in any form. Contrarily, we have contended that the healing and restoration offered in Christ does not, or at least should not, foster ableness normativity or marginalization in any form. In response to certain critical disability positions, as we move forward with our theological task, it is imperative to assert that any theory that denies our need for and access to God's redemptive love, restoration, and wholeness in Christ is incompatible with Christian teaching. In this regard, this work is unapologetically and confidently Christian and theological and yet humbly seeks redemption from our theological misspeaking or malpractice. We hope to accomplish that task through a humane and theological view of humanity and a balanced and nuanced concept of healing.

DEPRESSION AND THEOLOGICAL MEANING-MAKING

Depression can heavily shroud every facet of one's life—physical, mental, emotional, spiritual, relational, and other aspects. Often despondency comes in the form of multidimensional loss. One feels loss of self (e.g., identity, memory, ability, bodily coordination, energy, faith) and connection with others, the world, and God. As one's sense of self dissipates, everything seems to dissipate, and nothing holds together. Reality under depression becomes meaningless, purposeless, directionless. One doubts one's self and faculties as well as others, the world, reality, and even God. One feels helpless, worthless, hopeless, and abandoned to one's own gradual erasure, an existential slippage into an imploding and suffocating vortex of nothingness without escape.

Viktor Frankl, a Holocaust survivor and psychoanalyst, found that the will to pursue and make meaning in life, or Logos crafting,[7] is key to overcoming the lethal conditions bred by mental disorders and other trauma from war or imprisonment.[8] Frankl cites the vital human need for a logos, or a will to meaning, to counter the entropic pull of despair and to discover wholeness and peace in life. Meaning and purpose in life, for Frankl, become the metaphysical ground, gravity, stasis, raison d'être, *telos*, and overall logos for existence. The theological case we are making here is that the "logos" that ultimately fulfills these existential categories in their highest sense is the Logos made flesh, Jesus Christ.

The divine Logos, Emmanuel (God with us), is eternal meaning freely communicated to persons in depression. When nothing seems to hold together, God can provide that elusive meaning needed for the journey. In what seems to be a furnace of affliction, depression can be transformed by God into a crucible that forges new life and new meaning out of the ashes of anguish.[9] Melancholia can be a liminal, transcendent experience, an affective rite of passage that creates new meaning and order out of chaos, a Holy Saturday bringing resurrection from death. Such liminality may serve as a matrix to incubate an innovative vision of a new world, a new logos of creation out of chaos. Melancholia at its constructive best can function as a crucible where creativity excavates, inchoate, raw form from the bowels of chaos and disorder. Within the cocoon of depression, the will to live crafts and forges a reconfigured inner geometry for meaning making, a new shape of interpretive framework. This freshly minted hermeneutic has its own grammar and logic that articulates a new language to sing a new song. The melody interprets and gives meaning to the old reality and births the new, a metaphorical intimation of the eschaton. The place and power of transcendence in human experience, problem solving, growth, and evolution are vital to our perseverance.

With depression, persons need that metaphysical center or transcendent ground to uphold what seems to be a fading or dissolving reality. Persons feel unable to hold their self, their world, and their faith together. The malady feels like a toxic substance coursing rampantly through every crevice of their life, eroding every semblance of meaning, order, function, ability, relationship, and faith. The power of a theological response to depression is that God loves us even when we cannot love or feel love. God moves toward us when we feel inert. God upholds us, our world, and our faith, when we no longer have the strength to get out of bed in the morning. He carries us when we cannot walk. He is strong when we are weak and incapable. He sees us when we do not see him. And God is already restoring when we believe that all things are lost and cannot be recovered. Christ, our advocate, is the stasis and metaphysical anchor for persons with melancholia, so that they can moor their self, their world, and their faith to him when all seems to be spiraling out of control and vanishing. The theological response to depression begins with the *missio Dei*. Long before we seek God, the Almighty is already seeking us.

God's love finds us when we cannot find ourselves. The mission of God in the lives of those with depression is to reveal the meaning of the knowledge and love of God in Christ by his Spirit. The revelation of God with us (Christ) and in us (the Holy Spirit) generates a new creation; a new ground that upholds the unbearable weight and anxiety of being; a new center that holds our mental and cosmic world together with the gravity of his mercy and love; a new meaning, purpose, and way (*hodos*) of wisdom forged out of the aimlessness of angst and the disorder of despondency; a new stasis of his eternal presence that negates abandonment and presents the gifts of affirmation, approval, and acceptance to the self-disqualified and self-condemned; the gift of new life freely given not based on human knowledge, morality, or power but on God's grace and goodness; and a revelation of a new identity in the image of God in Christ etched indelibly on the mind that transcends depression's deception of perception that portrays God as absent and inaccessible. God in Christ by the Spirit is fully present in melancholia.

MISSIO TRINITATIS AND DEPRESSION

In this chapter we will build on chapter 4, critically interpreting the three theological types in terms of the missions of the Son and the Holy Spirit. We will focus specifically on the incarnation, including the atonement, and the sanctifying grace of the Spirit. How does Christ identify with the three relational states of the image of God, and how is that identification instrumental through the Spirit in carrying out our salvation, precisely in terms of addressing psychiatric disabilities? In the earlier chapters we established that there is a connection between the ontology of depression and philosophical anthropology. As a result, prior to identifying a theology of mental disorder, we recognized the significance of investigating theological anthropology in search of a lead into melancholia. Affirming but deconstructing and decentering traditional loci of theological anthropology such as rationality and ability on the humane grounds of demarginalization, we looked to the relational dimension of the image of God. If the image of God is relational and anthropology impacts ontology of depression, then melancholia and a divine response must be relational in some respect. We critically examined three relational states within human experience: creation, fall, and new creation. We also correlated these three states to the relational nature of depression and three theological types: natural, consequential, and purgative melancholia. In our critical analysis of these traditional theories on depression, some aspects of the theories were dismissed on philosophical, theological, or pastoral grounds. Other components of the theories that withstood scrutiny were maintained. One conclusion was that depression is relational as much as it is cognitive and/or somatic.

The *imago Dei*, traditionally defined by rationality and functionality, was examined relationally in terms of Jesus Christ the Son of God as the true *imago*. In this respect, the image of God in Christ is economically seen as relational with the goal of divine *familitas* (daughter/sonship). Further, when we think theologically of the image of God and relationship, we revert to its trinitarian grounding. Let us briefly review the classical understanding of Trinity and mission and their bearing on the relational image of God in humanity. The divine processions are intricately connected to the divine missions. We know that the economic *missio* is a modality of the immanent *processio*, and the processions result in the intra-trinitarian relations within the divine essence. These subsistent relations constitute the persons of the Trinity. Hence, distinction and plurality within the one divine essence are defined relationally. The eternal begetting of the Son (filiation) and the spiration of the Spirit (passive spiration) from the eternal origin of the Father (paternity) define the persons from relations of opposition. Corresponding to the relations are the processions (generation) of the Word (as the knowledge, wisdom, or image of God by intellection) and the Spirit (as the love of God by the will). The *processio ad intra* (in the divine essence) is causal and definitive of the *missio ad extra* within the *oikonomia*. The sending of the Son and the Spirit is the economic expression of the eternal processions. The Father sends the Son and the Spirit in mission to the world. Mission originates from the Father and is carried out through the Son and the Spirit, a *missio Trinitatis*. The two divine missions are the *visible*, temporal, economic sending of the Son in the incarnation for salvation and the *visible*, temporal, economic sending of the Spirit at Pentecost. The two *invisible* missions of the Son and the Spirit are their ongoing work in the life of the church and in the heart of the Christian.

In summation, the processions point to relations within the Trinity that constitute the persons, Word and Spirit. These processions of wisdom (Word) and love (Spirit) are revealed economically by God creating *adam* in his image. As the processions give rise to trinitarian relations *ad intra*, analogically, distinct yet similar, wisdom and love give rise and order to the relational nature of the image of God in us. The relational image of the Trinity is imprinted not only psychologically within us (intellection and will) but also socially and theologically as we relate to God, our origin, in whom we live and move and have our being. We exist through participation in God's existence (*analogia attributionis*). Our existence and personhood depend entirely on our relationship to our Creator. Our dependent I-Thou relationship with God is the foundation and context for the rational-volitional attributes that contribute to agency. Our relation with God, not our personhood, was marred by sin and the consequences of the fall, impacting all things, including our mental health. Christ took on human form to restore the image of God in us by restoring the relationship between God and humanity.

Through the mediation of the incarnation culminating with the atonement, Christ invites us in baptism to become daughters and sons of God, born again in his image in righteousness and true holiness (*theosis*). The Word became human to restore our relationship with the Father. In assuming our human condition, Christ also assumes our disabilities and our suffering as his own. It is not that he eradicates disability and suffering in this age. In becoming one with humanity, he identifies with the entirety of the human predicament. We are not alone. God is with us! Through the atonement offered by Christ and the work of the indwelling Spirit, God walks with us on a journey of healing and inspires new meaning regarding our melancholia. Along with other trials and tribulations in this life, the weight of melancholia is given to Christ as we learn to trust. In trusting, we come to learn what healing really signifies in a personal way. Melancholia itself is not a felicity or blessing, and neither is it a prerequisite for a blessing. Yet melancholia in the light of redemption and restoration is not a sentence handed out or a disqualifier of blessing. Mental disorders are not relegated to an exceptional place outside of salvation, untouched, as socially stigmatic emotional leprosy but, as part of the human condition, assumed and touched by salvation in Christ.

Christ assuming all of our humanity is to deify all of our humanity. The invisible missions of the Son and Spirit minister the *via salutis* to all willing persons through the sanctifying grace of God. We are all called to participate in the new life in Christ, which is a journey of healing. The Eastern church has long understood sanctifying grace as healing (*therapeia*) and restoring (*soteria*) the sin-sick soul. Our current human condition, including mental disorder, is in need of salvation, and we are qualifying salvation in terms of healing or *therapeia* of the *imago*. The missional work of the Spirit restores health and *shalom*, which is *soteria*. We are highlighting the connection between salvation as healing with the *telos* of the incarnation, *theosis*. True healing is to become like God. True health is Christlikeness.

The missions of the Word and the Spirit are woven in the interrelation of a Logos Christology, a Spirit Christology, a Christocentric pneumatology, and a charismatic ecclesiology at work in the missional *oikonomia*. The missions of the Word and the Spirit knit the entire integrity of the distinct persons and work together in a fully orbed, robust Christology that is Logos grounded (Logos Christology) and Spirit empowered (Spirit Christology). Likewise, the person and work of the Spirit witness and work based on the person and work of the Son (John 14–16), according to the *taxis* of the economy (a Christocentric pneumatology). The Word became flesh by the Spirit and was anointed with the Spirit for ministry.

Christ conceived and empowered by the Spirit in his incarnate life and ministry exemplifies a Spirit-filled life and ministry for the charismatic body of Christ, who, in turn, is baptized in the Spirit by Christ (Matt. 3:11-12).

Similarly, the missions shape our ecclesiology, as we are born of the Word (John 1:12-13) and the Spirit (John 3) and baptized by the Spirit into the one body, a charismatic community (1 Cor. 12:13).[10] Further, we are sanctified (John 17:17; 1 Pet. 1:2) and empowered (1 Pet. 2:2; Acts 1:8) by the Word and the Spirit with the Spirit witnessing and working based on the salvation offered in Christ, a Christocentric pneumatology (John 14–16). The Spirit, sent by the Father through the Son to us at Pentecost, constitutes, sanctifies, and empowers the church by baptism in Christ—in full identity with his death, burial, and resurrection. Because of the consubstantiality and economic functional unity between the Son and the Spirit, the person and work of the Spirit bear witness to the person and work of the Son, who carries out the will of the Father (John 14–16; Rom. 8).[11] As Vladimir Lossky declares, the Holy Spirit is "the image of the Son."[12] Only through the Spirit can we discern and receive the Son of God and the image of the Father that he bears.[13]

Thus, the work of redemption accomplished by Christ through his life and ministry, culminating in the atonement, is realized and executed by the Spirit in our hearts. Though these common divine roles, attributes, and features are ascribed as personal properties of the Son or the Spirit through appropriation, they are from the one nature and will of God at work in the world. In acknowledging the consubstantiality and conjunctive missions of the Son and the Spirit in this work, we reaffirm *opera Trinitatis ad extra indivisa sun*, the external works of the Trinity are undivided, working one divine will.

In asserting the triune mission of God, this work above all affirms that God is present in the lives of those who face depression. However, the challenge is that the symptomology and conditions that persons with depression face can mask the truth and prevent them from knowing that God is with them. Data collected from a study of those who experience depression report the following oppressive existential states: life as meaninglessness, global doubt, feelings of abandonment, failure of relationships, depleted energy or exhaustion, and a sense of being trapped or suffocated in life.[14] In that study, John Swinton notes that depression is a holistic experience, including a spiritual experience. Every aspect of the person is affected.[15] The hypothesis in his work is that spirituality, which has been a neglected approach, is a potential resource that can positively address the adverse conditions revealed in the study and offer hope, meaning, and purpose.[16] Our work supports this study and further contends that Christian Trinitarian theology speaks to these and other realties experienced by persons with depression.

In this chapter we will demonstrate how the missions of the Son and the Spirit mediate healing and salvation in the three relational states and their corresponding theological types of mental disorders. The triune mission of God speaks to our melancholia through (*empathic*) *advocacy*, *healing*, and *friendship*, as Christ and the Spirit take on these roles. Experiencing the journey of salvation is a transformation in the image of God that carries an eschatological tension of healed, healing, and will be healed. In this life healing is not always curative, though it can be. Healing is more often an eschatological trajectory of integrative restoration (*therapeia*) through which we learn to accept God's presence and peace and receive the daily renewing power of the Spirit regardless of circumstance. Healing occurs in the individual but also in the church. For the church, the Spirit's advocacy offers an example of what it looks like to be in ministry with the weak. The Spirit not only empowers persons with disabilities but also empowers the church by convicting its prejudice and oppression and redeeming it to work for and defend the rights of all people.

TYPE 1—NATURAL MELANCHOLIA: WORD AND SPIRIT AS MEDIATOR AND ADVOCATE

Maximus the Confessor affirms, "There exists such a relationship of polarity between God and man, that the incarnation of God and the deification of man condition each other mutually."[17] Through the person of Christ, divinity is mediated to humanity, and humanity is mediated to divinity. God becomes human, so humanity can become like God. He participates in our humanity that we may participate in his divinity (*metousia theou*). Jesus Christ our mediator reveals the face of divinity for the world to behold. He also bears the visage of true humanity. Christ is the presence of God, Emmanuel (God with us), and the presence, example, and advocate of true humanity. Not only does God show us what the divine looks like, but the divine shows us what it means to be truly human. In the cosmic descent of the universe's King to creaturely dependence, the High Priest from heaven condescends to feeble contingency to exemplify the covenant faithfulness of a Son through the wisdom of perfect love. In becoming truly human, he embraces our every weakness and gives "courage to be" in the face of anxiety. And in becoming truly human through Christ, we become truly divine.

The divine becomes truly human to clarify our vision. We are able to see that we are made to be truly human and what that fully involves. We observe the holy in daily life, obeying Torah (God's teaching), walking in the way of God by the Spirit, and loving neighbor and stranger. Christ clothed in the weakness of humanity becomes fully dependent on the Spirit of God, living the life of an obedient Son. In utter dependence, the divine nature clearly shines through the tinted glass of humanity. We are able to see the holy and be transformed in his image. Divinity has provided space for difference and hosts otherness (human nature) in the person of Jesus Christ, showing us the hospitality of God in the incarnation. "The Word made strange," as Milbank puts it,[18] in this case is made strange by uniting with an alien humanity. He joins with the stranger of otherness to fill the margins of creation to its center with the infinite dimensions of his boundless love (Eph. 3:18-19; Heb. 7:25).

When we embrace the weakness and limitation of not only our own humanity but also the humanity of the stranger (the other), then we learn to become human in all of its frailty, ready to host in our hearts the weakness of the other in all of their difference. In becoming truly human, we embrace the stranger and create space for our experience of depression and for theirs. In becoming truly human, we move toward becoming truly divine. We are transformed by Christ when we embrace the least of these, in whom Christ is hidden. In his weakness and brokenness, he uncovers our true nature, as it is before God. In terms of created being and existential melancholia (type 1), Christ takes on contingency and limitation. Christ, the suffering servant, has hidden his identity in the extreme margins of society and is clothed in the skin of the poor, the naked, the hungry, the sick, the prisoner, and the stranger (Matt. 25:31-46). Our love is measured by our love for the despised who disguise his presence. Our ontological poverty is made clear in Christ. The ontological difference is concretized through the hypostatic union in the person of Christ, what Balthasar calls the "concrete *analogia entis* itself."[19] The incarnation embodies that difference, which embraces all differences. Further, we are invited to be one with him to fulfill our humanity.

In the divine becoming fully human, God assumed our weakness in the disfigurement of the cross to reconcile and restore a broken people to God. Christ taking on cruciformity is God bearing the extremities of our temporal condition, taking on the feeble dust from which we came, as symbolized in Ash Wednesday—"Remember that you are dust, and to dust you shall return." Further, he dies, executed as a criminal, though innocent, and returns to dust in death on our behalf on Good Friday and in burial on Holy Saturday. The Paschal Triduum culminates with the Word taking on frail human form and being made sin for us. He dies our death for us, yet we are united with him. In the sacrament of baptism, we allow not only our disorder and brokenness but also our hubris and self-righteousness to join him in disfigurement on the cross that he may transfigure us in resurrection. The blood of the cross blots out our transgressions. We are made right in God's sight, adopted as sons and daughters and restored in his image. We are baptized into his fullness and made partakers of the divine nature through fellowship in his humanity. We learn (μανθάνω, manthano *to learn*, is the verbal form of μαθητής, mathētēs, *disciple*) to be human and thus divine, the process of discipleship. As μαθηταὶ, *mathētai* (disciples), we learn to fulfill our humanity through obedience, becoming like Christ, the exemplar, particularly in cruciformity. The shape of the cross captures human limitation, difference, depravity, disability, and disorder in all of its facets. God crucified in Christ is a conforming to our human form in all of its shapes. Through a theology of the cross, we learn who we really are. Like the apostle Paul pierced with an obstructing thorn (2 Cor. 12–13), we learn weakness in our melancholia, which leads to dependence on God and others. Unshackled from the Edenic lie of human autonomy, we find true life in God. We learn our human identity in Christ through life's vicissitudes, which illuminate and make us aware of our finitude and dependence. We learn from disability and disorder what it means to be human. As opposed to being objects of ministry, we become learners and teachers, humbly embracing limitations and abilities and finding sufficiency and even perfection in the grace of God.

Being truly human is not a liability but our deification. When we, by the Spirit, identify our limitation, our healing and sanctification begin. *Theosis* is our *therapeia*, or healing. In this life, cure sometimes occurs, but healing is always available. Healing is an eschatological trajectory that originates, points toward, and culminates in the resurrection, which is the redemption of all things, including our minds and bodies (Rom. 8:23). As we depend on the work of the Spirit, we experience the healing of sanctification, even symptomatically at times in our hearts, minds, and bodies, through the *shalom* of God, which provides and even surpasses the meaning making needed to cope and overcome (Phil. 4:1-9).

In realizing the kingdom's manifestations, the church can easily fall into an overrealized eschatology and even a false triumphalism that expects the alleviation of all suffering and the cure of all sickness. The healing that comes in salvation is not triumphalistic, though it can involve alleviation of symptoms and measurable progress toward wholeness. More so, healing within the dissonance of depression can also be marked by acceptance of a new emerging reality, the unyielding presence of the Spirit, who desires to bring new meaning and hope for the journey. In too many cases, those struggling with mental disorders, including depression, commit suicide. This is the harsh reality. Suicide is always a possibility lurking in the shadows for persons with mental disorders. The church needs to be educated on the risk of mental health symptoms and the possibility, the warning signs, ideation, and the various plans connected with the danger of suicide. On the other hand, the church should not address the symptoms of mental disorders hopelessly as if the good news of Christ does not offer God's presence and comfort and at times relief from such symptoms, especially when coupled with proper medical treatment. Contrarily, we all know persons who in spite of treatment and/or prayer have not been healed.

Why some experience healing as alleviation or relief of symptoms more than others may be related to many variables, known and unknown, the greatest being the mystery of God's providence. So much is unknown when considering these aspects of mental disorders. We are often left silent or in lament as we consider the mystery of suffering in our world. Nonetheless, whether in silence or voiced, God speaks to melancholia.

FACING THE ANXIETY OF FREEDOM AND TEMPTATION

As we analyze the natural or existential type of depression in light of the *missio*,[20] we are led to the front side of the cross, which is Christ's death and the road of freedom and temptation leading up to it. In the existential type of disorder, the possibility of melancholia is seen as structural to the human condition, attending freedom and temptation. Kierkegaard identified the anxiety that emerges from the dilemma of freedom. Tillich recognized the anxiety that emerges from the meontological threat that is rooted in our ontological difference. Balthasar identified that same anxiety as stemming from the space of temptation that God allows to test us. Evolutionary psychology looks at the developmental nature of the biological order and the logical possibility and adaptive benefits of melancholia. With type 1, depression can occur naturally, adaptively, or due to a probationary world.

Some things simply occur naturally in an incurably human world. They are structural. The second installment of the popular Matrix film trilogy, *The Matrix Reloaded*, reveals many of the enigmas of *The Matrix*, the first installment in the series.[21] The Matrix is a computer-generated world produced by machines to keep humans in blissful ignorance of the truth that they are being held in captivity by the machines. Their human energy is being harnessed and used as batteries to power the machine world and perpetuate machine control. The problem with this system is that the Architect of the Matrix, also a computer program, failed in its attempt to create a suitable world for humanity. The Architect's failure was that it created a perfect machine world and not a flawed human world. Imperfect humans could not adapt to a perfect machine world. The program created by the Architect was not sufficiently fallibly human. The Matrix world excluded necessary variables and factors that make our anthropomorphic world possible—namely, choice and love. In order to create a world that humanity would accept and thus allow the machines to maintain control, the Architect acquiesced and created an imperfect version of the Matrix program that accommodated human choice, love, uncertainty, and other variables. The problem with this imperfect Matrix is that owing to a mathematical anomaly it would inevitably generate a savior (the One, Neo) and a people who would choose to escape the Matrix, create their own city, and follow the One in rebellion against the machines. In an incurably human world of choice, choosing between the "red pill" and the "blue pill" in the Matrix engenders a seismic anxiety prior to, during, and following our existential choices. The Architect and humanity are forced to face the entire permutation of consequences that emerge naturally with the reality of freedom of choice. Similarly, in our world, we face such consequences of freedom, as the existentialists would have it. Even the divine, by choice, is not exempt. God willingly works with us in our world. In other words, in order to accommodate creaturely freedom, imperfection, and development, certain natural consequences are inevitable, including the possibility of evil, adversity, suffering, and even depression. From an evolutionary perspective, many of these same categories occur naturally in the order of things, to facilitate adaptation and survival.

When the Logos willingly became a contingent, created being, he was born into the entirety of these conditions. He assumed the states that allow for anxiety and depression to surface—the *nihil* of contingency, freedom to choose, temptation, and natural environmental conditions. Jesus was not exempt from these conditions, and neither are we. He faced them depending on his heavenly Father in the power of the Spirit, most notably in his temptation, resistance, and victory in the desert. He walks as a man in the Spirit, and as a man, he knows his identity. He is the Son of God and is aware of the mission related to his Sonship. He boldly faces Tillich's *nihil* of human contingency with the courage to be who the Father declares him to be at his baptism, the beloved Son. Yet the Father allows Christ the space of temptation with its attending anxiety and melancholia in the wilderness, as Balthasar had noted. Nonetheless, when persistently tempted as to his identify, he does not waver. The Son doggedly holds fast to his relationship with the Father when his identity is tempted. He knows that the Father is well pleased with him, and his favor stems from his relationship with the Father as opposed to something earned by his ministry performance—preaching, teaching, or healing—or by overcoming temptation when provoked in the desert. As a human person, Christ's "being" preceded his "doing," and his "doing" was derived from his "being." He did not become the Son of God through what he achieved. He eternally is the Son of God. The paralysis of performance and the despondency of failure are met in Christ's realization of relationship and identity. In Christ, our relationship with God trumps ability and performance and thus welcomes our weakness.

The empowerment of unconditional love and acceptance that comes from a relationship with the Father enabled Christ, the man, to face Kierkegaard's dizzying dilemma of freedom and temptation. Owning all of our susceptibility and weakness, Christ fronts our existential nascent type of mental disruption while remaining faithful to the Father by the Spirit. He is not spared its challenge or sting but is immersed in the depths of barrenness with nothing to depend on but the Word that proceeds from the mouth of God. Christ, in his high priestly role, serves as mediator, inspiration, and example: "Since he himself has gone through suffering and temptation, he is able to help us when we are being tempted" (Heb. 2:18). He does not shrink from death or into the fear of nonbeing, though he faces and tastes both. Christ's awareness and grounding of his identity and mission in the eternal Father communicated through the Word not only allow him to confront the haunting void of existence, freedom, and evil with fortitude and hope but also empower us to participate in the same courage to be.

With depression, people experience loss—loss of meaning, purpose, identity, faith, their sense of God, and connection with self and others. Christ stands firmly as human, as us, in the face of anxiety and loss. God is with us, grounding our existence with eternal courage through Christ. During depression, persons feel mentally and physically paralyzed. They question their purpose and worth in the midst of existential inertia. Self-disqualification spreads internally like wildfire. Yet God in Christ acts on our behalf unconditionally. As mediator, Christ breaks through the solipsism and abyss of depression, enabling access to the vital transcendence that restores meaning, purpose, identity. The personhood of disabled individuals and disability itself is affirmed, accepted, and incorporated into a saving relationship in Christ as a free gift rather than earned by performance. God's free grace and saving action toward us in our helplessness are evident in the sacraments of baptism and the Eucharist, in which divine agency ministers salvation to us when we are unable to save ourselves. Sacramental grace moves first in our life when we cannot. God is the agent of salvation. Liberation begins with the church understanding God's radical free grace for all. We frequently create the prejudices and barriers that keep persons from coming to God. We put up a hedge of moral, social, and ecclesial disqualifiers that prevent persons from fully participating in the blessing of God and the full life of the church. We are challenged to accept freely whom God has freely accepted and remove the obstacles that disable us from salvation and be like the friends who took off the roof of limitation (architectural and social) that prevented their paralytic friend from coming into the presence of Christ. And even when persons with disability cannot come to God, or there are no friends to make a way, God relentlessly comes to them.

We are reminded of the peculiar narrative from the Hebrew Bible of Mephibosheth, the grandson of King Saul.[22] The stirring account from 2 Samuel, in one reading, can be understood as a poignant illustration of how God relates to persons with disabilities. The story can also be a model for the church to follow today. When Mephibosheth was five years old, his father, Jonathan, and his grandfather, King Saul, died in battle. The nurse, in a panic, grabbed the child and hastily fled to save him. Most likely the nurse dropped the baby, leaving him a paraplegic. Later, when David became king, he sought out any living members from the house of Saul. He pursued Mephibosheth. David had made a covenant with Jonathan to show loving-kindness to his family forever (1 Sam. 18:3; 20:14-15, 42; 24:20-21). David wanted to offer Mephibosheth the *chesed* (loving-kindness and favor) of God that he had shown Jonathan. Once he found Mephibosheth, King David became the friend and servant (2 Sam. 9:6) of Mephibosheth and restored his name, honor, favor, estate, and inheritance and took him into his own palace. When Mephibosheth met King David, he referred to himself as a "dead dog" (2 Sam. 9:8). He viewed himself as an anonymity, an outcast without a name, without a people, and without an inheritance owing to his condition and being a family member of a former king. In some traditions, persons with disabilities were often viewed as cursed. Further, family members and the courts of former kings were often executed. They were seen as a potential threat. Perhaps Mephibosheth anticipated that the king found him in order to kill him. He was surely more than surprised at how the king welcomed him in his palace.

David, remembering the covenant he made with Jonathan, instead viewed himself as the servant of Mephibosheth, who in fact was a prince. He used his power to restore much that belonged to Mephibosheth as a person. More, he did not allow his king's status to separate him from Mephibosheth and his marginal status. Rather, he became his friend, fellowshipped with him, and shared regular meals, an intimate demonstration of closeness between friends. Scripture claims in 2 Samuel 9:13, "Mephibosheth lived in Jerusalem, because he always ate at the king's table." He lived in the holy, royal city in the king's palace and ate at the king's table, receiving the highest treatment. Later in the story, in return, Mephibosheth would show his faithfulness to David when his throne was threatened by Absalom. The story and history ultimately honor Mephibosheth by referring to him numerous times first by name[23] and only twice referencing to his disability as an aside. He was a person first. Secondarily, he had a disability, but it did not impede him from receiving God's loving-kindness, favor, and inheritance.

King David embodies God's *chesed* toward persons with disabilities and toward outcasts. The king zealously sought out Mephibosheth, when he could not seek out the king. God's grace and love are not based on our ability. When he found Mephibosheth, he restored his dignity by blessing him with what belonged to him by birth, his inheritance. God in Christ longs to restore our relationship with him and the blessings that follow. Mephibosheth was a grandchild of the king. Likewise, all persons with disabilities are children of the King. God freely bestows his inheritance of love, favor, and salvation upon them. This *chesed* is not based on our goodness or ability but on the covenant that God extends to us all. David restored Mephibosheth holistically in every aspect of his being, beginning with his wounded identity and outcast status. The acts of King David are not only representative of those of God but are also a model for the church to follow. We are exhorted to extend the unconditional favor and loving-kindness of God to persons with disabilities and restore their name, honor, and inheritance. Inheritance refers to all of the grace, promises, and blessings that pertain to the covenant that God offers to all in Christ, our mediator and advocate.

MEDIATOR AND ADVOCATE

Christ as high priest stands between God and humanity to mediate God's eternal covenant. As mediator, he stands as us and for us, but he also stands with us. He is our advocate. Immersed in the floods of life, we may fear drowning in the consuming vortex of our own *nihil*. As the funeral liturgy expresses, "In the midst of life we are in death." Yet Christ has overcome death, and we participate through baptism in his life-giving death. In the unity of the person of Christ, his humanity is forever united with divinity and with our frail humanity. Likewise, our humanity, immersed in Christ, is mysteriously moored through adoption to his unshakeable divine being. His divine essence is a *hyperousia*, which is transcendent, ever dissimilar, and impassible to the act of being and nonbeing. In him, we overcome in life and in death. The prophet prescribes, "Trust in the Lord always, for the Lord God is the eternal Rock" (Isa. 26:4). The immutability and immovability of divine being overcome, on our behalf, the haunting angst-ridden reverberations that echo from the analogical chasm of our nothingness, which threaten to swallow us into nonexistence.

Susceptibility and temptation, which are inherent to our frame of sentient dust, will not subside or terminate in this life, and neither will the conditions or possibility of suffering related to melancholia. Any combination of medication, counseling, prayer for divine healing, or spontaneous remission may or may not fully, partially, or temporarily relieve depression symptoms. The existential condition for melancholia does not subside in this life or because one is a praying, practicing Christian.[24] Christ takes on our existential somatic condition to be with us; no docetic appearance here. Passibility and freedom are what make us human. These conditions are integral to our becoming and will remain with us. Christ does not take away our humanity, but as our example, he reinforces it and embodies the true definition of it. Christ is true humanity as us, for us, and with us, even when circumstances do not change.

In Christ, the true image of God in flesh, we behold the finitude, frailty, and finality that are ours. However, human weakness need not fear the freedom (Kierkegaard) or temptation (Balthasar) that confronts and yet strangely invites a response of faith from us. Likewise, fear, with the shadow of death before us, does not have to be final or consuming, because he understands as us, for us, and with us what it means to be "exceedingly sorrowful even unto death." He assumed what is hyperhuman,[25] even its final form of death; "for only as a human being could he die, and only by dying could he break the power of the Devil, who had the power of death. Only in this way could he deliver those who have lived all their lives as slaves to fear of dying" (Heb. 2:14-15). In his death he swallows both death and the phobia and anxiety of death (sickness unto death), from which all anxieties spring forth.

As our mediator, Jesus Christ is high priest, self-offered sacrifice, and example of humanity divinely charged and baptized in the Spirit. He understands as us, and on our behalf, as he chose to abide in the will of God in the midst of pressing opposition and suffering. He also understands as us and for us to die and yet live. As the high priest of our testimony, Christ knows what it means to be alienated from God and others and rejected as a sociopolitical outcast, a victim of systemic injustice, a capital offender, a faithful servant, a suffering sacrifice, and a sorrow- and grief-stricken soul condemned to death. The Lord has laid on him the iniquity of us all (Isa. 53:6). His crucified form is the *Gestalt* of human weakness, injustice, heinousness, and aborted hope on display before the entire universe as a mirror to behold (*ecce homo*), the disabled God.[26] He assumes the suffering of the victim and the sin of the victimizer in his tortured flesh. Stripped, beaten, and humiliated, prophetically he embodies and exposes the disfigurement and grotesquery of our masquerading civility and justice. Yet also as our sacrifice[27] his stigmata not only reflect but share in our stigma and shame, even those associated with melancholia. Depression or any mental ailment is not excluded from the cross. Christ makes space and ministers solace for mental disorder.[28] He is crucified at the place of the skull, Golgotha, with a crown of thorns piercing his own skull, reeling with excruciating pain and mental anguish; "for our transgressions, he was crushed for our iniquities; the punishment that brought us peace was on him." His wounds become wells of healing from which we draw empathy and compassion and find peace: "By his wounds we are healed" (Isa. 53:5).

In identifying with our weakness, he gives strength to the powerless (Isa. 40:29). Depression's symptomatic triad of hopelessness, worthlessness, and helplessness is met and embraced by Christ's ministry of presence (Emmanuel) and by the sending and the indwelling of "another Paraclete" (Comforter, Counselor, Helper). The balm of "God with us" works through the third person of the Trinity, as "God in us," ἄλλον Παράκλητον (*allon Parakleton*—another Comforter—John 14–16). In this case, *allon*, unlike *heteros*, which is another of a different kind, indicates another of the same kind. The Spirit, who dwells within us, ministers the same comfort and counsel as Christ did to the disciples. The Spirit, who is consubstantial with the Son, is sent to reveal and bear witness to the Son, who is sent to reveal and bear witness to the Father. The unbearable void of loneliness is met with the immovable, impassible, eternal presence of God in us through his Spirit. The sanctifying medicine of the indwelling Helper is a balm of *shalom* to those whose minds are ridden with anxiety and depression. As an intercessor of comfort, the Spirit prays through us with suprarational groaning from the abyss of our despondency that transcends speech (Rom. 8:26) and reason (Isa. 26:2; Phil. 4:7). In the silence of our weakness, the Spirit our Advocate groans within us intercession that transcends language (Rom. 8:26).

The Spirit seeks to guard us against every ruminating wind of despair with his peace, a stilling power that silences all powers. As the Spirit of adoption (Rom. 8:15, 23), the Advocate redeems us from alienation and a state of desolation, making us God's children, no longer estranged from our Father and from others. The desolation and dissonance of loneliness so kin to depression are greeted by the Spirit of Life resident within the deepest recesses of our own spirit, Christ within us the hope of glory (Col. 1:27). The alienation, estrangement, and existential dissonance of depression are encountered by the presence of God. In God's seeming absence, he is advocating on our behalf and assures us he will never leave us or forsake us for all eternity. The Comforter, the presence of God in us, is the assurance and promise of hope that we will press on and along the trajectory of healing ahead through the depressive valley of the shadow of death and receive the fullness of our inheritance as children, which is dwelling in the house of God forever (Ps. 23; Eph. 1:14).

These words of exhortation and comfort from Scripture are promised to us in Christ. Yet they can be easily read as triumphalism, romanticism, denial, or even exclusivism. Although God's promises are "yes and amen" or affirmed, the fact is that many who suffer with mental disorder do not find relief, and the option of suicide always lurks in the shadows of desperation. Under such circumstances, suicide can seem like the best logical option, as jumping out of a burning building would seem like a better option than burning to death. Mental disorder can acutely alter our consciousness to the point where it creates a warping divide between what is real and what we perceive through the distorted filter of depression. Melancholia has a detaching effect, creating an alienating rift that separates our depressed worldview from other explanatory narratives arrived at by common sense, psychology, or theology. The disorder erects an impenetrable wall between one's imploding personal perception and the agreed-upon external world on the other side. Depression can shroud us in haunting absence, the absence of reality, meaning, friends, and even a perceived absence of the divine, leaving us silent. At times it seems like the only pastoral response is the ministry of nonanxious presence wrapped in the lament of mourning silence, a fitting apophatic response to the mystery of suffering and the divine, as we partake of seasons of grief together.

TYPE 2—CONSEQUENTIAL MELANCHOLIA: WORD AND SPIRIT AS MEDIATOR AND HEALER

Immediately following World War II, much of America experienced unprecedented prosperity. A weary but jubilant people were zealous to rebuild the nation for a hopeful and peaceful future. Two nuclear bombs were reluctantly dropped on Japan, leading to a swift end to the war. The fascist menace was defeated, the threat gone. Post–World War II offered great promise, touted as a golden age by some. But the gilding around our trophied society, under closer inspection, was a thinly veneered pop panacea that covered our underlying angst and inequity. The precarious house of cards we built in the 1950s would collapse. Its suppressed fears and tensions would soon shake the foundations. Fear of nuclear annihilation, the ensuing Cold War, the failure of the American Dream for all people, specifically African Americans, civil unrest, and the Vietnam War shattered the blind and feeble pursuit of a "father knows best" society.

The 1960s became an experimental and tumultuous period of protest, systemic violence, civil disobedience, conflict between the generations, and the dawning of a new Aquarian Age of turn on, tune in, and drop out.[29] Young people were charged to discover the Shambala of their choosing and pursue it by any means. Experimental drug use, free forms of sex, and exotic methods of expanding consciousness were some of the "far-out," "groovy" paths one could indulge on this magic carpet ride. Noble intentions. But the unbridled hedonism of the flower power generation ended with a bang at the conclusion of the 1960s. The Manson cult murders, the Altamont disaster, and the ongoing Vietnam War brought a violent closure to a tumultuous era that collapsed under a flimsy idyllic mantra of "peace and love."

The self-styled gurus of the flower power generation prescribed drug use and other perilous expressions of freedom in order to heal a generation lost in space, children wounded from the sins of their fathers. History is clear that the choices and sins of the fathers are compounded through consequences in subsequent generations. The excesses of the 1960s revealed the shortcomings, secrets, and sins of the suppressed 1950s. What was hidden or forbidden was now hip. No hang-ups. But the flower children would pay a grave price for eating Eden's fruit. A restless generation of teenagers heeded Leary's hypnotic message to "turn on." Syd Barrett (1946–2006) was one of many. The wunderkind lead guitarist and singer of Pink Floyd (in its early psychedelic phase) was a lyrical and instrumental genius, showing infinite promise.

Through use and abuse of LSD, Syd Barrett became no longer functional as a musical performer or as a person.[30] A casualty of mental disorder meets experimental drugs, Syd was seized by debilitating depression and mood swings and haunted by hallucinations and catatonia. It is debated whether Barrett had prior conditions of depression or schizophrenia before his life of addiction. Nevertheless, both conditions were evident during and after his drug use.[31] Barrett was forced by the other members to leave Pink Floyd. He would live the remainder of his life in seclusion, struggling with his demons. Some narratives claimed he found a short-lived reprieve in painting and gardening. He died of pancreatic cancer in 2006. Some of Pink Floyd's subsequent work, especially their best-selling album *The Dark Side of the Moon*, dealt openly and artistically with the issue of mental health and was a tribute to Barrett's struggle.[32] Why did such a tragedy befall this promising young man? Along with the mystery of evil working in this world that we cannot fully understand, I propose the ancient belief in a fallen world. A fallen world precipitates fallen choices and devastating consequences both direct and indirect and intentional and unintentional. The structural and generational sin of the fifties, the hedonism of the sixties, and Barrett's decision to pursue escape through harmful substances—all contributed to his ailing mental health. Sin impacts everyone. No one is left unscathed, and no one is innocent.

We noted in chapter 6 a second theological type of mental disorder that originates as a consequence of a fallen world. The consequential type asserts that mental disorders are the direct or indirect result of sin or sin's collateral damage. A self-constructed world and order apart from God results in cosmic chaos, a paradise lost. The ascetic monk Evagrius sought to diagnose and remedy the ailment. Acedia is the problem. Spiritual warfare is the solution. The desert father identified mental idleness instigated by supernatural demonic beings as one of the deadly sins, clearly linking sin and acedia. The way forward is to combat sinful thoughts with the truth of God's word.

Balthasar strictly correlates anxiety with one's relational status with God. He likewise views mental disorder as a consequence of sin. The case is not always so facile. There are detractors who make a challenging case against the univocal causation and totalizing indictment that mental disorder stems from sin.[33] We have also critically examined this simplistic diagnosis, identifying the complexity and problems with it. All have sinned. Yet only some have mental health issues. Why is God's judgment selective for the sin of some and not others? Is God's judgment just in such cases? Simply, Scripture does not make a clear univocal causal connection between sin and sickness, mental or physical. We have not excluded the possibility of correlating sin with sickness, since there are isolated instances in holy writ. There is a lack of consistency, though, to establish a rule or principle. On this point, Scripture and science are in agreement. Ultimate etiology is not clear according to the conclusions of the medical model of depression.

What we have crafted are three theological hypotheses from the data offered by select theologians and practitioners within the Christian tradition and our critical response. In this chapter, as opposed to offering an etiology, we are proposing a triune mission of healing and salvation as a response to the three theological types. How does Christ our Mediator and Savior address mental disorders, whether they are consequential or collateral to the fall? In this regard, we are making an unpopular assumption that the traditional view of humanity has fallen is accurate. This study will not go further into that controversy because of limited space. Our work assumes humanity has broken its relationship with God through disobedience. However, it does not signify that sin is necessarily causal to sickness.

We acknowledge the nexus between theological anthropology and ontology of depression. The relational image of God needs to be restored in order to heal the condition of humanity. Christ comes to forgive, justify, and sanctify us of our sin and restore us to right relationship with God and others as sons and daughters. Salvation restores relationships. Further, *theosis* is the full restoration of the relational *imago Dei* and a recapitulation of the plan of God. Restoring the image involves the transformation and wholeness of creation following the fall through a new creation. A cosmic transfiguration is God's vision for the healing and restoration of all things, a new heaven and a new earth (Eph. 1:10), *theosis* as healing.

As we think about healing and restoration, let us examine form. Forms (e.g., medicine) heal and need to be healed (e.g., bodies). We bifurcate and categorize our forms or constructs of normativity in terms of ability and disability, order and disorder. Ableism within mental health becomes our construct of normativity, our secular salvation. We establish our standards and measures of acceptance, our notions of right and wrong, good and bad, true and false, and able and disabled. Some of our constructed forms heal and others hurt. Yet God can use medicine or laws, for example. They are solutions offered from below, which is not necessarily to disqualify some of them from God's use. But there is also a response from above.[34] Christ, as the divine image, is the form that is lifted up before us as normative. And his form is the goal of our recovery, rehabilitation, and recapitulation. Though there are differences and distinctions to our forms, God universally restores all in Christ. Salvation approaches us equally. Regardless of our forms, abled and disabled or disordered and ordered, we need redemption. No one is innocent. No one is whole. We cannot fall into some simplistic totalizing indictment of any person(s) or group(s). This group is always right (the elect), and that group is always wrong (the demonized). This does not mean that we are not accountable for our wrongs and need not amend them. As our culture becomes more particularized and its narratives more diversified and specialized, we tend to draw boundaries, exclude, blame, and judge. Regardless of our unique location and experience, Christ is the form and measure of God's salvation offered to all.

We err not only in polarizing, but also in our fixing of the other. We presume that the other can be merely fixed, and that we can fix them. Our existing forms do not need to be modified or simply corrected of minor glitches here and there. Nor are we called to fix them. God does not even intend to "fix" us. In a fallen world, nothing will suffice but an entirely new creation. The whole of our semiotics and the systems we construct by them need to be completely renewed in the light of the transcendental signifier (Christ), as Balthasar put it. In light of the Christ form, we are all disfigured. Our violence, oppression, hate, and self-centered life have warped our image. Restoration as healing invites the world to be resignified in the light of his form—death, burial, and resurrection.

Christ becomes our eschatological sign language. He is God's sign to us that communicates healing and wholeness. He is God's Word that clarifies the divine image to our understanding. Through his language of divine holy love, Christ came to recreate our semiotic systems in line with his kingdom and heal our world. The holy love of God in Christ resignifies not only our theological forms and meanings but our sociopolitical forms as well. The kingdom of God reveals a new order of righteousness, peace, and joy. We are all called to turn from our self-centered lives and follow Christ who is the embodiment of the kingdom. The kingdom of God subverts the order of this cosmos, by judging it in his disfigured flesh. Christ identifies with our disfigured cosmos through his own cruciformity. At the cross, he takes on our disfigurement in order to transfigure it. He assumes our form to reconfigure and transfigure our (personal and social) forms in his righteous image by the empowering work of the Spirit. The *therapeia* of the Spirit restores and reshapes our world in alignment with God's kingdom, an order that empowers rather than marginalizes the weak.

Eastern Christianity has long recognized therapeutic and medicinal categories for both sin (soul sickness) and salvation (holistic healing).[35] Healing as a ministry has also been emphasized beyond Eastern Christianity in Holiness,[36] Pentecostal, and charismatic streams.[37] Even some sacramental traditions have embraced holistic[38] healing both in the Eucharist and in holy or extreme unction.[39] Although not a sacrament for Holiness, Pentecostal, and charismatic Christians, divine healing is both a doctrine and a practice or rite that includes the confession of sin, the anointing of the sick, the laying on of hands, and the prayer of faith (James 5:13-16). Healing, in the Holiness-Pentecostal-charismatic traditions, is virtually inseparable from salvation. It has also becoming more commonplace to see charismatics, like their sacramental sisters and brothers, claim holistic healing in the Eucharist.[40] These renewalist streams consider healing as normative because they see it as normative in the ministry of Jesus and the apostles. Renewalists view holistic healing, along with forgiveness, as part and parcel of the atonement (Matt. 8:17).[41] Healing becomes a benefit of salvation alongside forgiveness of sins and should be ministered regularly through anointing and prayer.

Perhaps divine healing is an instrumental component of salvation that we cannot afford to exclude from our theology. The affirmative position on divine healing in this book stands in a long line of Christian traditions that claim that God still heals spirit, soul, and body, as he did throughout the Scriptures. I have had this reality confirmed. In my own ministry over the past thirty-three years, I have witnessed countless persons healed by God of every type of ailment, from mental health issues, to cancer, to broken bones, broken marriages, to paralysis and a wide variety of other conditions.[42] Many of these cases involved family members, and so I walked through the healing process with them and can verify claims.[43] Although the medical field generally does not recognize God as a treatment or cure of an illness, there have been many medical studies and experiments recently that have sought to document the positive effects of prayer on the healing process.[44] Holistic healing needs to be taken seriously as an active component of salvation. The assumption of healing in this text does not reduce the act of healing to any one type, such as physical, spiritual, or mental. God is concerned for the whole person and cares for us holistically. Also, I do not support any healing strategy that seeks to control God by either telling God how to heal or when to heal. We cannot put God in our box or on own clock. The Lord can heal in any way and at any time from now to eternity. So, it is important to expect healing at any time and in any way, including immediately and entirely or gradually and partially and physically and/or spiritually.

HEALED: TO BE OR NOT TO BE

For so-called Spirit-filled churches and traditions, divine healing is a doctrine rooted in the finished work of Christ in the atonement and is available to all by faith.[45] However, at times, through lack of theological nuance, the doctrine can be proclaimed quite rigidly. "If you repent of all of your sins and have enough faith, only then you can be healed" comes close to Pelagianism. The onus of healing strictly depends on one's righteous living and faith. Thus, in these circles, when one is not healed, it is because they "lack faith," or they are in known, "unconfessed sin." Granted, unbelief or other unconfessed sin can separate one from God. In some instances in Scripture, though not uniformly, healing seems to be correlated to faith. "According to your faith be it unto you" is a phrase that occurs in pericopes from the synoptics. And in one reference (Mark 6:5), Christ worked only a few miracles in Nazareth because of their unbelief.

However, as we referenced earlier, the witness of Scripture is more polyphonic than monophonic regarding faith, righteousness, and healing. Sometimes the faithful suffer sickness as Job did, and the faithless are healed like the boy with the "mute spirit" (Mark 9:14-29). The story does not say the boy had faith. Rather, his father could only claim, "I believe; help my unbelief," and yet his son was delivered. There is a healing syllogism in these charismatic circles that goes something like this:

Premise 1: One of the benefits of the atonement is physical cure;
Premise 2: One accesses this benefit by faith;
Premise 3: One has faith;
Conclusion: Therefore, one is physically cured.

The argument is valid but not sound. If the premises are true, then that conclusion follows (valid argument). However, the premises are not always true, as in the second premise, which is reductive and not always the case (unsound argument). This line of reasoning goes counter to examples of faith healers who have died untimely deaths from sickness in spite of prayer and their faith. John Wimber (1934–1997) was such a case. Wimber was the founder and leader of the Vineyard movement and an influential teacher and practitioner of divine healing. Although he vehemently preached on divine healing, Wimber began to experience heart issues at the early age of forty-nine. He had a heart attack at fifty-one and was diagnosed with cancer eight years later. Two years following he had a stroke, and two years later triple bypass surgery. Sadly, he died that same year in 1997 at only sixty-three years of age. Wimber also struggled during that same time with depression.

The Vineyard founder is one of many examples of leaders who taught and practiced divine healing and yet died prematurely of illnesses in spite of prayer and faith. Faith does not always guarantee a specific healing or a cure. On a promising note, his health issues challenged his theology and faith, which led to a different type of healing. Wimber became more open to medical treatment and also to the fact that some do not receive the healing they request (in this sense a cure). He documents his struggle in *Living with Uncertainty: My Bout with Inoperable Cancer*. Wimber's story illustrates that healing comes from God as God sees fit. Even more problematic are groups (e.g., Christian Science or Jehovah's Witnesses) or individuals who have taught that doctors and modern medicine are contrary to God. They claim that if you seek medical care, then you are not demonstrating faith in God. In the healing revival following World War II, many faith healers like Jack Coe (1918–1956) and William Branham (1909–1965) preached against the use of doctors and modern medicine by Christians. Often parents influenced by such teaching fatally imposed their convictions on their own children and refused treatment. Many fatally refused it for themselves as well. It is not unusual for popular healing movements to see faith and science in diametric opposition.

The notion of healing proposed in this work is holistic and interdisciplinary. Medical science and faith are not always mutually exclusive. God's common, prevenient grace provides resources from his storehouse for all persons and through a variety of means. As the grace of God upon creation causes the sun to shine on the just and unjust, so also does the grace-filled created order of God allow for healing in creation through the internal healing mechanisms in our body, medical advancement, and the gifts of care in the health professions.[46] Healing can occur through supernatural, natural, and even artificial means, all under the providence of God. Too frequently popular theologies of healing are exclusive, reductive, and extreme. As a result, "nonsupernatural" means of healing are not attributed to the providence of God. And many are excluded from healing.

These extreme perspectives on healing are even more damaging to persons with disabilities and mental disorders. Often, they are made to feel culpable, guilty, and ashamed of their ailment, especially if they are not healed. The spiritual handicap we place on them is more crippling than the disability or disorder that they have learned to accept. Other persons who may be healed are held up as trophies and objects of our triumphant faith. Persons with disabilities and disorder become a means to our own ends. Whether healed or not healed, persons with disabilities or disorders are often objectified, minimalized, oppressed, and deflated of their humanity because of the spiritual disability of the church.[47]

Through work in theological anthropology, we learn that every individual is a person made in the image of God and in relationship with God and others. And all deserve love. Above all, we are persons not disqualified by our limitations, which we all have. The problem is not in our differences but in the way that we respond to our differences with injustice, oppression, and exploitation. Thus, healing, in this particular sense, is needed for the hermeneutically sick rather than those who experience mental disorders. Simply, a sound scriptural theology of divine healing is broad, integrative, balanced, and nuanced.

HEALING OR CURING: THE NUANCES OF HEALING

Prior to examining the nuances of healing, I want to identify a nuance within the notion of disease. As stated earlier, "illness," as opposed to "disease," indicates the subjective experience of disease, disability, and disorder, while "disease" designates the objective or biological correlate to the subjective experience. Many persons in these categories suffer needlessly because of externally inflicted restrictions and stigmas. These external factors contribute to the cultural impact of the illness on the individual. Various socially constructed "scarlet letters" inflict stigmas and devalue one's sense of personhood. Oppression often begins at the level of language. On the other hand, there are some who push back on social pressure and stigma. They find courage to embrace and redefine their physical or mental "limitation." As Amos Yong has claimed, many identify with their disability and even own it as their own abled construction of one's own self over against the identification, stigma, and objectification from society. In this sense, the powerless assume power over themselves by owning their narrative and overcome socially imposed shaming. Then there are others who have refused to identify with their disability and seek a cure. And still others are ambivalent.[48] Part of the mathetic process of healing is meaning making and constructing one's own self-narrative. Restoring the ability to define oneself and speak with one's own voice can bring healing to one's identity. It means learning a new language for a redeeming narrative. Liberation and healing are as much semiotic as somatic. And they are needed for the so-called abled as well as those who have disabilities.

Returning to our conversation on abusive teaching regarding healing, it is important to note that most of the faith healers or practitioners of divine healing today no longer hold to such extreme views that restrict medical treatment. For the most part, they have become more open to medical science and integrative approaches to healing. Many, just like John Wimber, have come to realize that God the healer is sovereign and chooses to define and work healing when and how he sees fit. Unbelief and sin may be an impediment at times, but God also can work in spite of us. God can work healing with or without faith and prayer. Further, divine healing may or may not involve cure of the ailment or suspension of the symptoms. This implies that illness and healing may not always be mutually exclusive. One who is facing cancer may be healed emotionally in spite of not being healed physically. In the larger scope of things, we need to acknowledge that even with prayer, faith, healing, or even a cure, we will not live in our mortal bodies forever.

As we continue to work out the nuances, we may find that our particular construct of healing may need redemption. Our concept of healing may stem more from the medical notion of curing than from a holistic and salvific notion of restoring. We are distinguishing healing from curing. Curing connotes a ceasing of the ailment, an alleviation of symptoms, and a full reversal of the area in question to "normal" function. A cure is the result of spontaneous remission or a medical or spiritual treatment that thoroughly eliminates the adverse medical or even spiritual condition, symptoms and all. On the other hand, healing, in our precise usage, is about being made whole in terms of Christlikeness. It is about restoration from sin-sickness. Healing is instrumental to *theosis*. With our definition, healing can occur without a cure, and a cure can occur without healing.[49]

Another important distinction that needs to be made is between relief and healing.[50] We have unpacked the meaning of healing. What about relief? In this distinction, relief is an alleviation of pain, symptoms, and the discomfort of suffering. Relief allows one to continue to live life and take on its daily tasks and functions without distress. Relief deals with symptoms. Healing deals with the underlying sickness. With our rabid pursuit of a commercial *eudaemonia*, relief becomes vital and all consuming, taking on the power of a valuable economic commodity. Such relief can be merely a cosmetic healing that never addresses the true problem and need. It can superficially reenergize and enable us to be more productive participants in a pragmatic results-driven society. Although we would all desire immediate relief from stress and discomfort, we would be amiss at times to not discern that painful somatic or mental symptoms may be signs of a deeper problem that may point to a spiritual ailment. In such a case, relief may not be the best or ultimate solution. Diagnosis and treatment of the underlying cause maybe discomforting and undesirable at first. But *therapeia* moves beyond relief to potential healing. The nagging question then is, "Do you want to be made whole?" The desire for relief from depressive symptoms may unveil the need for deeper restoration.

Beneath the cry for relief is a deeper cry for truth and healing. In my previous experience in pastoral counseling, I found this to be the case. Prior to effective treatment, many parishioners felt closer to God when they faced chronic depression than in any other period in their lives. The overbearing symptoms drove them to rely on God in an unprecedented way. In this sense, melancholia was used instrumentally by the Spirit and the individual to draw closer to God. Yet things do not always work out so well. In other cases, depression created despondency and doubt, drawing persons further away from God. Depression in one instance may better serve holiness than in another instance. Also, a cure in one case may better serve holiness than in another case. However, if there is a cure but no growth in holiness, then there is no healing. Consider a wealthy, dishonest, racist Wall St. investor who once had cancer. The cancer was treated. They run tests. The results come back. He has perfect physical health and soundness of mind. Even though he was physically cured of the disease, he is still a racist. He cheats on his taxes but gives 10 percent of his income to the poor. He would seem to be further from the kingdom of God than one with incurable paraplegia with chronic depression who radically loves God and others by spending a vast amount of her time visiting and praying for the little ones at the local children's hospital. The Wall St. investor has been cured but not healed, while this woman is being healed, even though she has not been cured. There can be healing without a cure, and a cure without healing.

The stark contrast between curing and healing can be seen in the "people professions." In my former life as a pastor, so many of us ironically sought to cure others of their problems while we were still in need of healing in our own lives. At best, we sought relief but were never healed. In Charlie Kaufman's award-nominated stop-motion animated film *Anomalisa*, customer service expert Michael Stone drudges through his banal life, mechanically putting on seminar after seminar on success.[51] On the inside he is dying. In daily life he is only going through the motions of listening and helping persons. In his eyes every person is perceived as a nameless and faceless entity that sounds and looks the same (a Fregoli delusion). Stone is lonely and probably clinically depressed. He needs self-help or help and healing from someone else. Help arrives with one of his conference attendees, Lisa. The effervescent Lisa stands out from his flat, insipid perceptual horizon and arises as a real person, arousing him from his insular, dehydrated, vapid existence. The physician is healed proverbially by the patient, as Lisa nurtures Stone back to life by awakening his humanity. The irony of the unhealed physician is proverbial and perennial, and its lesson needs to be heeded. The Christian church often finds itself in this predicament of faulty self-reference. The church, which would like to be relieved of the "burden" of the poor, the outcast, and those who experience disabilities, is in need of deeper healing. The church also claims to offer a "cure" for sin and society's ills. Yet the church is either guilty of the same sins or is one of the chief perpetrators of social ills, such as racism, classism, and ableism.[52] In this case the physician needs to heal herself first. Vision cleared of any obstacles, logs or otherwise, will then enable us to see unmistakably what the real problem is and attend to it.

In the ministry of healing, it is essential to parse correctly our ideas of relief, healing, and curing. Further, it is vital to recognize that, ultimately, any relief or cure or quest for these is temporal and incomplete. In the end there is no relief or cure for mortality, besides the resurrection, which is relief, healing, and cure. Healing, on the other hand, is the restoration of health. We are qualifying healing and health as holistic—the integration of spiritual, mental, emotional, physical, relational, and other aspects. Wholeness is defined by the image of God in Christ, which may or may not involve the curing of a disability or disorder.[53] The one guaranteed "cure" offered by Christ is resurrection.[54] Healing is the inner and relational experience of transformation proleptically stemming from the objective resurrection. The claim is that the resurrection, involving the redemption of our bodies, is the greatest and ultimate healing. This healing is even extended to the entire groaning creation,[55] which awaits its redemption, a new heaven and a new earth.

HEALING: AN ESCHATOLOGICAL TRAJECTORY TOWARD CHRISTLIKENESS

Divine healing is a semirealized eschatological trajectory of *imago* restoration, now and not yet. Healing originates, draws from, and is finalized in the resurrection. The healing and redemption of our bodies (our whole selves) are grounded in the work of the atonement, manifested through the Spirit in the ongoing transformation of the image of God and fully realized in glory following death. The *missio Christi* is summed in part in Acts 10:38, which tells us how "God anointed Jesus of Nazareth with the Holy Spirit and power, and how he went around doing good and healing all who were under the power of the devil because God was with him." Healing was a vital component of Christ's ministry. We note this truth rehearsed in the various formulae throughout the Gospels that list the works of Christ and his disciples, as exemplified in Matthew 10:7-8—"heal the sick, raise the dead, cleanse the lepers, drive out demons." The healing mission of Christ culminates with the atonement, which objectively establishes our salvation. The *missio Spiritus* is to execute and bear witness to the *missio Christi* (John 14:16-26; 15:26; 16:13-15). As Christ was filled with the Spirit and healed (Acts 10:38), so also, in the book of Acts, is the charismatic body of Christ anointed to minister healing.

Scripture does not make a univocal causal connection between sickness or mental disorder and sin. Disorder in general and its particular manifestations are part of the fall, though not necessarily linked to judgment or punishment.[56] Thus, the question of healing mental disorders and depression is part of a larger holistic healing of the image of God within us. Specifically, the healing is relational. Christ restores our relationships with God and others. The healing work of the Spirit continues through sanctification. The Spirit perfects Christ's image in us. We are reminded that the Spirit is attracted to our brokenness and works with us in our weakness. God allows adversity and suffering to function as a messenger that calls us to him. Paul the apostle heard such a call. He was sent a messenger. The thorn in his flesh was not removed but allowed by God. The adversity manifested Paul's weakness and moved him to depend on the perfecting grace of God. It is debated what the thorn specifically represented, but the point is clear that God works with our affliction and turns it into an occasion for sanctification. Weakness attracts grace.

In this case, healing is a manifestation of weakness that finds hope in Christ. Christ modeled the same dependence. In embodying our weakness, he relied fully on the Father through the power of the Spirit. His dependence instructs us to likewise. As God's power was revealed in Christ's weakness at the cross, so similarly God's power is revealed in our weakness. The revelation of God's power in human weakness is a sign (*semeion*) of the subverting power of the kingdom of God. Human power is toppled. A kingdom that values the weak decenters and supplants our binary power constructs of abled and disabled. Radical reversal is exemplified in the deliverance of the tormented Gadarene man. Christ delivered him from the torture chamber of a demon-plagued mind. He was given the gift of peace. After being healed and given a sound mind (σωφρονέω), he yearned to follow Christ. The healing that the Gadarene man experienced was a sign of the power, peace, and mercy of God. These coveted blessings attracted him to follow Christ. However, Jesus insisted that he not follow him back to the boat. Instead, he released him to his people as a wounded healer to share the goodness of God. The Gadarene man, who once afflicted himself because of his mental illness, was liberated physically and mentally. His bound and chained humanity was released. A free man, he no longer viewed himself through his mental illness, a powerless victim. He became a bearer of good news when he became good news at his deliverance. An identity transformed. In Christ, the weak are made strong.

Christ empowers persons with mental illness to shatter the confines of stigma and shame imposed by society, a reversal and healing of status. His unwavering presence is a gift of comfort and hope. The kingdom overthrows despair from within and rules in peace. The climate of inner turmoil is dissipated. The kingdom within then grows and manifests without. The reversal of this worldly order into one of *shalom* is the work of the kingdom of God (Rev. 11:15). A cosmic transfiguration requires nothing less. Healing advances from self to system, as the body of Christ works as a just agent to mend or transform the ailing and oppressive structures and systems of the world that afflict the weak and the mentally downtrodden.[57] The church must rigorously work for mental health justice at all levels, from ministering with persons to confronting the structures and systems that generate and perpetuate the conditions for mental disorder that disproportionately afflict the poor, women, racial and ethnic minorities, and the intersectionality of these.[58]

HEALING AND FORGIVENESS

Veteran of the Korean War and retired autoworker Walt Kowalski is one of the last of his generation and ethnic background living in his degentrified neighborhood, which was once working-class Euro-American. The auto factories are closed, and the housing stock is now teeming with young Latino, African American, and Hmong families. The movie *Gran Torino*, starring Clint Eastwood, opens with the death and funeral of Kowalski's wife. Alone, Kowalski, who is depressed because he lost his wife, his neighborhood, and his America, barricades himself in his unresolved past from the war with racial prejudice, distrust of strangers, and an overall comfortable, incurable curmudgeonry. All that Walt has left in his fading world is his '72 Ford Gran Torino, his alcohol, and his dog. He refuses his yuppie children's suggestion to move into a retirement community. He wants to make a final stand and die in his invaded neighborhood.

A multigenerational extended Hmong family moves in next door. Walt despises the family at first because of their different culture. He is also angered at Thao, the young Hmong boy living next door, who was coerced by a local gang to attempt to steal Walt's Gran Torino as an initiating rite into the gang. Thao gets caught, and his grandmother makes him pay off his debt by doing chores for Walt around his house and the neighborhood. As he works off his debt, he forms a close bond with Walt, who begins to develop affection and care for Thao, his sister Sue, and the rest of the family as well. Hmong kindness and hospitality and Thao's need for paternal direction, in the absence of a father, soften Kowalski's hard heart. He forgives Thao for trying to steal his car. In the process of forgiveness, he seems to release his anger toward Asian people in general. His rage and resentment, which represent a larger American prejudicial sentiment, were residual and leftover from the Korean and Vietnam Wars. Gradually, Walt is healed of his hatred, prejudice, and even his isolating depression as he finds new meaning in helping Thao. He teaches him how to work and to stay away from the pressure of gang recruitment.

When the gang fails to recruit Thao, they resort to violence and threaten him by raping his sister Sue. The violence against Sue is also a message to the family about what will happen if Thao refuses to join the gang. Walt, who has made the Hmong family his own, is infuriated and tempted to retaliate with force. He knows he has to stop the cycle of violence or the gang will kill members in Thao's family and eventually Thao. Walt has a plan. He knows he will not be around forever to protect Thao. He also knows that if he acts violently against the gang, he not only puts himself at risk but risks perpetuating the cycle of violence by drawing potential retaliation by the gang against Thao's family. Walt knows he has to let go of his consuming drive to take vengeance on the gang. He needs to forgive and even sacrifice his life for the future safety of Thao and his family.

Walt goes to the house of the gang members unarmed, though they do not know he is unarmed as they see him out in front of the house. The gang noted in the past that Walt brandished a weapon and was not afraid to use it. They are expecting him to be carrying a concealed weapon as he approaches the house. Walt expects them to expect as much. The gang members come outside to confront him. They are armed. Walt reaches for a lighter to light a cigarette that is already hanging from his mouth. Thinking he is reaching for a gun, they fire their weapons at Walt and kill him, an innocent, unarmed man. The police come and lock up the members of the gang. The kindness, forgiveness, and unconditional love shown by both the Hmong family and Walt toward each other have broken the cycle of violence and freed Walt's soul from depression, guilt, and unforgiveness. Prior to executing his plan, Walt finally confessed his sins to the young priest who had been trying to reach out to him throughout the story. Unconditional love and forgiveness can heal hate and depression and break cycles of prejudice and violence.

Unforgiveness can be a contributing factor to depression. Walt was overtaken by depression because he could not let go of the past. Unforgiveness can result in torment of the soul both eternally and temporally, as illustrated in Christ's teaching on the parable of the unforgiving debtor. We who have been forgiven often hold others in debt to our unforgiveness. In the end, both the indebted and the debtor are tormented by unforgiveness. Much has been documented medically and theologically about the power of forgiveness in terms of giving and receiving forgiveness from each other. The fruit of forgiveness is overall improved health, including mental health, as unforgiveness can foster and exacerbate depression and anxiety.[59] Unresolved injustices, relational transgressions, emotional wounds, pain, and anger that contribute to depression can be addressed therapeutically. Various types of forgiveness therapy help to uncover, communicate, process, and resolve possible issues around unforgiveness and its toxic consequences. Some of these treatments are integrative, working from the healing model of the atonement and applying forgiveness therapy, psychotherapy, or some form of CBT.[60]

We often unnecessarily inflict and are afflicted by unforgiveness, which can inflict depression and anxiety. Forgiveness is one of the most vital human needs and is a core blessing of the Christian faith. The cross of Christ is the primary locus for receiving forgiveness for transgressions against God (Luke 1:77; Eph. 1:7; Col. 1:14).[61] Partaking of the fruit of the cross is also a principal practice of the Christian church, celebrated at the eucharistic table, where the blood of God's covenant is poured out for the forgiveness of sins (Matt. 26:28). The cross is also the basis for giving and receiving forgiveness, a vital exchange that sustains human relations.[62] We are admonished throughout the New Testament, as highlighted in the Lord's Prayer, to forgive as we have been forgiven. The rhythmic exchange of giving and receiving forgiveness as a spiritual discipline among the communion of saints is the divine antidote to compounded and cyclical injustice, vendettas, rage, envy, jealousy, and hatred inflicted on each other in a fallen world. The church draws from the example of Christ, who was anointed with the Holy Spirit to bring good news that heals the brokenhearted and release those tormented in captivity (Luke 4:18-19). Modern therapy, of course, teaches us the finer psychosocial dynamics and nuances. These strategies involve seeking justice, forgiveness, and, if possible, reconciliation, which do not involve further enabling, denial, or abuse within the forgiveness process.[63] Receiving and offering release from mental and emotional "debts" through Christ-initiated forgiveness can foster healing. Pent-up depressive symptoms due to the somatization of unforgiveness can be released.

HEALING AND ADOPTION

Depression carries with it an overwhelming sense of radical alienation and depersonalization from one's self, the world, and even God. One can feel isolated, excluded, rejected, and even trapped, thinking no else experiences what they are experiencing. Someone with depression feels as if their mind is their own inescapable prison. They search for someone who could break through the solid walls and iron bars of despair that have them trapped. The good news is that God has broken into this world and breaks into our life to break us out of our own prisons and set us free. Persons with depression long for deliverance and belonging. The Good Shepherd seeks out and saves the lost and the rejected of this world. He binds their wounds and brings them back home to the fold. God adopts as his own those whom he has forgiven (Eph. 1:5). He calls them his own children (Rom. 8:14-16). He gives them a new name and place in the family of God. Healing of identity, or identity reformation, is grounded in God's grace in baptism, which initiates us into the family of God. Our new identity in Christ is realized and appropriated daily through faithful discipleship, catechesis, receiving the sacraments, living out the liturgy, and serving each other. New meaning emerges from a new identity in Christ. Those adopted into the body of Christ are an eschatologically reconstituted humanity, the redeemed people of God.

The estranged, the fatherless, the widow, refugee, immigrant, migrant, asylum seeker, the alienated, and the mentally anguished, all are welcome (Ps. 146:9). The doors of the church are to be pushed open as wide as the world. Unconditional belonging is what depressed persons long to find. The church is called to be a community of radical hospitality that not only opens its doors but goes outside its four walls to seek and save the lost. The *ecclesia* is a living witness of God's relentless pursuit of outcasts and marginalized persons, who find a home in God's heart. The church announces and works the justice of the kingdom of God with the stranger and with those in despair, inviting them to the family table. The healing of adoption also extends beyond human persons to creation care. The Spirit moves from people to the environment to promote *soteria* and *shalom* to the systems and structures that impact (mental) health. As the people of God become an icon of God, in all of its vertical and horizontal implications, its imprint on all of the cosmos will become visible. Salvation as *therapeia* of the *imago* in this sense renders the *via salutis*, as a way of health, with the *telos* being *theosis*, even a cosmic *theosis* extending to all of creation.[64]

TYPE 3—PURGATIVE MELANCHOLIA: WORD AND SPIRIT AS COMFORTER, COUNSELOR, AND FRIEND

In prior chapters we drew the correlation between an ontology of depression and anthropology. An analysis of theological anthropology has steered our course toward the importance of a relational understanding of human personhood and the nature of depression. We identified the human person in terms of the relational image of God as revealed in Christ, the Son of God. Next, we identified three relational states (creation, fall, new creation) that correspond to three classical theological types of melancholia (natural, consequential, purgative). Consequently, we examined the three relational states and types of melancholia in light of the redemption found in Jesus Christ. In the economy of salvation, the Son and the Spirit minister the *via salutis* along an eschatological trajectory of healing that not only positions us forensically in right standing with God but also treats our souls therapeutically, restoring us as daughters and sons of God in the image of Christ. In assuming the human condition, God relates with and redeems our brokenness. As our advocate, he stands on behalf of persons with mental disorders, ministering healing and power. He liberates from personal and social oppression and restores our identity and dignity as daughters and sons of God.

In the final relational state, we embark on the journey of sanctification. Sanctification, or *theosis*, is the eschatological trajectory of healing imparted by the Spirit into our lives. Through the energies of God, we are transformed in the image of Christ. The Spirit's work of purification and perfection is an ongoing dynamic, comprising movements of crisis and process along the *via salutis*. The Spirit of Pentecost is sent to us and received in chrismation as the *Parakletos*. As the Spirit of truth, he is the agent of both revelation and transformation. The Παράκλητος reveals Christ and sanctifies us in his image. The use of *paraclete* seems to include, but transcend, its forensic sense of legal advocate and points to the Jewish sapiential tradition. In this tradition, wisdom serves a greater soteriological function. Wisdom is the embodied practices that lead to salvation.[65] The Spirit becomes our wisdom, a helper or counselor on the way of salvation. Translated diversely as "advocate," "helper," "comforter," and "counselor," and the Paraclete, the semantic range is extensive and rich, adding to our understanding of the sanctifying work of the Spirit.[66]

As noted above, we have identified the person and work of the Spirit (John 14–16) as *Paraclete*, in light of the person and work of the Son. The Son and the Spirit are consubstantial with the Father. The work of the Spirit witnesses to the mediating work of the Son, as willed by the Father. By revealing and teaching what the Son has committed to the Spirit of truth, the *Paraclete* is revealing the person and work of Christ. The Spirit functions as the agent of revelation and salvation in the life of the church and in the world. Further, the Spirit mediates the work of Christ in the fullness of his ministry, culminating with the salvific import of the cross in Christ's death, burial, and resurrection. In sum, the Spirit as *Paraclete*, in its semantic range, is identified soteriologically in consonance with the salvation identified in Christ. The Spirit of truth mediates the sanctification that was secured for us in the offering of Christ (Heb. 10:10-14). We are washed in his blood, sanctified in the name of the Lord Jesus by the Spirit of God (1 Cor. 6:11), and set apart in holiness for his use. The Spirit of sanctification renews us daily in his image, inhabiting the recesses of the human heart as *Paraclete*. He intercedes through

advocacy, comfort, and counsel on our behalf. In these roles, the Spirit ministers the healing and saving work of Christ to us. Persons who experience the
alienation of depression are not abandoned to themselves, without counsel,
or left comfortless, but are promised that Christ will come to them, dwell in
them, and advocate for them by the Spirit (John 14:18).

MELANCHOLIA AND THE DARK NIGHT OF THE SOUL

Can the Spirit lead us through the darkness of depression? We identified the
third theological type of melancholia as the "dark night of the soul" (DN).
The DN is the liminal passage on the excursion of sanctification, where we
are arrested in our spiritual development by darkness and seemingly abandoned by God. Yet this perceived setback has been divinely designed. The
anguish of the DN purges us of our trust in sense and reason and is divinely
orchestrated to lead us into total dependence on God. The *missio Spiritus*
leads and guides the soul in all truth providing light in darkness and wisdom, counsel, and comfort in despondency. As *Paraclete*, the Spirit convicts
the world of truth in regard to sin, righteousness, and judgment. He leads us
away from autonomy to utter dependence on Christ and purges our hearts
of the proclivity toward inversion and self-service. In the DN, the purging
involves spirit-sensory deprivation. He temporarily suspends our spiritual
senses. We feel destitute and are pressed to walk by blind faith.

Prior to advancing our discussion of the Spirit, purgation, and melancholia, we need to be reminded once again of the ontological difference
between us and God. There is an infinite analogical *diastema* between divine
and created being. The hyperessence of God utterly transcends our capacity
for univocal correspondence. Our vast impeding limitations are both ontological and epistemological, rendering hyperessentiality unknowable. However, the incarnation, the personified *analogia entis*, is God in the flesh made
known to us. He is the full cataphatic embodiment of the deity revealing the
mystery of salvation (Eph. 3:1-10). Yet our doctrinal definition of the incarnation is hedged by apophatic language, which characterizes a rich tradition of
via negativa that precedes and follows Chalcedon.[67] Nonetheless, even in his
cataphatic energies, he can be *deus absconditus*, as in the DN or in depression.
Simply, the knowable God can "hide himself," making him unknown.

For persons with depression, the seeming absence of God from one's
experience becomes overwhelming. The apophasis of depression is often
identified in negative terms related to function. One feels spiritually paralyzed as in the DN, or one falsely interprets the spiritual impairment of
depression as divine punishment. On the contrary, the point of the DN is
purgation. The uncharted topography of the contemplative journey is leveled

of Pelagian morality, ability, and knowledge. As God hides, the wandering soul is rendered blind, deaf, numb, and speechless. No flesh can glory in his presence or pass through the aperture of this needle. The DN, the purgative process of sanctification, starkly discloses our spiritual disability and disorder. Frailty and powerlessness become normative in the light of divine darkness, warranting the advocacy of the Spirit. For those who experience melancholia, they need to be reminded that God is with them even though masked by the dullness of their senses. Depression, like the DN, can bring inner blindness and deafness. Under the imploding darkness, one feels abandoned.

DEPRESSION VERSUS THE DARK NIGHT OF THE SOUL

In chapter 7, we clarified that the DN and clinical depression are not synonymous but distinct. However, they can be comorbid and share similar phenomenology. In both spiritual and melancholic darkness, the mind suffers in affliction and torment.[68] In the DN and in major depression, irritability,[69] dysphoria, and anxiety are common symptoms that quench a person's sense of serenity. Such turbulence to the soul makes peace seem unattainable. In either case, God is present as Emmanuel. He dwells within us as Counselor to illuminate the way through the dark valleys. His light beams over our mindscape, revealing the hope of green pastures and still waters that comfort and restore the soul. The peace of God navigates us on the right path that leads to goodness and mercy in God's presence forever. The promise of the Spirit's fruit of peace is consistent throughout Scripture as God's counter to the suffocating atmosphere of anxiety (Isa. 26:3-4; Phil. 4:6-9). The peace of God is not circumstantial but is an attribute of God (*Adonai Shalom*) and can only be given by God. God's peace is in diametric opposition to the type of superficial peace found in this world's system and transcends the temporal relief we seek from depressive symptoms (John 14:27). God's peace does not depend on our capacity to understand it (Phil. 4:7), nor is it impeded by the inner turmoil characteristic of the melancholic life. God's peace provides the transcendence that persons with depression long for when they feel hopelessly trapped behind the locked doors of their own mind.

While our Western tendency is to think solely of peace as personal between God and an individual, Scripture extends the promise relationally and socially to others, even divided people groups (Eph. 2:14-18). *Shalom* is divine order for all people on earth as it is in heaven. God's people are identified as peacemakers, those who make, work, or create peace through creating just systems (Matt. 5:9). Social conditions and sociopolitical systems that foster mental disorder due to poverty, oppression, and tyranny must be addressed by the church through its educational and justice ministries. We are reminded that the Holy Spirit is the executor of the kingdom of God, ministering righteousness, peace, and joy (Rom. 14:17). The Spirit begins by convicting the church of sin and unrighteousness and its own shortcoming in working for *shalom*. We have often been used as an instrument of oppression in enabling and furthering semiotics and systems that have disabled rather than liberated. The Spirit teaches us how God sees each of us in his image, enabling the church to recover her sight and her mind. He opens our ears to the cries of injustice, heals our hearing, and gives us his heart for humanity. He heals our limbs to reach out. He then leads our feet to walk with him and with the oppressed on paths of righteousness. The *Paraclete* as Advocate works justice through the church individually and socially, empowering the marginalized and speaking truth and justice to the powers.[70] A church that rethinks and reworks power truly means good news for the poor. Structuring and operating from the bottom up denote that we all are made in the image of God and are weak and in need of mercy and goodness.

MELANCHOLIA AND THE STRANGER

One of the most debilitating symptoms of depression is alienation. Major depression can afflict persons with an eerie estrangement from others, everyday life, and even reality, a derealization. Persons with depression report an uncontrollable and overpowering sense of detachment. They feel hopelessly sealed off from the world, trapped in an impenetrable and inescapable, solipsistic bubble. Severe cases are usually related to trauma. Persons feels as if they are estranged from themselves, out of their own body and mind (depersonalization).[71] They no longer recognize themselves, and the things that they do are unfamiliar, not an amnesia but a dissociation from one's current depressed self. They vaguely recall the person that they used to be and vainly attempt to conjure up and recover that person. Inner and outer detachment were not uncommon experiences in the depressed persons that I counseled as a pastor. They felt that everything, including themselves, appeared distorted to their senses and mind. I am reminded of the 1960s rock group the Doors. In their song "People Are Strange," they uncannily described the syndrome when they sang, "People are strange when you're a stranger. Faces look ugly when you're alone."[72] When one is estranged inwardly from oneself, then outwardly everything else appears estranged. As a stranger to oneself, the person feels engulfed by a haunting, vacuous, and all-absorbing loneliness that acts as a black hole where one cannot be reached and from which one cannot escape. The holy strangeness of the *mysterium tremendum* works adeptly in this inner unfamiliar terrain. The numinous can awaken, capture, and rapture the imploding soul into transcendence and liberation.

God knows something about strangers and being a stranger. God came into the world as a stranger and abides with both the poor and the stranger. We are called to love not only our neighbor as ourselves but also our enemies and strangers. Even so God loved his people, Israel, when they were strangers (Lev. 19:33-34). As a pillar of cloud by day and a pillar of fire by night, he was with them to guide and comfort. When Christ came to bring good news to the poor, he came as a stranger. He created the universe, but the universe did not know him. There was no place he called home, but he preached as an itinerant from town to town. He was rejected and scorned by the common person and elite alike for his message of repentance and the kingdom of God. Though he was far from heaven, heaven was within him on earth. The Father declared his favor on his beloved Son and sent him the Holy Spirit. He was equipped by the Spirit for his ministry to the lost house of Israel and the estranged Gentiles. Subsequently, the Spirit led him to the cross and the grave and justified him in the resurrection. The Spirit of Pentecost is sent as a stranger to the Gentiles, for the Gentiles were estranged from the covenants, blessings and promises of God's people (Acts 10; Eph. 2:12). The Spirit comes as a stranger to the stranger to dwell with her as friend. The Holy Spirit as gift and guest identifies with the stranger and the outcast. For John of the Cross, the weary, wandering traveler transcends the dark of night by scaling the ladder of ascent, which is the love of God. Through the Spirit, God turns the tables. He makes the stranger his home.

He dwells with us, modeling radical, holy hospitality for the church to emulate. Love is not only the bond of *familitas* that is expressed between the Father and the Son in the procession of the Spirit, but also the *chesed* (lovingkindness and mercy) for the outcast that seeks and saves the lost and the discarded.[73] Thus, the love we need in order to love the stranger actually stems from the stranger, who is inhabited by the Holy Spirit. For the Spirit loves the stranger. In the end, we need the *other*, who teaches us to be and love like Christ.[74] Christ is in the other. Christ is in the marginalized and the estranged, and we are judged by how we respond to the least of these. Those with disabilities and mental disorders are empowered to teach the church hospitality. The estrangement of melancholia is met through the democratization of the Spirit, who has broken down all constructed barriers of young and old, female and male, Jew and Gentile, and free and slave (Acts 2). We are all called to break down barriers and embrace the outcast because we are all strangers to someone.[75]

DIVINE FRIENDSHIP

What happens when radical hospitality is reversed and the stranger makes room for us and becomes friend? Many literary works and films have captured this twist on welcoming, but perhaps none so endearing as the 1994 Academy Award–winning classic *Forrest Gump*, loosely adapted from the 1986 novel of the same name.[76] The film is a flesh-and-blood story of how a person (an anti-everyman) who is marginalized and estranged because of his intellectual disabilities (probably on the autism spectrum) becomes a friend and a healer through his radical hospitality to Jenny, who was sexually traumatized as a child, and to Lieutenant Dan, who suffered PTSD and depression from the Vietnam War. Forrest Gump does not seek healing but is a healer. Gump, although an outcast because of his condition, is healed of marginalization by simply accepting himself as he is and giving himself to others. He heals others by being himself. He is a stranger to everyone's world, but when he enters into everyone's world, he becomes their friend because there are no barriers to his hospitality. There are no handicaps to his friendship.

In the previous section we realized how God comes to his own as stranger. The Comforter not only identifies as stranger but ultimately as divine friend, as Christ called his disciples friends (John 15:9-17). Being estranged from self and the world is innately connected to isolation and loneliness, which are idiosyncratic of the depressed life. Suffocating symptoms of loneliness can saturate one's world. The strangeness of depression can transfer to one's self-concept, impacting identity. One becomes estranged from one's self and thus from the world. One does not feel at home in one's own body and mind, let alone with others. Depressed persons need to be reconciled with strangeness on three levels: God's, their own, and the other's, in that order. God seems far off or a figment of our imagination. Yet he embraces our awkward alienation, teaching us acceptance and trust at new levels. Epiphany and new revelation break us out of the solipsism of depression. When depressed persons give themselves and their experiences permission and affirmation, they can learn new meaning about themselves, God, and the world around them. They learn that God loves them and accepts them in the middle of their feelings of estrangement and absence. Their faith is lifted to a new level. They walk in confidence through the desert of their mind even when there seems to be no evidence of God. They learn that God transcends one's feelings and remains God, even a present God. Instead of fighting the waves of doubt, they learn to surf them. Being unconditionally embraced teaches them to embrace God, themselves, and others. God disciples through depression. His immovable, inviting presence, which tabernacles with us in the desert of despair, teaches persons to be at home with God, the universe, and themselves.

When we fearlessly embrace "the strange," we ultimately discover that the stranger is our friend. Uncreated divine being is indeed strange to created human being. We cannot comprehend an eternal and infinite nature with its omni-attributes, including being all loving and all powerful. The strange becomes familiar as God becomes human, and we see the face of the Father when we behold Christ. Christ calls his disciples his friends. The Spirit is the bond of friendship between Christ and his disciples.[77]

The love of God works beyond the contingency and accidents of our estrangement and alienation. God's gratuitous love flows from his infinite, boundless, and immutable goodness for the benefit of others and not for himself. Aquinas defines divine friendship by contrasting it with the familiar. He makes the distinction between the love of concupiscence and the love of divine friendship.[78] The good that I desire for the person I love is the love of concupiscence, either self oriented or other oriented.[79] This type of love, which is human and limited, even at its best seeks its own fulfillment even in desiring the good, while, on the other hand, the divine love of friendship does not need to pursue and increase its own goodness because the love of God flows from an infinite source of goodness.[80] Unlike our conditioned love, the gratuitous, perfect love of God is without condition and is true friendship. Likewise, divine friendship yields unrelenting compassion and mercy for humanity in its suffering and mental anguish. We are reminded that such pathos is unlike our imperfect sadness and sympathy, which attempt to empathize and alleviate suffering. Divine friendship stems from a perfect and infinite healing love that is untouched by evil but overcomes it.[81] Through "divine friendship we are made lovers of God and raised up into the mystery of God's own Trinitarian life."[82] We can come to God with our strangeness, our shadow side, uncertainties, and imperfections and transparently give them all to him. Out of our clay he crafts an exquisite new vessel that is truly human. As a new creation, we are no longer disabled by a false identity of sin. Once aliens but now welcomed as friends, we are called to do likewise.

The power of divine friendship offered by the Spirit to the church can be vital to building the type of relationships and communities that can foster healing. In the name of God, the church has alienated persons with psychiatric disabilities and failed to minister to those who are estranged and imprisoned in deafening loneliness due to mental health struggles.[83] Being present even as the Spirit is always present creates a consistent ministry of presence and friendship that allows for hope in all seasons. We learn the craft of friendship, beginning with being a nonanxious presence as the Spirit is a nonanxious presence. He teaches us to embrace and abide with *difference*. The *shalom* of God allows us to be a safe and stabilizing presence of hospitality and companionship amid the chaos and calamity of life's storms. Mental disorders are taxing, especially over time. They wear out both you and the support around you. Resources, both human and financial, begin to dry up. Those experiencing melancholia and other mental health struggles soon learn over time how either thin or limited the help from family and friends can be. Among persons with depression, there is a real need for thick, durable friendships. The *familitas* of God exemplifies the faithfulness and depth of true love in action. *Amicizia*, true friendship, begins with being present just as Christ, sent by the Father in the Spirit, is present with the ones the world calls the lost, the lowest, and the least. The forgotten and the voiceless need advocacy, not only the type that speaks on their behalf but also that empowers them to speak on their own behalf, which is a *charism* of the witness of the Spirit (Acts 2). As inhabitants of the Spirit of God, we, with and without mental disorders, become witnesses of the presence and work of the kingdom, living epistles declaring the goodness and faithfulness of God.

CONCLUSION

There is a strong correlation between how we understand what it means to be a human person and how we understand the nature of depression. A biological definition will correlate to a chemical understanding and treatment of depression. A semiotic definition will correlate to a sociocultural understanding and treatment of depression. As theological creatures, as well as biopsychosocial creatures, it is imperative that we address mental disorder and our relationship with the divine. How does theological anthropology come to terms with being human? We examined the widely held notion in the Christian tradition of the *imago Dei* and its various interpretations. Defining the human person solely by reason and/or ability is detrimental to those with disabilities. Human reason and power need to be defined relative to our relationship with God. Although acknowledging the traditional rational-volitional notion of the image of God, we recognized that this construct is situated in a larger relational, trinitarian context that is purposed for deification. Further, we were directed to the incarnation to divulge the full intent and clearest portrait of the image of God in Christ and the goal of salvation.

Identifying the image of God as relational, and its goal *theosis*, we located our relationship with God in three fundamental states along the *via salutis*: creation, fall, and new creation. With a relational notion of theological anthropology, we were able to retrieve from the Christian tradition three related theological types of mental disorder (natural, consequential, purgative) that correspond to the three relational states. Further, we examined the relationship between these three states and the *missio Trinitatis*. How are mental disorders or melancholia related to or met in the missions of the Son and the Spirit? We began with the obvious, the (in)ability of God to suffer.

Upholding the traditional view and yet allowing the furthest stretches of the hypostatic union, we maintained that God assumes our deepest suffering and pain in the truest way, as human, and yet encounters it in the most perfect way in divine love. The divine-human person Jesus Christ takes our sin, ailments, and suffering upon himself that we may be healed.

Mental disorder in its three states is addressed through the way of salvation. The work of Christ and the Holy Spirit as *advocate*, *healer*, and *friend* mediates the redemption of God at various junctures along the *via salutis*. The way of salvation is viewed in one sense as a larger work of *therapeia* of the *imago*. Salvation as healing and divine healing, including healing of melancholia, operate jointly in a semirealized eschatological trajectory of *imago* restoration, now and not yet, that originates, draws from, and is finalized in the resurrection. Thus, in this life healing is not always cure, and a cure may not involve healing. The healing of the Spirit and the mind are not compartmentalized. Healing as cure and cure as healing are realized in *theosis* of the entire person in the resurrection.

Although a theological framework is asserted in this study, an integrative approach that includes theological work and correspondence with other relevant fields is prescribed for future study. The holistic and analogical epistemology of this study requires it. What is presented here is depression under the bright light of hope on this side of glory, yet as seen through a glass dimly. We are promised the hope of resurrection. Healing occurs in many forms, though symptomology may subside or remain, but the presence and peace of God abides forever: "I will never leave you or forsake you" (Heb. 13:5).

Notes

PREFACE

1 Psychiatric disability is defined by the Americans with Disabilities Act (ADA) as a "mental impairment that substantially limits one or more of the major life activities of an individual; a record of impairment; or being regarded as having such an impairment."

CHAPTER 1: INTRODUCTION

1 Medieval scholasticism spilled much ink debating whether the incarnation would have happened if there were no fall. I would argue that there would have been an incarnation even if the fall did not occur, per Duns Scotus.

2 Augustine, *Enchiridion* VIII, in *Confessions and Enchiridion*, trans. Albert C. Outler (Philadelphia: Westminster, 1955).

3 Thomas Aquinas, *Summa Theologiae* 3.1, 3. Quotations are from *Summa Theologica of St. Thomas Aquinas: English Dominican Province Translation* (Notre Dame, Ind.: Christian Classics, 1981).

4 Hans S. Reinders, *Disability, Providence, and Ethics: Bridging Gaps, Transforming Lives* (Waco, Tex.: Baylor University Press, 2014), 12.

5 For example, in the case of disability, the ableist worldview and its grammar are the ones primarily adopted by society. William Gaventa asserts, "Similar to many of the assumptions underlying the medical model of disability (i.e., disability is an aberration), the ableist societal worldview is that the able bodied are the norm in society and the ones with the authority to name difference. . . . A disability is thus a 'bad' thing that must be overcome, rather than a simple consequence of human diversity, akin to race, ethnicity, sexual orientation, or gender." William C. Gaventa, *Disability and Spirituality: Recovering Wholeness*, Studies in Religion, Theology, and Disability (Waco, Tex.: Baylor University Press, 2018), ch. 1.

6 Contrary to popular opinion there is no single cause for depression. Neither are we aware of any direct neurobiological cause, though there are neurobiological correlations that have been identified. For example, see the article "What Causes Depression?" Harvard Health

213

Publishing, Harvard Medical School, June 2009, accessed June 3, 2020, https://www.health
.harvard.edu/mind-and-mood/what-causes-depression.

7 The commitment to the Trinity and incarnation is steady throughout the book.

8 "Depression: A Global Public Health Concern," World Health Organization, 2012, accessed
January 20, 2016, http://www.who.int/mental_health/management/depression/en.

9 Paul E. Greenberg, "The Growing Economic Burden of Depression in the U.S.," MIND
Guest Blog, *Scientific American*, February 25, 2015, https://blogs.scientificamerican.com/
mind-guest-blog/the-growing-economic-burden-of-depression-in-the-u-s/.

10 I am acknowledging the current multi-issue debate as to whether Adam and Eve really
existed; whether Adam and Eve are figures; whether Adam and Eve were the first or sole
original parents; whether Adam and Eve were among the first population of people. A few
texts that have recently tackled the issue are John H. Walton, *The Lost World of Adam and
Eve* (Downers Grove, Ill.: IVP Academic, 2015); Dennis R. Venema and Scot McKnight,
Adam and the Genome: Reading Scripture after Genetic Science (Grand Rapids: Brazos, 2017);
and William T. Cavanaugh and James K. A. Smith, eds., *Evolution and the Fall* (Grand
Rapids: Eerdmans, 2017).

11 However, animal models of depression are in use in which the disorder is identified and
tested by endophenotypes that can be reproduced and evaluated in animals. See V. Krishnan and E. J. Nestler, "Animal Models of Depression: Molecular Perspectives," in *Molecular
and Functional Models in Neuropsychiatry*, ed. Jim J. Hagan, Current Topics in Behavioral
Neurosciences 7 (Berlin: Springer, 2011), https://doi.org/10.1007/7854_2010_108.

12 In *Melancholy and the Otherness of God*, Alina Feld often uses the term "hypostases" to
describe the various manifestations of depression. Feld, *Melancholy and the Otherness of God:
A Study of the Hermeneutics of Depression* (Plymouth, UK: Lexington Books, 2011).

CHAPTER 2: ONTOLOGY OF MELANCHOLIA

1 There are Christian theologians and scholars—Nancey Murphy, Joel Green, and Malcolm Jeeves, among others—who hold to a nonreductive physicalist position on the
human person and clearly incorporate theological resources, though many do not claim
the existence of the soul. However, the tendency in the medical and broader scientific
community with a biomedical model is to hold to a reductive physicalist position that
often squeezes out the need for serious faith considerations and theological resources.
On the other hand, there are tendencies to create social constructivist reductions of the
human person and specifically intellectual disabilities. Heather E. Keith and Kenneth D.
Keith, *Intellectual Disability: Ethics, Dehumanization and a New Moral Community* (West
Sussex, UK: Wiley, 2013), xiv.

2 Stanley W. Jackson, *Melancholia and Depression: From Hippocratic Times to Modern Times*
(New Haven, Conn.: Yale University Press, 1986), 3.

3 Jackson, *Melancholia and Depression*, 3.

4 Jennifer Radden, *Moody Minds Distempered: Essays on Melancholy and Depression* (Oxford:
Oxford University Press, 2009), 20, 52, 64–67, 75–90.

5 Radden, *Moody Minds Distempered*, 77.

6 Radden, *Moody Minds Distempered*, 77.

7 Jennifer Radden, *The Nature of Melancholy: From Aristotle to Kristeva* (Oxford: Oxford
University Press, 2000), ix.

8 Jackson, *Melancholia and Depression*, 5.

9 Jackson, *Melancholia and Depression*, 5. However, while Jackson tends to interpret the
uniformity of melancholic manifestations, Jennifer Radden in *Moody Minds Distempered*

documents the divergence in the nineteenth century of the trajectories of melancholia and melancholy, with the former becoming more regarded as a disease and abnormal, while melancholy retained the notion of "subjective suffering as a condition of poets, artists, and men, as a part of normal human experience" (52).

10 Radden, *Moody Minds Distempered*, 52, 64.

11 The bifurcation of depression into normal and abnormal iterations is a common interpretation of the divergent manifestations based on symptomology, intensity and functionality. Although specific criteria validating bifurcation have varied across analyses, the tendency is to divide the condition, depression as well as anxiety, broadly into normal adaptive and pathological responses. It seems intuitive to distinguish the "black sun" of Julia Kristeva from "the blues" of B. B. King. Julia Kristeva, *Black Sun* (New York: Columbia University Press, 1987).

12 Kristeva, *Black Sun*. Jackson, *Melancholia and Depression*, 7.

13 Clark Lawlor, *From Melancholia to Prozac* (Oxford: Oxford University Press, 2012), 19.

14 Jackson, *Melancholia and Depression*, 4, 7.

15 See Jackson, *Melancholia and Depression*, 7, and Lawlor, *From Melancholia to Prozac*, 25, 27.

16 Feld, *Melancholy and the Otherness of God*, xviii.

17 Feld, *Melancholy and the Otherness of God*, xviii, xx. Feld also identifies two distinct complexes and two corresponding trajectories emerging out of the nature of melancholy—a depressive (acedic) complex of sloth-boredom-emptiness and a melancholic complex of sublime-tragic-non-being, which she tracks and unfolds in her detailed hermeneutical analysis.

18 Feld, *Melancholy and the Otherness of God*, 43. In her analysis, Feld sees Ficino weaving together several traditions in his topography of the melancholic genius: "the Greco-Roman myth of Cronos-Saturn, the astrological symbol of the planet-god Saturn, the metaphysical theory of the four elements, the medical theory of the corresponding humors, as well as Plato's theory of divine madness."

19 Or most likely Pseudo-Aristotle or one of his followers who authored the *Problemata*. See Lawlor, *From Melancholia to Prozac*, 33. The melancholic genius in Pseudo-Aristotle also echoes the notion in Plato that epilepsy, which was impacted by black bile, was somehow a "sacred disease" or divinely inspired.

20 In an attempt to link the temperaments cosmologically, writers in the medieval and Renaissance periods often depicted melancholia in astrological terms of its interrelationship with the sign and planetary motion of Saturn. Radden, *Nature of Melancholy*, 9.

21 Marsilio Ficino, *Three Books on Life*, trans. Carol V. Kaske and John R. Clark (New York: Medieval and Renaissance Texts and Studies, 1989).

22 Emil Kraepelin, *Textbook of Psychiatry*, ed. George M. Robinson (Edinburgh: E. & S. Livingstone, 1920).

23 Aaron T. Beck's *Depression: Causes and Treatment* (Philadelphia: University of Pennsylvania Press, 1967) is a key work outlining his philosophy of depression.

24 Albert Ellis' *A Guide to Rational Living* (Englewood Cliffs, N.J.: Prentice Hall, 1961) exemplifies his work.

25 American Psychiatric Association, *Diagnostic and Statistical Manual of Mental Disorders*, 5th ed. (Arlington, Va.: American Psychiatric Association, 2013). Hereafter cited as *DSM-5*.

26 Jackson, *Melancholia and Depression*, 5.

27 *The Oxford American Dictionary and Thesaurus* (Oxford: Oxford University Press, 2003), 379.

28 Robert Burton, *The Anatomy of Melancholy*, intro. William H. Gass, ed. Holbrook Jackson (New York: New York Review Books, 2001), 21.

29 As referenced in Jackson, *Melancholia and Depression*, 145–46.

30 Jackson, *Melancholia and Depression*, 6.

31 Jackson, *Melancholia and Depression*, 6.

32 Kraepelin as cited in Jackson, *Melancholia and Depression*, 6. See Emil Kraepelin, *Psychiatrie: Ein kurzes Lehrbuch für Stuirende und Aerzte*, 2nd ed. (Leipzig: Abel, 1887).

33 Lawlor, *From Melancholia to Prozac*, 150.

34 Radden, *Moody Minds Distempered*, 79.

35 The *DSM-5* outlines the following criteria to make a diagnosis of depression. The individual must be experiencing five or more symptoms during the same two-week period, and at least one of the symptoms should be either (1) depressed mood or (2) loss of interest or pleasure.

   1. Depressed mood most of the day, nearly every day.
   2. Markedly diminished interest or pleasure in all, or almost all, activities most of the day, nearly every day.
   3. Significant weight loss when not dieting, or weight gain, or decrease or increase in appetite nearly every day.
   4. A slowing down of thought and a reduction of physical movement (observable by others, not merely subjective feelings of restlessness or being slowed down).
   5. Fatigue or loss of energy nearly every day.
   6. Feelings of worthlessness or excessive or inappropriate guilt nearly every day.
   7. Diminished ability to think or concentrate, or indecisiveness, nearly every day.
   8. Recurrent thoughts of death, recurrent suicidal ideation without a specific plan, or a suicide attempt or a specific plan for committing suicide.

   To receive a diagnosis of depression, these symptoms must cause the individual clinically significant distress or impairment in social, occupational, or other important areas of functioning. The symptoms must also not be a result of substance abuse or another medical condition.

36 For example, in a particular, more recent iteration, as opposed to the generic sense, melancholia is classified in the *DSM-5* as a subtype featured or specified in some cases of major depression, i.e., melancholic depression. In previous DSMs, melancholia was categorized as a distinct disorder. See Gordon Parker, Georgia McClure, and Amelia Paterson, "Melancholia and Catatonia: Disorders or Specifiers?" *Current Psychiatry Reports* 17 (2015): 536, https://doi.org/10.1007/s11920-014-0536-y.

37 Alina Feld works with the term "melancholy" with some similarity to the way I am employing "melancholia." See Feld, *Melancholy and the Otherness of God*.

38 John Swinton, "Theology or Therapy? In What Sense Does Depression Exist?" *Philosophy, Psychiatry, & Psychology* 22, no. 4 (2015): 295–98.

39 Radden, *Nature of Melancholy*, 36.

40 It is noteworthy that traditional disability studies and critical disability studies differ vastly in how they understand a social approach to disability, with the latter following critical theory to its logical consequences by deconstructing normativity to its furthest extent in society, culture, economics, language, gender, sex, and other domains. See Melinda C. Hall, "Critical Disability Theory," in *The Stanford Encyclopedia of Philosophy*, ed. Edward N. Zalta, winter 2019 ed., https://plato.stanford.edu/archives/win2019/entries/disability-critical/.

41 Gaventa, *Disability and Spirituality*, 25.

42 John Swinton's thesis in *Spirituality and Mental Health Care: Rediscovering a "Forgotten" Dimension* (London: Jessica Kingsley, 2001) is that the field of spirituality—I use the term *theology* or *theological* in this work—is grossly neglected in the research, diagnosis, and treatment of mental disorders and needs to be factored significantly into an integrative approach to mental health care. This writer concurs.

43 Hippocrates, *Works of Hippocrates*, trans. and ed. W. Jones and E. Witherington, 4 vols. (Cambridge, Mass.: Harvard University Press, 1923–1931). Aristotle, book 30 of *Aristotle: Problems*, vol. 16, trans. W. S. Hett, Loeb Classical Library (Cambridge, Mass.: Harvard University Press, 1957). Galen, *On the Affected Parts*, ed. and trans. Rudolph Siegel (Basel: Karger, 1976).

44 Evagrius and John Cassian, embodying the desert monastic tradition. Evagrius Ponticus, *The Praktikos and Chapters on Prayer*, trans. John Eudes Bamberger (Kalamazoo, Mich.: Cistercian, 1972). John Cassian, *The Conferences*, trans. Boniface Ramsey (New York: Paulist, 1997).

45 Burton, *Anatomy of Melancholy*.

46 The Florentine Neoplatonism of Marsilio Ficino. Ficino, *Three Books on Life*.

47 Blaise Pascal, *Pensées*, trans. W. F. Trotter (New York: Random House, 1941), 21–28. Pascal merely picks up on the Evagrian theme of boredom as a means of contemplation of the true condition of humanity apart from God. For Heidegger it is a means to discover the groundlessness of *Dasein*. Feld, *Melancholy and the Otherness of God*, 125–31.

48 Viktor E. Frankl, *Man's Search for Meaning* (New York: Simon & Schuster, 1959), 121–31.

49 Sigmund Freud, *On Freud's "Mourning and Melancholia,"* ed. Thierry Bokanowski, Leticia Gloser Fiorini, and Sergio Lewkowicz (New York: Routledge, 2010).

50 As embodied in some of the writing and characters of existentialist literature, such as Dostoevsky, Camus, Kafka, Sartre, and above all Samuel Beckett. See Beckett's *Waiting for Godot* (Estragon), *The Unnamable* (the narrator), and *Endgame* (Hamm and Clov), among others.

51 *DSM-5*, 20. The *DSM-5* classifies it as a disorder rather than a disease. Claiming it as a disease would point to a neurobiological or neurophysiological correlation or cause (biological or mental mechanism), which the *DSM-5* does not intend to do. According to the *DSM-5*, "A mental disorder is a syndrome characterized by clinically significant disturbance in an individual's cognition, emotion regulation, or behavior that reflects a dysfunction in the psychological, biological, or developmental processes underlying mental functioning." Syndrome in this context is understood as a set of symptoms. Although the DSM is the gold standard in the industry, critiques of the underlying philosophy of the DSM are not wanting, ranging from philosophical to social and political to even psychiatric and psychological polemics.

52 The *DSM-5* from the American Psychiatric Association represents the biomedical model always extending toward a biopsychosocial approach to counter the biomedical tendency to reductive materialism.

53 Cognitive distortion or irrational beliefs around the triad of self, world, and future according to Aaron Beck, pioneer in cognitive behavioral therapy. Aaron Beck, *Cognitive Theory of Depression* (New York: Guilford, 1987).

54 Piotr Gałecki and Monika Talarowska, "The Evolutionary Theory of Depression," *Medical Science Monitor* 23 (2017): 2267–74, doi: 10.12659/MSM.901240.

55 Michael L. Raposa, *Boredom and the Religious Imagination* (Charlottesville: University of Virginia Press, 1999).

56 Dan Blazer's *The Age of Melancholy: Major Depression and Its Social Origins* (New York: Routledge, 2005) examines the social origins of major depression.

57 Jerome C. Wakefield defines a mental disorder as harmful dysfunction: when the mental function fails to perform what is expected in its evolutionary adaptation (dysfunction), and the dysfunction is harmful and not beneficial to the individual as deemed by the culture. Jerome Wakefield, "Disorder as Harmful Dysfunction: A Conceptual Critique of DSM-III-R's Definition of Mental Disorder," *Psychological Review* 99, no. 2 (1992): 232–47. Allan V. Horowitz and Jerome C. Wakefield, *All We Have to Fear: Psychiatry's Transformation of Natural Anxieties into Mental Disorders* (Oxford: Oxford University Press, 2012).

58 "Driven by New Therapeutic Drug Classes, Depression Drug Market to Grow to $7.3 Billion by 2024," Pharmaprojects: Track pharma R&D, *Pharma Intelligence*, October 8, 2017, accessed September 16, 2020, https://pharmaintelligence.informa.com/resources/product-content/depression-drug-market-to-grow.

59 For an overview of scientific realism and other competing approaches from an antirealism standpoint, see Anjan Chakravartty, "Scientific Realism," in *The Stanford Encyclopedia of Philosophy*, ed. Edward N. Zalta, summer 2017 ed., https://plato.stanford.edu/archives/sum2017/entries/scientific-realism/.

60 See Bas Van Fraassen, *The Scientific Image* (Oxford: Oxford University Press, 1980) for a comprehensive treatment of scientific realism and Fraassen's own response in constructive empiricism.

61 Lawlor, *From Melancholia to Prozac*, 24.

62 Radden, *Moody Minds Distempered*, 79.

63 Biological theories of depression can be, in their most radical expressions, but are not always, types of reductive physicalism or even eliminative materialism that seek a purely neurological etiology for depression that rules out appeal to mental states.

64 Radden, *Moody Minds Distempered*, 79.

65 Radden, *Moody Minds Distempered*, 83.

66 *DSM-5*, 749–59.

67 Dr. Allen Frances, concerning overdiagnosis, was quoted as stating, "Normality is an endangered species" owing to "fad diagnoses" and an "epidemic" of overdiagnosis, as cited in the blog post by John Grohol, "Overdiagnosis, Mental Disorders and the DSM-5," *PsychCentral*, July 8, 2018, accessed September 16, 2020, https://psychcentral.com/blog/overdiagnosis-mental-disorders-and-the-dsm-5/.

68 Thomas S. Szasz, *The Myth of Mental Illness: Foundations of a Theory of Personal Conduct* (New York: HarperCollins, 1974), xii. Szasz' groundbreaking work calls for the elimination of the concept of mental illness since it cannot be detected and proven from a "materialist-scientific definition of illness." In other words, until mental illness can be located in physical causes in the brain, such diagnoses should not be made. For Szasz, the field of psychiatry has been given legitimacy through the legislation and medicalization of the field, which has standardized mental disorder diagnoses as a form of sociopolitical control, as the American Psychiatric Association "contain[s] the imprimatur of the federal and state governments" (x).

69 Blazer, *Age of Melancholy*, ix, 4, 8.

70 For example, note the strong connection between social factors (socioeconomic background, gender, education, and ethnicity) and intellectual disabilities from Indian researcher Ram Lakhan, "Profile of Social, Environmental and Biological Correlates in Intellectual Disability in a Resource-Poor Setting in India," *Indian Journal of Psychological Medicine* 37, no. 3 (2015): 311–16, doi: 10.4103/0253-7176.162957. See also Eric Emerson, "Poverty and People with Intellectual Disabilities," *Mental Retardation and Developmental Disabilities Research Reviews* 13, no. 2 (2007): 107–13, Special Issue: Public

Policy Aspects of the Developmental Disabilities, https://doi.org/10.1002/mrdd.20144. Eunice C. Wong, Rebecca L. Collins, Jennifer Cerully, Rachana Seelam, and Beth Roth, "Racial and Ethnic Differences in Mental Illness Stigma and Discrimination among Californians Experiencing Mental Health Challenges," *Rand Health Quarterly* 6, no. 2 (2017): 6. I would also further note the factors of gender and race in mental disorders and the impact they have on women and racial minorities in oppressed contexts and the related stigmas and biases in treatment. See Joel Rennó Jr., Gislene Valadares, Amaury Cantilino, Jeronimo Mendes-Ribeiro, Renan Rocha, and Antonio Geraldo da Silva, eds., *Women's Mental Health: A Clinical and Evidence-Based Guide* (Cham, Switzerland: Springer Nature Switzerland AG, 2020). See also the World Health Organization's article "Gender and Women's Mental Health," accessed December 26, 2019, https://www.who.int/mental_health/prevention/genderwomen/en/. For a thorough analysis of the impact of racism on mental health and treatment and justice solutions, see also Suman Fernando, *Mental Health, Race and Culture*, 3rd ed. (London: Springer Nature, 2010), and Monnica T. Williams, Daniel C. Rosen, and Jonathan W. Kanter, eds., *Eliminating Race-Based Mental Health Disparities: Promoting Equity and Culturally Responsive Care across Settings* (Oakland, Calif.: New Harbinger, 2019).

71 George W. Brown and Tirril Harris' *Social Origins of Depression* (London: Routledge, 1978) examines social and environmental factors in depression, specifically life events.

72 Edward Shorter, *Before Prozac: The Troubled History of Mood Disorders in Psychiatry* (Oxford: Oxford University Press, 2009). Medical historian Edward Shorter painstakingly discloses the modern development of pharmacology and psychopharmacology as a power play, uncovering the political and economic influences, particularly of the FDA and the American Psychiatric Association that constructs the DSM, that mark the landscape of the industry.

73 Erick Ramirez, "Philosophy of Mental Illness," in *Internet Encyclopedia of Philosophy*, accessed September 16, 2020, https://www.iep.utm.edu/mental-i/.

74 Arthur Kleinman, *Social Origins of Distress and Diseases: Depression, Neurasthenia, and Pain in Modern China* (New Haven, Conn.: Yale University Press, 1986). Arthur Kleinman, *The Illness Narratives: Suffering, Healing, and the Human Condition* (New York: Basic Books, 1988), 100–120.

75 Arthur Kleinman, *Rethinking Psychiatry: From Cultural Category to Personal Experience* (New York: Simon & Schuster, 1981).

76 Kleinman, *Rethinking Psychiatry*, 7–8.

77 Arthur Kleinman, *Patients and Healers in the Context of Culture: An Exploration of the Borderland between Anthropology, Medicine, and Psychiatry* (Berkeley: University of California Press, 1980), 72.

78 Radden, *Moody Minds Distempered*, 83.

79 Arthur Kleinman and Byron Good, "Introduction: Culture and Depression," in *Culture and Depression: Studies in the Anthropology and Cross-cultural Psychiatry of Affect and Disorder* (Berkeley: University of California Press, 1985), 7. Some, like Jennifer Radden and Carles Keyes, note that Kleinman has shifted somewhat on his position, probably more toward disorder as a cultural interpretation and construction.

80 For more on the cultural impact of intellectual disability, see William C. Gaventa Jr. and David L. Coulter, *Spirituality and Intellectual Disability: International Perspectives on the Effect of Culture and Religion on Healing Body, Mind, and Soul* (New York: Routledge, 2014).

81 Byron J. Good, *Medicine, Rationality, and Experience: An Anthropological Perspective* (Cambridge: Cambridge University Press, 1994), 53.

82 Good, *Medicine, Rationality, and Experience*, 54.

83 Good, *Medicine, Rationality, and Experience*, 65.

84 Good, *Medicine, Rationality, and Experience*, 66.

85 A semiotic approach is based on sign systems used to construct and interpret mental disorders, along with the hermeneutics applied to interpretation and the meanings we construct about our experience of mental disorders.

86 Good, *Medicine, Rationality, and Experience*, 89.

87 Lawlor, *From Melancholia to Prozac*, 199.

88 See Geoffrey M. Reed, "Toward ICD-11: Improving the Clinical Utility of WHO's International Classification of Mental Disorders," *Professional Psychology: Research and Practice* 41, no. 6 (2010): 457–64.

89 Conor Cunningham and other so-called Radical Orthodox proponents posit the theory that a created order grounded in its own autonomy and univocity of being, which is grounded in nothingness, accounts for itself apart from the divine and any analogical participation in the divine, thus operating out of a logic of nihilism. The takeaway is the need to recognize that the contingent order participates and finds reference in the transcendent, in the divine. Without a transcendent reference, created being implodes on its own groundlessness or nothingness. Such is the case for all autonomous, closed systems, including biologically closed systems (e.g., nature) and culturally closed systems. See Conor Cunningham, *Genealogy of Nihilism: Philosophies of Nothing and the Difference of Theology* (New York: Routledge, 2002).

90 Jackson, *Melancholia and Depression*, 13–14.

91 For an extensive treatment of naturalism in philosophy of disease, see Élodie Giroux, *Naturalism in the Philosophy of Health: Issues and Implications*, History, Philosophy, and Theory of the Life Sciences (New York: Springer, 2016).

92 Elselijn Kingma, "What Is It to Be Healthy?" *Analysis* 67, no. 294 (2007): 128–33. Kingma offers a thorough critique of Boorse based on the evaluative construct of "reference classes."

93 Jerome C. Wakefield, "The Concept of Mental Disorder: Diagnostic Implications of the Harmful Dysfunction Analysis," *World Psychiatry* 6, no. 3 (2007): 149–56.

94 Wakefield, "Concept of Mental Disorder." For Wakefield, "A condition is a disorder if it is negatively valued ('harmful') and it is in fact due to a failure of some internal mechanism to perform a function for which it was biologically designed (i.e., naturally selected)." Further, harmful dysfunction (HD) analysis qualifies harmful as a negative value judgment "by sociocultural standards," and "dysfunction" as a factual scientific term, referring to "failure of biologically designed functioning."

95 Hong Lee, "Biological Functionalism and Mental Disorder" (PhD diss., Bowling Green State University, 2012), https://scholarworks.bgsu.edu/philosophy_diss/22/. Lee offers an accessible overview of the various biological or naturalist theories of disorder, paying specific attention to the concept of dysfunction. This work even-handedly critiques the theories of both Boorse and Wakefield among others.

96 Brülde Bengt, "Wakefield's Hybrid Account of Mental Disorder," *World Psychiatry* 6, no. 3 (2007): 163–64.

97 Karl Popper (1902–1994). See his work *Objective Knowledge: An Evolutionary Approach* (Oxford: Oxford University Press, 1972); and "Three Worlds," a Tanner Lecture on Human Values given at the University of Michigan in 1978, https://tannerlectures.utah.edu/_documents/a-to-z/p/popper80.pdf.

98 Critical realism (CR) is quite multivalent, extending from diverse proponents such as Michael Polanyi and Roy Wood Sellars in philosophy; Ian Barbour, John Polkinghorne, and Arthur Peacocke in science and theology; Roy Bhaskar in the social sciences; Bernard Lonergan, N. T. Wright, Wentzel van Huyssteen, and Alister McGrath in theology; and

Paul Hiebert in missiology. A version of CR proposed in this work is a broad model that would accommodate external, mind-independent causal ontology (a real world that supports and makes scientific inquiry possible) and mediating contextual epistemologies, as opposed to positivism, instrumentalism, idealism, and antirealism. CR does not claim to be value free but rather value aware. Thus, models are not literal but representative, analogical, comparable, and modifiable. See David Pilgrim and Richard Bentall, "The Medicalisation of Misery: A Critical Realist Analysis of the Concept of Depression," *Journal of Mental Health* 8, no. 3 (1999): 261–74. This article offers critical realism as a *via media* or middle way between "medical naturalism" and "social constructionism."

99 Roy Bhaskar, *A Realist Theory of Science* (New York: Routledge, 2008), 36–37, 47.

100 For Paul Hiebert, both supracultural revelation and contextual theologies are validated in a critical realist model. See the work of Paul Hiebert, including *The Missiological Implications of Epistemological Shifts: Affirming Truth in a Modern/Postmodern World* (Harrisburg, Penn.: Trinity, 1999); *Transforming Worldviews: An Anthropological Understanding of How People Change* (Grand Rapids: Baker Academic, 2008); and *Anthropological Insights for Missionaries*, 17th ed. (Grand Rapids: Baker Academic, 1986). Drawing from Ian Barbour, who draws from Ernan McMullin, Hiebert finds an alternative in critical realism to positivism (hard scientific realism), instrumentalism, and idealism. Ian G. Barbour, *Religion and Science: Historical and Contemporary Issues* (San Francisco: HarperCollins, 1997), 110, 117–20.

101 Pilgrim and Bentall, "Medicalisation of Misery," 262.

102 Pilgrim and Bentall, "Medicalisation of Misery," 271.

103 Swinton, *Spirituality and Mental Health Care*, 98.

104 Swinton, *Spirituality and Mental Health Care*, 131–33.

105 Swinton, *Spirituality and Mental Health Care*, 132.

CHAPTER 3: MODELS OF THEOLOGICAL ANTHROPOLOGY AND DEPRESSION

1 Granted, this is the prevailing approach in the Enlightenment. Nonetheless, there were exceptions within evangelical pietism. See Julius H. Rubin, *Religious Melancholy and Protestant Experience in America* (Oxford: Oxford University Press, 1994).

2 Joel B. Green, *Body, Soul, and Human Life: The Nature of Humanity in the Bible* (Grand Rapids: Baker, 2008), 28–32. Green defines many of the current positions in philosophy of mind. Also, for an interactive roundtable of four Christian perspectives in philosophy of mind, see Joel B. Green, ed., *In Search of the Soul: Perspectives on the Mind-Body Problem*, 2nd ed. (Eugene, Ore.: Wipf and Stock, 2005).

3 Eliminative materialism takes the radical position that commonsense notions of mind, consciousness, and qualia either do not exist or are reducible to matter (reductive materialism) or in this case the brain. Paul and Patricia Churchland are examples of this position.

4 Physicalism is the monistic view of reality that holds that all things are or are ultimately reduced to (reductive) or supervene on (nonreductive) one substance, the physical. Ernest Nagel, a philosopher of science, represents the reductive physicalist position. Philosopher Nancey Murphy is a strong proponent of nonreductive physicalism. There are a variety of monistic views that hold to one thing: substance (physical or immaterial-idea, mind, or spirit) exists; one existent (existence monism); one property (property monism); one category (genus monism-being); two sides of one coin (dual aspect monism-mind and body).

5 In philosophy of mind, property dualism is the position that there is one substance (the physical) with dual supervenient properties such as the physical and the mental. Saul Kripke and David Chalmers are well-known property dualists. Some hold that mind

including consciousness is an emergent property (emergent property dualism) from the brain through upward causation. Others further would claim that the mind acts back on the brain through downward causation.

6 Substance dualism, held by Plato, Augustine, and Descartes, claims that reality is ontologically made up of two independent substances, mental and physical. Interactive substance dualism holds that the two substances causally interact and impact each other. Radical dualism is the position that the soul and body are separate and act separately without relation. Parallelism holds that each substance causes its own effects without interaction (Leibniz). Occasionalism states that all causation is divine, using the natural order as occasion for divine agency (Malebranche).

7 Panpsychism signifies that everything has mind (thought and/or conscious experience). Spinoza and William James espoused panpsychism.

8 Philip Clayton, *Adventures in the Spirit: God, World, and Divine Action* (Minneapolis: Fortress, 2008), 244–55.

9 Amos Yong, *The Spirit of Creation: Modern Science and Divine Action in the Pentecostal-Charismatic Imagination* (Grand Rapids: Eerdmans, 2011), 196–225.

10 For a genealogical account of the Western fall from transcendence to nihilism stemming from a Western epistemological crisis and deflationary ontology, see Peter J. Bellini, *Participation: Epistemology and Mission Theology* (Lexington, Ky.: Emeth, 2010). This work provides a thorough critique of the problem with a closed Enlightenment worldview. See also Charles Taylor's *A Secular Age* (Cambridge, Mass.: Harvard University Press, 2018), which addresses the disenchantment of the modern self and world.

11 Jaegwon Kim, *Supervenience and Mind: Selected Philosophical Essays* (Cambridge: Cambridge University Press, 1993), 280. There are also weak versions of physical causal closure as well.

12 Clayton, *Adventures in the Spirit*, 118–32. There are a variety of process theologians, scientist-theologians, and even Eastern Orthodox theologians that hold to some version of panentheism as a solution to many of the problems presented by causal closure. See Philip Clayton and Arthur Peacocke, eds., *In Whom We Live and Move and Have Our Being: Panentheistic Reflections on God's Presence in a Scientific World* (Grand Rapids: Eerdmans, 2004). Traditional Christian orthodox views of God as Trinity (one substance and three persons) creating the universe ex nihilo are often abandoned by process and panentheist theologians in order to accommodate modern scientific understanding of the universe.

13 Science itself abandoned strong foundationalism beginning with Einstein's theory of relativity, Heisenberg's uncertainty principle, the Copenhagen interpretation of quantum, and Kuhn's paradigm shifts and Lakatos' research programs.

14 We can speak theologically from cataphasis as to the existence and nature of God. Yet, there is the apophasis of God that transcends our theological analysis and construction and is suprarational. For Rudolf Otto "the Holy" is a numinous reality, and our apprehension of it is precognitive (moral, ethical, etc.). The numinous is a primary, nonderived, sui generis, self-evident, and self-defining datum that is experienced as *mysterium tremendum* and when conceptualized and theologized is thinned out and dissipates into nothing—not that the knowledge of the divine vanishes but the apophatic awe and overpowering gravitas of the wholly other is deflated from our experiential knowledge. Rudolf Otto, *The Idea of the Holy* (Oxford: Oxford University Press, 1923), 5–9, 25–27.

15 Arguments for the existence of God are not wanting in the history of philosophy and theology. From Aristotle to Alvin Plantinga and beyond a baffling host of types (i.e., a priori or a posteriori) and options (ontological, cosmological, teleological, etc.) are available. Many of these types of arguments are traditional and foundationalist, while other

types are non- and post-foundational. See Alvin Plantinga's *Warrant* trilogy (Oxford: Oxford University Press, 1993, 2000) for the claim of the existence of God and other Christian beliefs as basic, rational, and warranted without the need of foundationalist argumentation by appealing to the "proper function" of cognitive faculties according to their design plan and their operation in a conducive environment. Plantinga draws from both Aquinas and Calvin to construct his model. Plantinga and others like William Lane Craig, who has a modified version, lay claim to the tradition (Aquinas, Calvin, and others) of *sensus divinitatis*, or divine sense, that all humans have an innate sense of the existence of God that is a basic belief and is not derived a posteriori. However, because of the fall, sin can impair the proper function of our cognitive faculties (noetic effects of sin), and our sense of God may be fallible. Craig's modification relies on the reality of the *testimonium spiritu sancti internum* (the inward witness of the Spirit) as a self-authenticating, immediate reliable witness to our spirit, not the analogical proper function of our cognitive faculties, which may be impaired. For an overview of these positions, see William Lane Craig's chapter entitled "Religious Epistemology," in *Philosophical Foundations for a Christian Worldview*, by J. P. Moreland and William Lane Craig, 2nd ed. (Downers Grove, Ill.: IVP Academic, 2017). Of course, there are many counterarguments to and detractors of each of these types and options. See David Hume, Immanuel Kant, Martin Heidegger, Jean-Paul Sartre, and, more formally, William Clifford, J. L. Mackie, Douglas Gasking, Daniel Dennett, and Richard Dawkins, among others.

16   The author is not proposing an epistemology that sees no need for argument or evidence, thus inviting a retort of fideism, but understands that such foundationalist approaches often require a bar too high for any field to meet, even empirical fields. No longer do the sciences require such a bar—even the standard of falsification is up for debate—and principles of indeterminacy and uncertainty are integral to quantum dynamics. However, the *sensus divinitatis* is rarely a monologue but rather is in conversation with other evidences and arguments that can strengthen and confirm its testimony ontologically, cosmologically, teleologically, evidentially, cumulatively, morally, supernaturally, experientially, and in other ways as well.

17   The space of this work limits engaging the needed philosophical theology and epistemology of theology to speak further to the existence of the divine, divine agency, and divine action. For a thorough investigation and affirmation of an open concept of divine action, see William J. Abraham, *Divine Agency and Divine Action*, 3 vols. (Oxford: Oxford University Press, 2017–2018).

18   One way forward would be Aquinas' use of primary cause (God) working in conjunction with secondary causes (in the universe). For a thorough treatment, see Michael J. Dodds, *Unlocking Divine Action: Contemporary Science and Thomas Aquinas* (Washington, D.C.: Catholic University of America Press, 2012). For Aquinas, "God not only causes each thing to exist but also endows each with its own proper causality" (190). God has "gifted each creature with its own proper causality according to its nature, his influence does not interfere with the proper causality of the creature, but is rather its source" (191).

19   See John Milbank's groundbreaking work *Theology and Social Theory: Beyond Secular Reason*, 2nd ed. (Malden, Mass.: Blackwell, 2006); and Peter Bellini's *Participation* for a thorough critique of the autonomous individual and the need to recognize our participation in God.

20   The pathology of an amoral, self-absorbed, gratifying culture is the thesis of Christopher Lasch's modern classic *The Culture of Narcissism: American Life in an Age of Diminishing Expectations* (New York: Norton, 1979).

21   Elisabeth Lasch-Quinn introduces Philip Rieff's classic *The Triumph of the Therapeutic* with "we embrace a gospel of personal happiness, defined as the unbridled pursuit of impulse. Yet,

we remain profoundly unhappy." Philip Rieff, *The Triumph of the Therapeutic: Uses of Faith after Freud*, 40th anniv. ed. (Wilmington, Del.: Intercollegiate Studies Institute, 2006), vii.

22 See the Lasch-Quinn and Rieff texts referenced above.

23 A critique with a long genealogy beginning with Thomas Szasz.

24 Some of the work of Emmanuel Levinas, such as *Alterity and Transcendence* and *Otherwise Than Being or Beyond Essence*, have captured well the phenomenological perspective that we are defined and called by the other, turning outward horizontally and gazing at the face of the other.

25 The Enlightenment promised many versions of a New Atlantis advanced by rational human beings. Following, even Nietzsche envisioned the Übermensch who has murdered God and now lives beyond good and evil.

26 Hans Reinders' work *Receiving the Gift of Friendship* in part critiques any philosophical anthropology that is grounded in human agency.

27 Nineteenth- and twentieth-century existentialist literature has best captured the dark anti-hero specter that haunts the age of reason's quest to create a new man that will inhabit the New Atlantis or some other *Brave New World* utopia and reveals the stranger within slouching toward a promised wasteland. Camus' *The Stranger* and *The Myth of Sisyphus*; Sartre's *Nausea*; Beckett's *Godot, Endgame*, and *The Unnamable*; Kafka's *Metamorphosis* and *The Castle*; among others, have captured well the looming character of angst and alienation that drives us to face the absurd rather than the rational, positivistic mechanics of the Hegelian system or any other totalizing progressive system of idea, matter, technology, or other. Existentialism forces us to consider a reality that is not so rational and to question the nature of the absurdity and even depravity within us.

28 Likewise, postmodern apostles, such as Derrida (no presence outside of the text), Foucault (power is knowledge), Lyotard (no metanarratives), and Baudrillard (simulacra as hyperreality), through their unique proclamations have attempted to deconstruct the rational and positivist foundations and authority that undergird the Enlightenment project of progress.

29 Dylan Reaves, "Peter Berger and the Rise and Fall of the Theory of Secularization," *Denison Journal of Religion* 11, art. 3 (2012): 5–8.

30 See Peter Berger's *A Rumor of Angels: Modern Society and the Rediscovery of the Supernatural* (New York: Anchor, 1970).

31 Andrew Newberg, Mario Beauregard, James Ashbrook, and Mark Robert Waldman, among others, seek to locate and understand the neurological basis for religious beliefs and practices, with several holding to an evolutionary view that such beliefs are adaptive.

32 Danah Zohar and Ian Marshall, *SQ: Spiritual Intelligence: The Ultimate Intelligence* (New York: Bloomsbury, 2000), 68–77. The authors allege that through the synchronicity of oscillating neurons at the frequency of 40 Hz, transcendence can occur.

33 Physicist turned philosopher Michael Polanyi proposed that science is not an objective, positivist account of the universe but, like all knowledge, is approached through a priori fiduciary commitments. The knower participates in the known when knowing. See Michael Polanyi, *Personal Knowledge: Towards a Post-critical Philosophy* (Chicago: University of Chicago Press, 1958, 1962).

34 A so-called theological turn, though not predominant, has been evident over the past century in many fields, including phenomenology (see Jean Luc Marion, Michel Henry, Paul Ricoeur, Kevin Hart, Merold Westphal, and others), sociology of religion (Peter Berger, Rodney Stark, Roger Finke, and William Bainbridge, among others), and the hard sciences (Ian Barbour, Arthur Peacocke, John Polkinghorne, Robert J. Russell, and Francis Collins, among others).

35 *Analogia entis*, or analogy of being. Making a theological analogy between the divine being and the human being is often thought of in terms of similarity and even great dissimilarity, as established in the Fourth Lateran Council of 1215: "For between creator and creature there can be noted no similarity so great that a greater dissimilarity cannot be seen between them." The *analogia entis* proposed in this theological anthropology stands not merely or primarily on rational grounds or based on the transcendental (e.g., the one, the true, the good, the beautiful), though it surely encompasses these, but considers functional and relational aspects as they relate to Christ as the image of God and humanity as purposed in the *imago Christi*. Balthasar, in fact, viewed Christ as the concrete *analogia entis*. The incarnation is God in the flesh and the will of God fulfilled in humanity. Theologically, the image of God is found and fulfilled in the union of divine and human substance and their relation between God and humanity and the soteriological purpose carried out through Christ.

36 See F. LeRon Schults, *Reforming Theological Anthropology: After the Philosophical Turn to Relationality* (Grand Rapids: Eerdmans, 2003), 175–78. Stanley J. Grenz, in *Theology for the Community of God* (Grand Rapids: Eerdmans, 2000), 160–63, argues that Scripture offers a holistic view of the human person rather than a partite one.

37 See Green, *Body, Soul, and Human Life*, for a nonreductive physicalist interpretation. Also see Joel Green, ed., *In Search of the Soul: Perspectives on the Mind-Body Problem*, for a current debate between four different positions on the issue: substance dualism, emergent dualism, nonreductive physicalism, and the constitutional view of persons.

38 The trend today is to deny or condemn any form of essentialism either in metaphysics, sociology, or anthropology, especially in regard to the nature of reality, human nature, race, ethnicity, gender, sexuality, and ability, and categorize these as social constructs or constructivism.

39 Joel Green identifies the tendency to oversimplify the biblical material addressing human anthropology and to draw caricatured conclusions as to the Hebraic, Greek, or biblical view of human nature. See Green, *In Search of the Soul*, 18–21.

40 See Grenz, *Theology for the Community of God*, 156–64, for a thorough analysis and conclusion.

41 See Plato, *Phaedo*, for his view on the body and the soul.

42 Malcolm Jeeves and Warren S. Brown, *Neuroscience, Psychology, and Religion: Illusions, Delusions, and Realities about Human Nature* (West Conshohocken, Penn.: Templeton, 2009), 25.

43 Jeeves and Brown, *Neuroscience, Psychology, and Religion*, 25.

44 Aristotle, *De Anima (On the Soul)*, trans. Hugh Lawson-Tancred (London: Penguin Classics, 1987), 3.3:427a19–427b9.

45 For the roots and problems of the social construction of reason as the Western grounds for marginalization and exclusion of persons with intellectual disabilities, see Tim Stainton, "Reason and Value: The Thought of Plato and Aristotle and the Construction of Intellectual Disability," *Mental Retardation* 39, no. 6 (2001): 452–60. See also Stanley J. Grenz, *The Social God and the Relational Self: A Trinitarian Theology of the Imago Dei* (Louisville, Ky.: Westminster John Knox, 2001).

46 I.e., Philo.

47 I.e., Justin Martyr.

48 Aquinas, *Summa Theologiae* 1.29.

49 Boethius, *Liber De Persona et Duabus Naturis Contra Eutychen et Nestorium, Patrologia Latina*, ed. J. P. Migne (Paris, 1878–1890), 271.

50 René Descartes, *Meditations on First Philosophy* (Indianapolis: Hackett, 1993), "Meditation 6," 47–59.

51 Many popular Christian philosophers, such as J. P. Moreland, William Lane Craig, and Stewart Goetz, hold to mind-body type substance dualism. See Stewart Goetz and Charles Taliaferro's work entitled *Naturalism* (Grand Rapids: Eerdmans, 2008). This view is also implicitly held by popular evangelical thinkers and writers, especially those who promote a pretribulation, premillennial view of the rapture, i.e., Tim LaHaye, which allows for the survival of the soul following the death or rapture of the body.

52 There are multiple ways to measure reason and intelligence and multiple intelligences, including emotional and cultural. See Keith and Keith, *Intellectual Disability*, 99.

53 For the debate on the nature of rationality see Edward Stein, *Without Good Reason: The Rationality Debate in Philosophy and Cognitive Science* (New York: Oxford University Press, 1998).

54 On the history, analysis, and problems of intelligence testing see Keith and Keith, *Intellectual Disability*, 40–52.

55 Keith and Keith, *Intellectual Disability*, 51.

56 For example, currently the Netherlands, as part of its national screening program, offers noninvasive prenatal testing for Down syndrome, with the purpose of limiting the financial burden to society, imposing financial consequences for parents who choose to carry Down syndrome babies to full term.

57 Postmodern thinkers like Emmanuel Levinas claim there is a priori violence implied in the entire methodology of prioritizing ontology ahead of ethics. The project of ontologizing the other is a totalizing project of violent rationality that colonizes the other. See Emmanuel Levinas, *Otherwise Than Being or Beyond Essence*, trans. Alphonso Lingis (Pittsburgh: Duquesne University Press, 1981) and *Alterity and Transcendence*, trans. Michael B. Smith (New York: Columbia University Press, 1999).

58 See J. Wentzel van Huyssteen's *The Shaping of Rationality* (Grand Rapids: Eerdmans, 1999) as an example of a modest proposal for the interdisciplinary construction of rationality that works with theology and science.

59 Antonio R. Damasio, *Descartes' Error: Emotion, Reason, and the Human Brain* (New York: Avon Books, 1994), 247–52.

60 Damasio, *Descartes' Error*, xii–xiii. See also Antonio Damasio, *The Feeling of What Happens: Body and Emotion in the Making of Consciousness* (San Diego: Harcourt, 1999), for an analysis of the somatic neural ontology of consciousness and how it defines the emerging self.

61 Schults, *Reforming Theological Anthropology*, 169–74, also traces this history. I am working from his analysis as well as my own.

62 Reformed thinking (total depravity), Wesleyanism (universal grace partially restoring freedom), Catholicism (original sin and guilt inherited), and Orthodoxy (free will with a proclivity to sin) all recognize the impact of sin on the human will to some extent.

63 See Dale M. Coulter and Amos Yong, eds., *The Spirit, the Affections, and the Christian Tradition* (Notre Dame, Ind.: University of Notre Dame Press, 2016) for a comprehensive treatment of the historical role of the affections in various traditions of the church.

64 For elaboration on the term "pious self-consciousness" in Schleiermacher, see Schults, *Reforming Theological Anthropology*, 99–116.

65 See Kenneth Collins and John Tyson, eds., *Conversion in the Wesleyan Tradition* (Nashville, Tenn.: Abingdon, 2001) for various essays from the Wesleyan perspective on aspects of conversion, including conversion of religious affections.

66 The following are key sources representative of a larger corpus of reference on these renewal movements: Allan Heaton Anderson, *An Introduction to Pentecostalism: Global Charismatic Christianity*, 2nd ed. (Cambridge: Cambridge University Press, 2014); Donald W. Dayton, *The Theological Roots of Pentecostalism* (Grand Rapids: Baker Academic, 1987); Vinson Synan, *The Holiness-Pentecostal Tradition: Charismatic Movements in the Twentieth Century* (Grand Rapids: Eerdmans, 1997); John L. Peters, *Christian Perfection and American Methodism* (Nashville, Tenn.: Abingdon, 1956); among others.

67 For example, for a thorough philosophical critique, see Keith and Keith, *Intellectual Disability*.

68 Georg Northoff, "Brain and Self: A Neurophilosophical Account," *Child Adolescent Psychiatry Mental Health* 7, art. 28 (2013), doi: 10.1186/1753-2000-7-28. Resonating with the neurological reflection model of the self are the various postmodern views of the self. These models assert a deflationary, deconstructed, and decentered notion of a stable substantial self. Postmodern perspectives destabilize the modern construct of self. Among such voices are Derrida, Foucault, Lyotard, and Baudrillard. E.g., see Kenneth Allan, "The Postmodern Self: A Theoretical Consideration," *Quarterly Journal of Ideology* 20, nos. 1–2 (1997): 3–24. Yet, in the midst of the assault on the self, the Western autonomous individual has not been pronounced dead but seeks to rise from the grave, showing that postmodernity is in one sense hypermodernity, and attempts still to carry out the positivist potential of the Western autonomous individual through the commodification of commercial *eudaemonia* and other myths of the American dream. See Jay Lifton's *The Protean Self: Human Resilience in an Age of Fragmentation* (Chicago: University of Chicago Press, 1993); opposed to Christopher Lasch's *The Minimal Self: Psychic Survival in Troubled Times* (New York: W. W. Norton, 1984); and Kenneth J. Gergen's *The Saturated Self: Dilemmas of Identity in Contemporary Life* (New York: Basic Books, 1991).

69 There have been some interesting constructs of the image of God in history. For example, John Wesley, the father of Methodism, defined the image of God according to two attributes, the natural and moral image, and one function, the political image of God. "'And God,' the three-one God, 'said, Let us make man in our image, after our likeness. So God created man in his own image, in the image of God created he him:' (Gen. i. 26, 27:)—Not barely in his *natural image*, a picture of his own immortality; a spiritual being, endued with understanding, freedom of will, and various affections;— nor merely in his *political image*, the governor of this lower world, having 'dominion over the fishes of the sea, and over all the earth;'—but chiefly in his *moral image*; which, according to the Apostle, is 'righteousness and true holiness.' (Eph. iv. 24.) In this image of God was man made." John Wesley, Sermon 45, "The New Birth," in *The Works of John Wesley*, vol. 6, *Sermons on Several Occasions: First Series Concluded. Second Series*, ed. Thomas Jackson (London: Wesleyan Conference Office, 1872), 66, available online via HathiTrust at https://hdl.handle.net/2027/njp.32101075386605. However, the notion that the human person is defined by agency or capacity disregards human persons who because of disability may not possess or experience these faculties in any conventional way and yet are still human. Such conditions have always been present throughout history, though only recently have we begun to address the civil rights and equality of those who have impairments and the social oppression that contributes to disability.

70 J. Richard Middleton, *The Liberating Image: The Imago Dei in Genesis 1* (Grand Rapids: Baker, 2005), 24.

71 Middleton, *Liberating Image*, 44, 48.

72 "Image" and "likeness" are *tslem* and *demuth* in Hebrew, *eikon* and *homoiosis* in Greek, and *imago* and *similitude* in Latin. The theologian Stanley Grenz thoroughly parses the Old and New Testament terms around "image" and the related debate in *The Social God and the Relational Self*, 184–222. Although he engages a variety of sources on the topic, his conversation with the Hebrew terms is primarily with Claus Westermann, Edward Curtis, D. J. A. Clines, Gerhard von Rad, Werner Schmidt, and Phyllis Bird. The consensus seems to be that although the respective prepositions (*be-* and *ke-*) differ in meaning, the words *selem* (image) and *demuth* (likeness) are virtually synonymous (187–89). Although there seems to be no scholarly consensus as to what the terms mean, the consensus appears to be that they are more functional terms than ontological or attributive. The sense is of the human representation of the divine in the world for some specific function, i.e., to rule, take dominion, or to relate or partner (relationship, companionship, counterpart) (190–203).

73 Craig Keener, *The Mind of the Spirit: Paul's Approach to Transformed Thinking* (Grand Rapids: Baker, 2016). Keener offers a comprehensive Pauline theology of the mind (*nous*) and its relation to the Christian life. As is typical of Keener, he proficiently engages ancient Near East, rabbinic, Greco-Roman, and patristic sources to provide background and interpretation for the Pauline usage of key notions, such as mind, flesh, sin, passions, virtue, vice, wisdom, renewal, and Spirit. The work repeatedly emphasizes the Pauline prescription for a mind subjected to and controlled by the wisdom and power of the Spirit for holy living. Such a mind is exemplified in the mind of Christ.

74 For the roots and problems of the social construction of reason as the Western grounds for marginalization and exclusion of persons with intellectual disabilities, see Stainton, "Reason and Value." For further investigation into other problems of reason and dehumanization in Plato, Aristotle, Augustine, Aquinas, Descartes, and Kant, and into the modern era, see also Keith and Keith, *Intellectual Disability*, 60–64: "Aristotle then, like Plato, established a scale of beings that puts the gods at the top (eudaimonia is a reference to god-like goodness), with rational humans next and nonhuman animals further down the line. Humans who are not, due to birth or disease, able to fully actualize a eudaimonic life through phronesis and nous fall somewhere closer to nonhuman animals and certainly outside the range of moral engagement (and apparently outside the range of moral concern, as evidenced by Aristotle's remarks about infanticide)."

75 Shults, *Reforming Theological Anthropology*, 221.

76 Grenz, *Social God*, 144. However, Grenz also makes a case that some form of the structural *imago Dei* remained within Protestantism long after the Reformation (170–82).

77 Grenz, *Social God*, 145.

78 Grenz, *Social God*, 147.

79 Grenz, *Social God*, 149.

80 Grenz, *Social God*, 150.

81 Maximus the Confessor held a doctrine of the *logoi* that were divine ideas that embodied the mind, wisdom, purpose, order, and will of God for each distinct part of creation, including humanity, to participate and find their end in the one *Logos*. Thus, the *logos* in Maximus was rational—but more than merely rational—and volitional but also relational and functional in terms of mediating *theosis*.

82 Grenz, *Social God*, 150–61. For those working out of Eastern Christianity, such as Irenaeus, Athanasius, and Clement, the *telos* was *theosis*, or divinization. David Cairns, *The Image of God in Man* (New York: Philosophical Library, 1953), ch. 7.

83 Grenz, *Social God*, 153–56. Grenz is quoting and interpreting from Augustine's *De Trinitate*.

84 Cairns, *Image of God in Man*, 110.

85 Grenz, *Social God*, 170–73. In fact the Reformation offered more of a hybrid model, adding a relational dimension to a modified structural model that understood reason and righteousness to be marred to a greater degree than estimated by patristic and medieval doctors of the church.

86 Middleton, *Liberating Image*, 27.

87 Shults, *Reforming Theological Anthropology*, 231–32; Grenz, *Social God*, 190–99; Amos Yong, *Theology and Down Syndrome: Reimagining Disability in Late Modernity* (Waco, Tex.: Baylor University Press, 2007), 173.

88 Middleton, *Liberating Image*, 28.

89 Such thorough biblical scholarship is represented well in J. Richard Middleton's *The Liberating Image*. Middleton interacts with the immense amount of biblical scholarship generated over this topic that has often been neglected by theological and philosophical approaches. He notes the conspicuous absence of references to the body and the visible from historical, theological, and philosophical accounts of the term (24–25).

90 Middleton, *Liberating Image*, 60, 88, 264.

91 This is not in the scope of Middleton's text, however.

92 See H. Richard Niebuhr's classic *Christ and Culture* (New York: Harper & Row, 1975) for his framing of the problem and the solution as seen through five different models.

93 For example, see Alistair Kee, *Constantine versus Christ: The Triumph of an Ideology* (Eugene, Ore.: Wipf and Stock, 2016).

94 With a theological reading of Scripture, sacred text is read as a theological document in light of the doctrine of the Christian tradition.

95 A case does not have to be laid out and justified for the connection between ecclesial power, corruption, colonization, exploitation, racism, slavery, and a vast array of social injustices exacted against the other. See Yong, *Theology and Down Syndrome*, 175.

96 International Classification of Functioning, Disabilities and Health.

97 Gaventa, *Disability and Spirituality*, 19, citing the *International Encyclopedia of Rehabilitation* entry on the ICF model.

98 "Ableism," according to one critical disability theorist, is "a network of beliefs, processes and practices that produce a particular kind of self and body (the corporeal standard) that is projected as the perfect, species-typical and therefore essential and fully human. Disability, then, is cast as a diminished state of being human." Fiona A. Kumari Campbell, "Inciting Legal Fictions: 'Disability's' Date with Ontology and the Ableist Body of Law," *Griffith Law Review* 10 (2001): 42–62 (44). Campbell elsewhere states, "Key to a system of ableism are two elements: the concept of the normative (and the normal individual); and the enforcement of a divide between a 'perfected' or developed humanity and the aberrant, unthinkable, underdeveloped, and therefore not really human. The notion of ableism is useful for thinking not just about disability but also about other forms of difference that result in marginality or disadvantage." Fiona Kumari Campbell, "Ability," in *Keywords for Disability Studies*, ed. Rachel Adams, Benjamin Reiss, and David Serlin (New York: New York University Press, 2015), 12–14 (13–14).

99 For example, see the work of French phenomenologist Michel Foucault.

100 I believe such a cultural cold war is going on in the West between the old controlling institutions that have been critiqued as oppressive and hegemonic (i.e., patriarchy, capitalism) by the neocritical intersectionalist, often with the same exclusion, intolerance, violence, and binary categories that were employed by the old regime. Hypocrisy is as near to us all as our own true selves.

101 Mental health issues such as major depression disorder and anxiety disorders can be comorbid with intellectual disabilities.

102 American Psychiatric Association, *Diagnostic and Statistical Manual of Mental Disorders*, 4th ed. (Washington, D.C.: American Psychiatric Association, 1994), xxi.

103 Gerben Meynen, "Free Will and Mental Disorder: Exploring the Relationship," *Theoretical Medicine and Bioethics* 31 (2010): 429–43, doi: 10.1007/s11017-010-9158-5.

104 For more on the various views of free will and the connection between mental disorder and free will, see Meynen, "Free Will and Mental Disorder." Meynen claims that the *DSM-4* does not expound on the meaning of freedom and what its "important loss" conveys (429); he notes that according to forensic psychiatry and the philosophy of free will, mental disorders "compromise free will and reduce responsibility," specifically in regard to criminal responsibility (429). Meynen identifies three ways (there are more) in which one can be free in defining free will: "The first element is that to act freely, one must be able to act otherwise." Then, "second, acting freely can also be understood as acting (or choosing) for a reason." Finally, "third, free will requires that one is the originator—(causal) source—of one's actions" rather than being manipulated or having one's mind altered by an external agent (429). In the first instance, temporarily and within context, a person with a mental disorder may be irresponsible, as a forensic psychiatrist may ascertain, when committing a crime as the disorder manifests (437). Also, according to Meynen regarding the second sense, except for "tics in Tourette's" and catatonic states, the criterion of "acting for reasons" per se will not lead to considering psychiatric disorders in general as potentially undermining free will (436). In such scenarios, Tourette's or catatonia are temporary states and do not negate agency permanently, though they are a problem nonetheless. However, the writer also cites first-person cases of Tourette's syndrome in which "the majority of tic-disorder patients reported that their tics were voluntary" (439). In fact, "because of the apparent intentional nature of some of the tics, it was hypothesized that cognitive behavioral therapy . . . might be beneficial" (438). First-person studies also show that during manic or psychotic episodes persons do not experience a compromise of freedom (438). Regarding the third case, one can temporarily lose control and accountability, for example in a delusional or bipolar episode, and commit a crime. Thus, while some studies show that mental disorder may compromise free will, some first-person reports indicate the opposite.

The free will debate is extensively treated in theology, philosophy, and science and often revolves around the notions of freedom, compatibility, and determinism. Various theological positions have assumed all three: determinism (some forms of Calvinism), compatibility (free grace and free response in Wesleyanism), and freedom (libertarianism). Neuroscience tends toward physicalism, which offers no real free will; our choices are determined by impulses in the brain. If determinism is the case, then all persons, those with disabilities and those without, are equally determined and not free. In this case, capacity-based notions of the image of God are irrelevant if we have no real agency or moral responsibility. In terms of psychiatric disability, the question is often framed morally. Do persons with addictions, obsessions, compulsions, neuroses, etc. have free will, and then are they morally and legally responsible for their actions? Meynen addresses this age-old problem and also provides extensive references on the topic.

105 Meynen, "Free Will and Mental Disorder," 438. Meynen concludes, "It might be that various mental disorders result in different degrees of 'compromised' free will."

106 Catatonic states can accompany schizophrenia, bipolar disorder, major depressive disorder, post-traumatic stress disorder, narcolepsy, and other mental disorders as well as autoimmune, neurological, and other metabolic disorders, and also head trauma. With catatonia,

a person still has agency, though fully or partially hidden (not empirically expressed). However, catatonic states rarely last for a few weeks at a time.

107 Jann E. Schlimme, "Impairments of Personal Freedom in Mental Disorders," in *Handbook of the Philosophy of Medicine*, ed. T. Schramme and S. Edwards (Dordrecht: Springer, 2016), https://doi.org/10.1007/978-94-017-8706-2_24-1. The person with depression lives in a dialectic with their symptoms and their bearing on their prereflective world and choices and on their reflective responses. For more on phenomenological autonomy and depression (prereflective and reflective autonomy), see Jann E. Schlimme, "Lived Autonomy and Chronic Mental Illness: A Phenomenological Approach," *Theoretical Medicine and Bioethics* 33, no. 6 (2012): 387–404, doi: 10.1007/s11017-012-9235-z.

108 Those with temporary impairment of free will nonetheless have some of the same challenges as those with no agency. The difference again is that those impairments are most likely temporary.

109 Hans S. Reinders, *Receiving the Gift of Friendship: Profound Disability, Theological Anthropology, and Ethics* (Grand Rapids: Eerdmans, 2008), 20.

110 Reinders states that PID "indicates a developmental stage of mental development that has not gone beyond a toddler's stage of development. Whatever is true of these human beings, it is quite unlikely that one will find them advertised as 'being successful' in the way persons with mild intellectual disabilities—the proverbial 'happy kid with Down syndrome'—are sometimes advertised in the media." Reinders, *Receiving the Gift of Friendship*, 48.

Persons with profound intellectual disability often have congenital syndromes. These individuals cannot live independently, and they require close supervision and help with self-care activities. They have very limited ability to communicate and often have physical limitations. See J. M. Sattler, *Assessment of Children: Behavioral and Clinical Applications*, 4th ed. (San Diego: J. M. Sattler, 2002).

According to the National Institute of Health's NCBI, persons with PID often have "congenital syndromes" and physical and speech limitations; 1.5% of all intellectual disabilities are profound intellectual disabilities. According to the *DSM-4* criteria IQ is less than 20. *DSM-5* criteria based on daily skills say they require 24-hour care. AAIDD criteria state there is "pervasive support needed for every aspect of daily routines." SSI criteria state one has a PID if one has "a valid verbal, performance, or full-scale IQ of 59 or less." See table 9-1 in section 9, "Clinical Characteristics of Intellectual Disabilities" of *Mental Disorders and Disabilities among Low-Income Children*, by the Committee to Evaluate the Supplemental Security Income Disability Program for Children with Mental Disorders; Board on the Health of Select Populations; Board on Children, Youth, and Families; Institute of Medicine; Division of Behavioral and Social Sciences and Education; National Academies of Sciences, Engineering, and Medicine, ed. Thomas F. Boat and Joel T. Wu (Washington, D.C.: National Academies Press, 2015), accessed September 21, 2020, https://www.ncbi.nlm.nih.gov/books/NBK332877/table/tab_9-1/?report=objectonly.

111 Reinders, *Receiving the Gift of Friendship*, 24–28.

112 Reinders, *Receiving the Gift of Friendship*, 17.

113 Reinders, *Receiving the Gift of Friendship*, 47.

114 Reinders, *Receiving the Gift of Friendship*, 25.

115 Reinders, *Receiving the Gift of Friendship*, 27.

116 Reinders, *Receiving the Gift of Friendship*, 90. See also the Vatican's *Donum Vitae: Instruction on Respect for Human Life in Its Origin and on the Dignity of Procreation* (London: Publications for the Holy See, 1987).

117 Reinders, *Receiving the Gift of Friendship*, 91–100.

118 Reinders, *Receiving the Gift of Friendship*, 101.

119 Reinders, *Receiving the Gift of Friendship*, 101–2.

120 Reinders, *Receiving the Gift of Friendship*, 227.

121 Reinders, *Receiving the Gift of Friendship*, 154, 280–84.

122 Reinders, *Receiving the Gift of Friendship*, 155.

123 Reinders, *Receiving the Gift of Friendship*, 238–44.

124 Reinders, *Receiving the Gift of Friendship*, 249–63.

125 Reinders, *Receiving the Gift of Friendship*, 256. Reinders does not defend Zizioulas' hotly contested interpretation of the Cappadocian fathers, but he does agree with it as a general truth. He also judiciously deals with many of the problems with the interpretation and cites the arguments against Zizioulas' view (263–72). I will not be taking up this argument in this text, as it goes beyond the scope of my intentions. My interaction with Reinders is to address his theological anthropology that has removed agency from its definition. However, I also have included his work because he confirms our direction to define the image of God relationally.

126 Reinders, *Receiving the Gift of Friendship*, 256–57.

127 Reinders, *Receiving the Gift of Friendship*, 258.

128 Reinders, *Receiving the Gift of Friendship*, 248, 254.

129 Reinders, *Receiving the Gift of Friendship*, 275.

130 Reinders, *Receiving the Gift of Friendship*, 273.

131 Reinders, *Receiving the Gift of Friendship*, 260, 267.

132 In the United States less than 5 percent of the population has an intellectual disability. See the National Disability Navigator's Population Specific Fact Sheet at https:// nationaldisabilitynavigator.org/ndnrc-materials/fact-sheets/population-specific-fact-sheet -intellectual-disability/, accessed May 25, 2020. Those with profound intellectual disabilities make up 1.5 percent of all cases those with intellectual disability. See again table 9-1 in section 9 of "Clinical Characteristics of Intellectual Disabilities" (link above). Disability conditions surely existed in the time when Scripture was written and when the Christian tradition developed. However, proper awareness and advocacy were not always present. Although current disability studies with its language, terms, and related laws, policies, and practices is a modern phenomenon, disability has been a condition that we have always had to face throughout time and across various sociocultural contexts. The canons of the church, including Scripture and writings of the saints, martyrs, confessors, and theologians, to our condemnation have been often too silent or prejudiced on these matters. Holy writ and the tradition need to be liberated from disabling constrictions they have socially placed on persons, and hermeneutically revisited in a new light that graciously shines on all persons. Even so, this approach would still involve accounting for the human experiences that stem from those who have rational-volitional agency and those who do not.

133 Miguel J. Romero, "Aquinas on the *Corporis Infirmitas*: Broken Flesh and the Grammar of Grace," in *Disability in the Christian Tradition: A Reader*, ed. Brian Brock and John Swinton (Grand Rapids: Eerdmans, 2012), 67–100.

134 Romero, "Aquinas on the *Corporis Infirmitas*," 89.

135 Romero, "Aquinas on the *Corporis Infirmitas*," 89.

136 Romero, "Aquinas on the *Corporis Infirmitas*," 89, in response to Reinders and citing Aquinas (contra Reinders, *Receiving the Gift of Friendship*, 22; cf. Aquinas, *Summa Theologica* 1.78.4, *response*).

137 Romero, "Aquinas on the *Corporis Infirmitas*," 89.

138 Romero, "Aquinas on the *Corporis Infirmitas*," 90.

139 Romero, "Aquinas on the *Corporis Infirmitas*," 87, citing Thomas Aquinas in the *Summa Theologica* (3.9; cf. *Summa Theologica* 1.45.7).

140 Romero, "Aquinas on the *Corporis Infirmitas*," 91.

141 Romero, "Aquinas on the *Corporis Infirmitas*," 87–88.

142 Romero, "Aquinas on the *Corporis Infirmitas*," 92.

143 Romero, "Aquinas on the *Corporis Infirmitas*," 96.

144 Romero, "Aquinas on the *Corporis Infirmitas*," 88.

145 Romero, "Aquinas on the *Corporis Infirmitas*," 89.

146 Romero, "Aquinas on the *Corporis Infirmitas*," 94.

147 Romero, "Aquinas on the *Corporis Infirmitas*," 94.

148 Romero, "Aquinas on the *Corporis Infirmitas*," 96 (3.26; *Summa Theologica* 1.45.7, *response*; 2–2.45.5; 3.4.1, reply 2; 3.6.2, *response*).

149 Romero, "Aquinas on the *Corporis Infirmitas*," 96–97.

150 Romero, "Aquinas on the *Corporis Infirmitas*," 99–101.

CHAPTER 4: THE RELATIONAL IMAGE OF GOD

1 Vladimir Lossky, *In the Image and Likeness of God* (Crestwood, N.Y.: St. Vladimir's Seminary Press, 1985), 115–22.

2 Marion's notion of saturated phenomena is developed throughout much of his corpus. See Jean-Luc Marion, *Being Given: Toward a Phenomenology of Givenness* (Stanford, Calif.: Stanford University Press, 2002); and *In Excess: Studies of Saturated Phenomena* (New York: Fordham University Press, 2004).

3 Classical liberalism is a case in point of a theological tradition that trusted in scientism and higher criticism to a level that it deflated its view of revelation. In turn, classical liberalism placed its epistemic weight on modern autonomous rationalism and its ethics on a Kantian deontological imperative to build the kingdom of God through social effort, resulting in deflated theologies that embraced low views of Scripture, Christology, soteriology, and other orthodox doctrines held by the Great Tradition.

4 The ontological difference is between uncreated being and created being.

5 Nor are we claiming that disability is solely social and never pathological and in need of medicine, help, healing, or any other form of amelioration, as we see in radical circles of the neurodiversity movement. We need to critique and change social structures that contribute to disability and mental disorders and provide accommodations, advocacy, and training to assist in moving toward higher function. Yet, to avoid all clinical aspects of intellectual, physical, and psychiatric disability and refuse treatment can result in negligence, malpractice, suffering, and further harm. Granted, not all persons with disabilities suffer or have a condition that is unwanted, but in many cases healing of all sorts is needed, wanted, and can be provided. For a critique of the neurodiversity perspective on autism, see Pier Jaarsma and Stellan Welin, "Autism as a Natural Human Variation: Reflections on the Claims of the Neurodiversity Movement," *Health Care Analysis* 20, no. 1 (2012): 20–30, doi: 10.1007/s10728-011-0169-9.

6 Hyperhuman states are those in which our radical weakness is revealed. Hyperhuman is really what it means to be truly human. However, we do not notice our weakness and need except in these hyperhuman conditions, or revelations of our true state as sentient dust. Hyperhuman states simply make clear what is always there—weakness and need for divine dependence. I am not using the description hyperhuman to refer to hyperrationality or to other human superlatives or to power structures, but rather, the opposite, as a description

of our frailty and our radical dependence on God. Christ in taking on created being touches us in our weakest and truest states in our humanity. Our true state as human is weakness where the camouflage and pretense of ability is disabled and removed. When God assumes flesh, he is assuming the furthest reaches and full expressions that make us human, including weakness, suffering, and death. Thus, ultimately our humanness is revealed in our frailty and even in death. Thus, we all are bearers of the hyperhuman, though many refuse to recognize it. The term merely means truly human without our fabricated fig leaves of power, knowledge, and ability to hide us.

7   The *epektasis* (Gregory of Nyssa) of approaching the infinity of God in our diastemic difference of created being has no limits. We are forever approaching.

8   Of course, Heidegger, probably most prominently, brought the notion of "ontological difference" to our attention. He distinguished between being (*Dasein*, or being there) and beings (*Das Seiende*). "Being is essentially different from a being, from beings." For Aquinas, the difference was between *that* something is and *what* something is—existence and essence.

9   Grenz, *Social God*, 204–5.

10   Grenz, *Social God*, 214. Grenz is citing Arthur Patzia.

11   Grenz, *Social God*, 208–9. Grenz is interpreting NT scholar J. B. Lightfoot.

12   Grenz, *Social God*, 209. Grenz is citing Kittel in his *Dictionary of the NT*, 2:395.

13   Grenz, *Social God*, 214. Grenz is citing F. F. Bruce, *Colossians, Philemon, Ephesians*, 57–58.

14   Randall E. Otto, "The *Imago Dei* as *Familitas*," *Journal of the Evangelical Theological Society* 35, no. 4 (1992): 503–13 (506). Otto gathers support from the Hebrew Bible and builds on Barth's relational view of the *imago*. He sees the second person as the image of the Father from eternity. He makes a case for the image of God ultimately in terms of *familitas*. The image of God is the eternal distinctions in the persons of the Father and the Son. The Father-Son relation is the "divine archetype of the image in mankind [*sic*]."

15   Aquinas, *Summa Theologiae* 1.28 and 35.1–2.

16   David Coffey understands that Aquinas holds a relational view of human personhood via participation existentially in divine being, a transcendental relation to God. Coffey, *Deus Trinitas: The Doctrine of the Triune God* (New York: Oxford University Press, 1999), 76–80.

17   I.e., "We might therefore summarize our 'Trinitarian concept of person' by saying that a person—whether divine or human—is an ontologically discrete, responsible subject of thought, act, and relationship, endowed with understanding and will, and therefore consciousness." Thomas R. Thompson and Cornelius Plantinga Jr., "Trinity and Kenosis," in *Exploring Kenotic Christology: The Self-Emptying of God*, ed. C. Stephen Evans (Vancouver, B.C.: Regent College, 2010), 181.

18   Augustine identified vestiges of the Trinity in the mind (*logos*), such as knowledge and love.

19   Maximus identified vestiges of the Trinity in the human spirit, such as knowledge and love.

20   Lars Thunberg, *Microcosm and Mediator: The Theological Anthropology of Maximus the Confessor*, 2nd ed. (Chicago: Open Court, 1995), 130–31.

21   It is debated which trinitarian model (social or psychological) is most conducive to a relational model. A social model of the Trinity is often thought of as more of a relational model but has its own controversies.

22   I am using *logos* in this context and often subsequently in the sense that Maximus the Confessor used the term in his doctrine of the *logoi*. The *logoi* were the divine ideas from the *Logos* that expressed the wisdom, reason, will, and purpose of God in every aspect of creation with each created being having its own *logos*. Yet, each *logos* comes from (*exitus*) and returns (*reditus*) to the one *Logos*. Throughout the *Philokalia* (texts 3–6), Maximus elaborates on how

human nature and the cosmos inhere or participate in the *Logos*. Human nature has a dependent, relational, participatory ontology that is the theme of the theological anthropology proposed in this work. The image of God involves participation in divine sonship.

23 Theological anthropologies that are accommodating and accessible for persons who experience disability and disorder rightly identify the problems with a structural *imago Dei* that is based on reason-volition or a functional model. These categories as the basis for determining a priori what is human create oppressive binaries that wrongfully qualify and disqualify. An inclusive definition of the human person cannot be based on human capacities that are not empirically universal. However, as a result there is often an overreaction and an attempt to disregard or eliminate a rational or functional component to our understanding of human experience for agentive persons. The position in this work is to acknowledge the qualities of reason, freedom, and moral agency as gifts to the image of God but to decenter these faculties as instruments of autonomy and achievement as ends in themselves and to relocate them in terms of virtue (humility) and their renewal in relation to the true *imago* Jesus Christ as sons and daughters born of the Spirit.

24 In Greek mythology, the Titans were the second-generation race of deities who preceded the Olympians. Some sources credit the Titans for creating the human race. Others account that humans were created out of the ashes of the Titans, inheriting their "titanic nature." In Plato it is seen as the evil disposition or proclivity in humans.

25 See James 3:13-18 for the fruit and virtue that accompany heavenly wisdom.

26 He identifies with those we have placed last in terms of reason (children), status (the poor), race (Gentiles, the excluded), morality (the worst of sinners), and ability (persons with disabilities).

27 For instance, Maximus the Confessor connects the mind (*nous*) as well as the will with image and the *logos* with likeness in the sense of fulfilling God's *logos* (God's wisdom, idea, purpose, and will) for humanity through *theosis*. Maximus draws from the Alexandrian school and Origen in seeing the image and likeness pointing to Sonship and sonship in us. For Maximus, the image and likeness refer to the whole person—specifically mind and will—but as subservient to a relationship in Christ that functions as a means to *theosis* that further serves as a function to mediate cosmic *theosis*. See Thunberg, *Microcosm and Mediator*, 78, 117, 122, 126.

28 Although this work is not about class or race and ethnicity (but at places intersects these), it is necessary to mention that Christ comes not only as disabled, disfigured, and disordered but also as poor and racially marginalized even as the black Christ. He identifies with what the world has oppressed and rejected. In terms of the blackness of God and Christ and its significance, see, for example, Kelly Brown Douglas, *The Black Christ* (Maryknoll, N.Y.: Orbis Books, 1993); James Cone, *A Black Theology of Liberation* (Maryknoll, N.Y.: Orbis Books, 2010); *The Cross and the Lynching Tree* (Maryknoll, N.Y.: Orbis Books, 2013); and Cornel West, *Prophesy Deliverance!* (Louisville, Ky.: Westminster John Knox, 2012).

29 Kevin J. Vanhoozer, "The Trials of Truth: Mission, Martyrdom, and the Epistemology of the Cross," in *To Stake a Claim: Mission and the Western Crisis of Knowledge*, ed. Kevin J. Vanhoozer and J. Andrew Kirk (Maryknoll, N.Y.: Orbis Books, 1999), 136–39.

30 Keener, *Mind of the Spirit*, 189–95.

31 Gregory Nazianzus, *Epistle 101*. The context in the epistle, though, is the controversy with the heresy of Apollinarius and his assertion that Christ did not have a rational human mind. The point is that Christ fully assumes all that is entailed in the human nature, so that we can be fully healed and redeemed.

32 "Transcendental signifier" is the term used by Hans Urs von Balthasar.

33 For more on the *analogia entis*, see the seminal work by Erich Przywara, *Analogia Entis*, trans. John R. Betz and David Bentley Hart (Grand Rapids: Eerdmans, 2014). See also Thomas Joseph White, ed., *The Analogy of Being: Invention of the Antichrist or the Wisdom of God?* (Grand Rapids: Eerdmans, 2010).

34 Hans Urs von Balthasar, *Theo-drama: Theological Dramatic Theory*, vol. 3, *Dramatis Personae: Persons in Christ* (San Francisco: Ignatius, 1992), 220–29.

35 *Enhypostasis*: (being or existing) in a hypostasis or person; participation or inherence; that which subsists. Derived from Shults, *Reforming Theological Anthropology*, 150; and Alexi Nestruk, "The Universe as Hypostatic Inherence in the Logos of God," in Clayton and Peacocke, *In Whom We Live and Move and Have Our Being*, 172.

36 Paraphrasing Athanasius, *On the Incarnation* (Yonkers, N.Y.: St. Vladimir's Seminary Press, 1993), 54.

37 We see this relational turn beginning with Buber's *I and Thou* and Levinas' notion of the Other and alterity. See also Shults, *Reforming Theological Anthropology*, for a thorough account of the theological turn to relationality. He reviews historical and existing models for theological anthropology, but stakes a claim for a relational perspective, tracing its historical roots and working deeply with Barth and Pannenberg.

38 See Keith and Keith, *Intellectual Disability*, 87, 90–95; George Herbert Mead, *Mind, Self and Society*, ed. C. Morris (Chicago, Ill.: University of Chicago Press, 1934). Heather Keith and Kenneth Keith, intellectual disability scholars, stress the need to return to a relational notion of the human person and its emphasis on empathy. They trace this relational turn to the symbolic interactionism of George Herbert Mead. Mead contended that we are social beings that are formed and relate through the social construction, interaction, and interpretation of meaning mediated through symbolism. Empathy arises when one takes on the attitude of another that informs one's own self-construction. Social relationships form the person. For Mead, the self is not autonomous but emerges out of social relationships, and primarily the family, which is more evident, for example, in Asian cultures that build the notion of person on family and the larger society. Engagement, especially moral engagement, that considers the human person and disability needs to be grounded in relationality over rationality (Keith and Keith, *Intellectual Disability*, 110, 135).

39 Grenz, *Social God*, 162–66.

40 Shults, *Reforming Theological Anthropology*, 117.

41 Shults, *Reforming Theological Anthropology*, 118.

42 Shults, *Reforming Theological Anthropology*, 120–23. Interpreted from Barth, *Church Dogmatics*, III/1, cf. note 670.

43 This class debate between Barth and Brunner on natural theology and between Barth and Erich Przywara and Hans Urs von Balthasar on the *analogia fidei* vs. *analogia entis* reflects a classic tension between models of revelation and metaphysics. Because of the former, Barth sees no room for the latter. Barth's interlocutors, Przywara and Balthasar, likewise claim the primacy of revelation but in light of the analogical structure and ontological difference between uncreated being and created being. It is important to note that even Przywara and Balthasar slightly differed in their version of the doctrine. See White, *Analogy of Being*; and Emil Brunner and Karl Barth, *Natural Theology* (Eugene, Ore.: Wipf and Stock, 2002). Erich Przywara's *Analogia Entis* is his magnum opus and also reflects his ongoing debate with Karl Barth on the subject.

44 Shults, *Reforming Theological Anthropology*, 124–27.

45 For a contemporary and erudite interpretation of the *analogia entis*, see David Bentley Hart, *The Beauty of the Infinite: The Aesthetics of Christian Truth* (Grand Rapids: Eerdmans, 2002), 241–49.

46 For a good introduction to the topic, see the essay by John Betz entitled "After Barth: A New Introduction to Erich Przywara's *Analogia Entis*," in White, *Analogy of Being*.

47 Balthasar, *Theo-drama*, 3:220–22.

48 Erich Przywara and Hans Urs von Balthasar spent considerable time in dialogue and correspondence with Barth on this point, trying to clarify what they considered his misunderstanding of the *analogia entis*. Barth never conceded but in part developed and modified his *analogia fidei* in respect to those conversations. For continued contemporary debate on the topic, see White, *Analogy of Being*.

49 See the translator's introduction, in Erich Przywara's *Analogia Entis*, 106. Betz, reflecting on Przywara, declares, "Creation is a revelation."

50 Maximus the Confessor understood the revelation of the *logos* in creation as an anticipation of the *Logos* that would become flesh. In *Ambiguum* 33, Maximus interprets a phrase from Gregory of Nazianzus, "The Word becomes thick," as referring to three manifestions of the Word revealed through the *logoi* in creation. These three "manifestations" are seen as revelations even prefiguring, or serving as types of, the incarnation. Maximus understood the Word taking on form through the *logoi* in creation (the spiritual essence of created beings), through the *logoi* of Scripture, and in the flesh in Jesus Christ. All of creation is designed and directed proleptically by the *Logos* to lead up to the incarnation. Lars Thunberg called it a "threefold-incarnation" and later a "threefold-embodiment," and Paul Blowers, "three incarnations" (cited in Tollefsen, *Christocentric Cosmology*, 67n). Tollefsen understands these manifestations as a gradual revelation of the mystery of Christ, and I concur. He claims, "The divine economy, according to Maximus, is expressed and fulfilled by a threefold presence of the Logos: in the cosmos, in Scripture, and in the historical person of Jesus Christ." Tollefsen is careful to use the term "embodiment" and "incarnation" figuratively for the *Logos* in creation and Scripture and notes that this "is a metaphorical usage of the terms." These "embodiments" are "effected" through the *logoi*. Torstein Tollefsen, *The Christocentric Cosmology of Maximus the Confessor* (Oxford: Oxford University Press, 2008), 66–67.

51 Jordan Daniel Wood, "Creation Is Incarnation: The Metaphysical Peculiarity of the *Logoi* in Maximus Confessor," *Modern Theology* 34, no. 1 (2018): 82–102, doi: 10.1111/moth.12382.

52 Hart, *Beauty of the Infinite*, 242.

53 Stephen Lawson, "The Incarnation in the Theology of Maximus the Confessor" (paper given at Stone-Campbell Journal Conference, April 14, 2012), https://www.academia.edu/1964198/The_Incarnation_in_the_Theology_of_Maximus_the_Confessor.

54 Thomas Joseph White, "Through Him All Things Were Made (John 1:3)," in White, *Analogy of Being*, 249–50. Lawson, in "Incarnation in the Theology of Maximus the Confessor," cites Blowers' *Spiritual Pedagogy*, 118. On the connection between the *Logos* of creation and the *Logos* of incarnation, Blowers states, "The historical incarnation is not merely another provisional economy but carries in itself, from the beginning of time, the eschatological key both to the destiny of creation and the fulfillment of Scripture."

55 John Zizioulas, *Being and Communion* (Yonkers, N.Y.: St. Vladimir's Seminary Press, 1997).

56 Zizioulas, *Being and Communion*, 39.

57 Zizioulas, *Being and Communion*, 50. Defining the human person is a tense and complex debate. In this work we are defining the image of God relationally and integrally. In terms of the human person, the biological minimum is that the human person is a living organism with the biology that we have distinguished as human and at the center a human brain that has activity (brain waves) that is ultimately needed for consciousness and all of the biological functions and processes of embodied consciousness. Some define the biological

minimum of the human person in terms of when life begins, which is ardently debated. At what point does the organism have the intrinsic powers for self-development? Positions range from fertilization (zygote), to brain waves, consciousness, sentience, breathing, autonomous breathing, or some other degree of development. We debate when life begins, but legally we know that life ends when brain waves cease, brain death. Some assert the converse, then, that life begins with brain waves, while others debate this assertion. They claim that the significance and quality of fetal brain waves and adult brain waves are not synonymous. Regardless, we need to acknowledge that all life develops and is in development. Development does not disqualify life but qualifies it.

58   Zizioulas, *Being and Communion*, 106.

59   Zizioulas, *Being and Communion*, 106.

60   Zizioulas, *Being and Communion*, 107.

61   Zizioulas, *Being and Communion*, 91.

62   Levinas, *Otherwise Than Being or Beyond Essence*.

63   The analogy is along the line of love between the persons. The utter dissimilarity of humanity in relation and divinity in relation is noted in the nature of subsistent relations within the divine being as opposed to the relationship between contingent persons.

64   Philipp W. Rosemann, *Peter Lombard* (Oxford: Oxford University Press, 2004), 113.

65   See Amos Yong's *Theology and Down Syndrome* and his argument that intellectual and other disabilities, which define one's identity, may remain following the resurrection (261–92).

66   The argument goes that eschatological healing will not change our fundamental identity. For example, having Down syndrome is strongly connected with someone's identity, sense of themselves, and the experience that others have of them. To change this condition is to change the person's fundamental identity. I believe that to be the nature and purpose of salvation—to change us from the old creation to the new creation in which it is no longer I that live but Christ that lives in me. In terms of mental disorders, though not all suffer, most do not want the experiences that such disorders bring internally and externally. They seek healing. Also, though there is genetic influence, a mental disorder usually does not manifest at birth. Disorders manifest later in life, brought on by environmental factors. One is not born with these conditions. Further, regardless of the ailment, Christ came to heal. His normative response to all persons afflicted by sin or other ailments was healing.

67   See Andrew Louth, *Maximus the Confessor* (New York: Routledge, 1996), *Ambiguum* 41, 155–62; and Maximos (Maximus) the Confessor, *On Difficulties in Sacred Scripture: The Responses to Thalassios* (*Quaest. ad. Thal.*), trans. Fr. Maximos Constas (Washington, D.C.: Catholic University of America Press, 2018), 48 and 63.

68   *Différance* is Jacques Derrida's coining for the difference and deferral of meaning, which I interpret more as shared meaning rather than as an infinite deferral of meaning with no yield.

69   Although ability is not normative, this text uses the term *disability* for facility of use because of its familiarity, not seeking to introduce new nomenclature in this work. We all have limited ability. Thus, all of our ability and disability is relative.

70   For a thorough treatment of disability from a medical and social standpoint, see David Wasserman, Adrienne Asch, Jeffrey Blustein, and Daniel Putnam, "Disability: Definitions, Models, Experience," in *The Stanford Encyclopedia of Philosophy*, ed. Edward N. Zalta, summer 2016 ed., accessed November 1, 2019, https://plato.stanford.edu/archives/sum2016/entries/disability/.

71   For a moderating view between a medical and a social model of disability, see T. Koch, "Disability and Difference: Balancing Social and Physical Constructions," *Journal of*

Medical Ethics 27, no. 6 (2001): 370–76. See also Sara Goering, "Rethinking Disability: The Social Model of Disability and Chronic Disease," *Current Reviews in Musculoskeletal Medicine* 8, no. 2 (2015): 134–38, doi: 10.1007/s12178-015-9273-z.

72 While the traditional view of creation has been *creatio ex nihilo*, attempts have been made to reconcile these accounts with the laws of physics, resulting in a denial of the doctrine. Others deny the doctrine by claiming it is unbiblical and stems from attempts in the second century to respond to Gnosticism and Middle Platonism. Some would hold that creation has always come from something preexistent and that the universe is still cocreating alongside God in a panetheistic universe (*creatio continua*). For a variety of perspectives on the subject see Thomas Oord, ed., *Theologies of Creation: Creatio Ex Nihilo and Its New Rivals* (New York: Routledge, 2015). Often in these essays the concept of "nothing" or "nothingness" is redefined to account for cosmologies found in modern physics. Theological problems arise with creation from preexistence, such as the origin of anything preexistent. From where did it come? Can something exist without God creating it? Is that something eternal? Is that something divine? Is the universe divine (pantheism)?

73 Kallistos Ware, "God Immanent yet Transcendent," in Clayton and Peacocke, *In Whom We Live and Move and Have Our Being*, 159–61. Philip Clayton, "Kenotic Trinitarian Panentheism," *Dialog* 44, no. 3 (2005): 250–55, https://doi.org/10.1111/j.0012-2033.2005.00265.x. This author does not hold to an open view of God or a panentheism held by these authors but hypothesizes perhaps a metaphorical kenosis in creation as a nondualistic, preontological *nihil* from which God kenotically makes space for creation. God is over both being and nonbeing. Others, such as Isaac Luria (from Jewish Kabbalah) and Jürgen Moltmann, hold a view called *zimsum* or *zimzum* that is God's self-contraction and limitation, in which God withdraws God's self to make space, the *nihil*, for created beings to exist. See Jürgen Moltmann, *God in Creation: A Theology of Creation and the Spirit of God* (New York: Harper & Row, 1991), 86–93. Regardless, any type of kenosis cannot violate the nature of divine simplicity and immutability.

74 See Kierkegaard's *Concept of Anxiety*.

75 See Sartre's notion from *Being and Nothingness* that man [sic] has no essence prior to his existence, and so in order to be he must nihilate his essence of nothingness by choosing to become.

76 See Derrida's famous dictum that "nothing exists outside of the text."

77 Meontology is the philosophical study of nonbeing. In one sense, in the ontological difference, God's being is nonbeing from our perspective. God is what we are not.

78 Speaking of God in terms of being is analogical. In one sense God is actually above being and nonbeing, as hyperousia, hyperessence, or supraessence.

79 Throughout Scripture there are at least two kinds of fear. The first type as referenced in Hebrews 2:15 speaks to the fear of death and condemnation upon the one who has not received pardon and justification, owing to the judgment of sin. The second type of fear is a holy respect and awe of God that inspires obedience.

80 We will examine the natural etiology of mental disorder through the work of Søren Kierkegaard and Paul Tillich in the next chapter.

81 This is the language used by John Wesley to describe human depravity.

82 This is is a term coined by Martin Luther (Heidelberg Disputation, 1518) that became one of the primary lenses through which Luther understood the various loci of theology. A theology of the cross refers to how we know God. We truly only know God as he is revealed as the suffering and crucified One. We do not know him through a theology of human glory, expressed in human reason, power, and ability. A theology of glory holds that humans can

still choose and do good, and that human reason can still function to know God without the need of being transformed by God's grace.

83 See Nancy L. Eiesland, *The Disabled God: Toward a Liberation Theology of Disability* (Nashville, Tenn.: Abingdon, 1994) for a modern post–Civil Rights treatment of disability justice in light of the crucified God.

CHAPTER 5: THEOLOGICAL TYPE 1—THE NATURAL

1 Søren Kierkegaard, *The Concept of Anxiety*, ed. and trans. Reidar Thomte (Princeton, N.J.: Princeton University Press, 1980), 61.

2 Rollo May, *Man's Search for Himself* (New York: Norton, 1953), 40.

3 Kierkegaard, historical introduction to *Concept of Anxiety*, xii–xiii.

4 Kierkegaard, "Papirer II A)" (May 1839), 420, quoted in Kierkegaard, *Concept of Anxiety*, xiii.

5 Kierkegaard, *Concept of Anxiety*, xvi.

6 Kierkegaard, *Concept of Anxiety*, xvi.

7 Kierkegaard, *Concept of Anxiety*, 44–45.

8 Kierkegaard, *Concept of Anxiety*, 54.

9 Kierkegaard, *Concept of Anxiety*, 77.

10 Is it improper, inhuman, or unethical to suggest that suffering or mental disorder can be pedagogical? Or further, is it unethical that those who suffer from any disability should be viewed as an object for the teaching or inspiration of others, specifically the abled? In this case, Kierkegard puts all of humanity in the same category. There is no "us and them." Existential anxiety is a universal condition that we all must face and learn from or fall to, according to Kierkegaard.

11 Kierkegaard, *Concept of Anxiety*, 156.

12 Kierkegaard, *Concept of Anxiety*, 156.

13 Kierkegaard, *Concept of Anxiety*, 157.

14 Kierkegaard, *Concept of Anxiety*, 158–59.

15 Kierkegaard, *Concept of Anxiety*, 159.

16 C. S. Lewis, *The Problem of Pain* (San Francisco: HarperCollins, 1940), 91.

17 Lewis, *Problem of Pain*, 93.

18 The bifurcation of depression into mild and major types, or similar iterations, will be identified throughout this work. The former is often understood as potentially constructive, adaptive, and even educative, while the latter is destructive, maladaptive, and detrimental.

19 Carl T. Bergstrom and Frazer Meacham, "Depression and Anxiety: Maladaptive Byproducts of Adaptive Mechanisms," *Evolution, Medicine, and Public Health* 2016, no. 1 (2016): 214.

20 Bergstrom and Meacham, "Depression and Anxiety," 214.

21 For more on Augustine's interpretation of Romans 5, see Benjamin Myers, "A Tale of Two Gardens: Augustine's Narrative Interpretation of Romans 5," in *Apocalyptic Paul: Cosmos and Anthropos in Romans 5–8*, ed. Beverly Roberts Gaventa (Waco, Tex.: Baylor University Press, 2013), 39–58.

22 A thesis of a theology of genetic science is that the course of natural selection itself is responsible for the transmission of original sin, and redemption involves the human ability to act counter to natural selection. See Christian de Duve and Neil Patterson, *Genetics of Original Sin: The Impact of Natural Selection on the Future of Humanity* (New Haven, Conn.: Yale University Press, 2012).

23 This notion is also the thesis behind Matthew S. Stanford, *The Biology of Sin: Grace, Hope, and Healing for Those Who Feel Trapped* (Downers Grove, Ill.: InterVarsity, 2010). This work seeks to show the neural correlates for sinful behavior, defining sin in terms of biblical prohibitions.

24 Stanford, *Biology of Sin*, 136–37. In my years as a pastor, I had counseled persons whose sinful choices to be angry and violent contributed to their anxiety and depression in terms of living with the consequences of domestic violence. I have counseled others whose OCD and bipolar disorder contributed to a lack of impulse control that fed into addictive-sinful behaviors that had further damaging consequences, hijacking the nucleus accumbens (the so-called pleasure center) and the hippocampus (responsible for memory and learning), hence the neuroscience of addiction.

25 There are various theological interpretations of original sin or ancestral sin. For example, Eastern Orthodox tradition holds to a notion of ancestral sin that does not involve seminal or federal participation in Adam's sin, nor does it hold to the view that humanity is culpable, guilty, and punished for Adam's sin. Adam and Eve are alone fully responsible for their choice. The inherited consequence is a proclivity to depravity or rather moral sickness. For an Eastern Orthodox view of the fall, see Clark Carlton, *The Faith: Understanding Orthodox Christianity, an Orthodox Catechism* (Salisbury, Mass.: Regina Orthodox Press, 1997), 79–90. John Wesley adapted Augustine's view of original sin from more of a federal headship standpoint. Wesley believed that through prevenient grace, the universal benefits of the atonement granted that humanity be cleansed of the guilt of original sin by the merits of Christ's atoning death. See Wesley's "Treatise on Baptism," sermon 44 "Original Sin," and his work *The Doctrine of Original Sin*, all from *The Works of the Rev. John Wesley*, ed. Thomas Jackson, 14 vols. (London: Wesleyan Conference Office, 1872). For a theological history of the doctrine of original sin, though primarily from a Western perspective, see Tatha Wiley, *Original Sin: Origins, Developments, Contemporary Meanings* (Mahwah, N.J.: Paulist, 2002).

26 For an examination of Scripture regarding the connection between sin and sickness, see Yong, *Theology and Down Syndrome*, 21–44.

27 For a thorough critique of the thesis that sickness is the result of sin and judgment, see Fredrick Lindstrom, *Suffering and Sin: Interpretations of Illness in the Individual Complaint Psalms* (Uppsala: Almqvist & Wiksell, 1994).

28 Marcia Webb in *Toward a Theology of Psychological Disorder* (Eugene, Ore.: Wipf and Stock, 2017) makes the claim that the exorcisms performed by Jesus in the Gospels alleviated physical illnesses rather than mental ones. Although she addresses the case of the Gadarene demoniac in the Synoptics, she does not make the specific connection that after Jesus expelled the demons, it was said that the man was "clothed and in his right mind," *sōphronounta*, σωφρονοῦντα, meaning "a sound mind." At least the narrator's assessment was that mental instability was part of the problem but now was no longer an issue (Mark 5:15 and Luke 8:35). One of the main apologetic arguments in Webb's work is to disconnect mental disorders from selfishness, sickness, or demonic activity, either by causation or correlation. I believe the scriptural evidence makes it difficult to identify any one single cause or correlation or even a single rule of interpretation as to causation or correlation because it seems to give mixed (i.e., a variety of) readings. However, I think it is just as difficult to rule out absolutely any causation or correlation based on scriptural grounds as well.

29 Yong, *Theology and Down Syndrome*, 25. Yong holds that "Jesus' healing narratives served to perpetuate, at least implicitly, the ancient Hebraic beliefs regarding the connections between 'disability' and sin, impurity, and disorder."

30 William L. Lane, *The Gospel of Mark*, New International Commentary on the New Testament (Grand Rapids: Eerdmans, 1974), 331. Lane confirms that the illness was most likely epilepsy but that the illness was connected to demonic influence.

31 For a thorough treatment of the possible existence of the demonic, the need for exorcism, and discerning between demonic manifestations and mental health issues, see Peter J. Bellini, *Unleashed! The C1-13 Integrative Deliverance Needs Assessment: A Qualitative and Quantitative Probability Indicator* (Eugene, Ore.: Wipf and Stock, 2018).

32 Marcia Webb in *Toward a Theology of Psychological Disorder* cites the Job narrative as an exception to the absolute claim that sickness is due to judgment for sin, thus relativizing the claim.

33 I believe John Christopher Thomas comes to a similar conclusion in ch. 8 of his work *The Devil, Disease, and Deliverance: Origins of Illness in New Testament Thought* (Sheffield, UK: Sheffield Academic, 1998), 296–309, specifically 296–97.

34 Webb, *Toward a Theology of Psychological Disorder*, 47.

35 Webb, *Toward a Theology of Psychological Disorder*, 48–50.

36 Webb, *Toward a Theology of Psychological Disorder*, 55–57.

37 See several notes above on Marcia Webb.

38 Yong, *Theology and Down Syndrome*, 158–69.

39 Yong, *Theology and Down Syndrome*, 158–69.

40 For example, this case is made by Thomas in *The Devil, Disease, and Deliverance*, 297–309. Yong, in *Theology and Down Syndrome*, 21–28, also notes that both the Old and New Testaments often perpetuate the idea that disabilities are connected with the divine, sin, or the demonic, though Yong is not advancing that connection in his theology. He also recognizes that the Scriptures bless and honor persons with disabilities. They are "made special objects of divine care" and are welcomed in the kingdom as well.

41 Reinders, *Disability, Providence, and Ethics*, 9.

42 Reinders, *Disability, Providence, and Ethics*, 9–13. Religion, and particularly Christian theology, has often not fared well in trying to address the issues of disability and divine providence.

43 Kierkegaard, as well as Nietzsche, Heidegger, Sartre, and other existentialists, influenced Tillich's understanding of existential anxiety.

44 For a further analysis of Tillich's notion of existential anxiety, see Carl F. Weems, Natalie M. Costa, Christopher Dehon, and Steven L. Berman, "Paul Tillich's Theory of Existential Anxiety: A Preliminary Conceptual and Empirical Examination," *Anxiety, Stress & Coping: An International Journal* 17, no. 4 (2004): 383–99.

45 E.g., Madeline Kretschmer and Lance Storm, "The Relationships of the Five Existential Concerns with Depression and Existential Thinking," *International Journal of Existential Psychology & Psychotherapy* 7, no. 1 (2017).

46 Rollo May similarly holds that anxiety is structural to being human. His view is comparable to modern perspectives in evolutionary psychology that understand anxiety as essential for survival and growth in challenging environments. Proper response to anxiety fosters human self-realization. His classic treatise *The Meaning of Anxiety* covers the modern evolution of the term and its treatment from both philosophical and psychological perspectives. Rollo May, *The Meaning of Anxiety*, rev. ed. (New York: W. W. Norton, 2015).

47 Tillich's work is also understood as foundational to the genesis of the new field experimental existential psychology that holds that, for persons struggling to deal with the larger existential questions of life, such questions drive how they think and act. Such work analyzes core and peripheral threats in life and how one responds to and copes with such existential threats. Daniel Sullivan and Mark Landau, "Toward a Comprehensive Understanding of Existential Threat: Insights from Paul Tillich," *Social Cognition* 30, no. 6 (2012): 734–57 (734–35).

48 Meontology is the philosophical study of nonbeing.
49 Paul Tillich, *The Courage to Be* (New Haven, Conn.: Yale University Press, 1952), 32.
50 Tillich, *Courage to Be*, 35.
51 Tillich, *Courage to Be*, 35.
52 Tillich, *Courage to Be*, 39.
53 Sullivan and Landau, "Toward a Comprehensive Understanding," 737.
54 Tillich, *Courage to Be*, 35.
55 Tillich, *Courage to Be*, 38.
56 Sullivan and Landau, "Toward a Comprehensive Understanding," 738.
57 Sullivan and Landau, "Toward a Comprehensive Understanding," 738.
58 Tillich, *Courage to Be*, 39.
59 Tillich, *Courage to Be*, 41.
60 Tillich, *Courage to Be*, 66. See also Susan Iacovu, "What Is the Difference between Existential Anxiety and So-Called Neurotic Anxiety?" *Existential Analysis: Journal of the Society for Existential Analysis* 22, no. 2 (2011): 356–67.
61 Tillich, *Courage to Be*, 66.
62 Tillich, *Courage to Be*, 66.
63 Sullivan and Landau, "Toward a Comprehensive Understanding," 738.
64 Kierkegaard, *Concept of Anxiety*, 159. Tillich, *Courage to Be*, 69.
65 Tillich, *Courage to Be*, 72.
66 Tillich, *Courage to Be*, 87–88.
67 Tillich, *Courage to Be*, 89.
68 Paul Tillich, *Systematic Theology*, vol. 1 (Chicago: University of Chicago Press, 1951), 176.
69 Tillich, *Systematic Theology*, 1:171.
70 Of course, Tillich's version of theism deviates from the orthodox notion that we have accepted and have been working with throughout this work.
71 Tillich, *Courage to Be*, 186–87.
72 John Macquarrie and Laurence Paul Hemming have both noted the influence. Stuart Elden, "To Say Nothing of God: Heidegger's Holy Atheism," *Heythrop Journal* 45, no. 3 (2004): 344–48, https://doi.org/10.1111/j.1468-2265.2004.00259.x. See also Thomas F. O'Meara, O.P., "Tillich and Heidegger: A Structural Relationship," *Harvard Theological Review* 61, no 2 (1968). Also, John Caputo, in *Transcendence and Beyond*, 214–15, cites more classical influences like Augustine, Meister Eckhart, Kant, Hegel, and Schelling, among others. See Caputo, *Transcendence and Beyond: A Postmodern Inquiry*, ed. John D. Caputo and Michael J. Scanlon (Bloomington: Indiana University Press, 2007).
73 Tillich, *Courage to Be*, 155.
74 Tillich, *Courage to Be*, 39.
75 Tillich, *Courage to Be*, 66.
76 Sullivan and Landau, "Toward a Comprehensive Understanding," 745.
77 Tillich, *Courage to Be*, 66.
78 Tillich, *Courage to Be*, 171–86.
79 Tillich, *Courage to Be*, 184.
80 Tillich, *Courage to Be*, 185.
81 Problems with modern and postmodern epistemology of theology and their various deflationary ontologies (metaphysical, epistemological, and semantic problems with reality or the real) have been addressed by a variety of schools, including Radical Orthodoxy, Canonical Theism, and others. See also Bellini, *Participation*.

CHAPTER 6: THEOLOGICAL TYPE 2—THE CONSEQUENTIAL

1 Gabriel Bunge, *Despondency: The Spiritual Teaching of Evagrius Ponticus on Acedia* (Yonkers, N.Y.: St. Vladimir's Seminary Press, 2011), 11.

2 Bunge, *Despondency*, 12.

3 Bunge, *Despondency*, 13.

4 Bunge, *Despondency*, 13.

5 Bunge, *Despondency*, 14.

6 Bunge, *Despondency*, 14.

7 Controversy remains around the condemned teachings, regarding whether they were actually Origen's or only associated, rightfully or not, with Origen.

8 Feld, *Melancholy and the Otherness of God*, 15. Raposa, *Boredom and the Religious Imagination*.

9 Evagrius Ponticus, *The Praktikos and Chapters on Prayer*, trans. John Eudes Bamberger, 2nd ed. (Kalamazoo, Mich.: Cistercian, 1972), 16–17.

10 Bunge, *Despondency*, 24.

11 Bunge, *Despondency*, 26.

12 Feld, *Melancholy and the Otherness of God*, 16.

13 Since the Scientific Revolution and the Enlightenment following, the church in the West has been reticent to give credence to the supernatural and so has not worked out of supernatural categories, including demonology. However, with the explosion of the church in the global South and East, there has been a rise in spirit worldviews. A spirit worldview would be one in which the existence of an invisible spirit world inhabited by spirit beings, such as angels, demons, gods, God and the like are affirmed. In many of these regions of the world modernity has not influenced worldview as much as in the West with its reliance on reason and science. It will be interesting how Western impact on the South and the East through globalization will affect majority worldviews in the future and vice versa. Yet even in the West certain traditions in the church still acknowledge the reality of the supernatural, e.g., Pentecostalism, Roman Catholicism, and Eastern Orthodoxy. These traditions hold a worldview that integrates both spirit and matter and the invisible and visible in one overall reality. The justification may be from a literal reading of Scripture or a literal reading of Scripture coupled with a theology that has been influenced highly by metaphysics as in versions of Thomism.

14 *De vitiis quae opposite sun virtutibus* [On the vices that are opposed to the virtues], quoted in Bunge, *Despondency*, 65.

15 Bunge, *Despondency*, 65–85.

16 Bunge, *Despondency*, 69.

17 George Tsakiridis, *Evagrius Ponticus and Cognitive Science: A Look at Moral Evil and the Thoughts* (Eugene, Ore.: Wipf and Stock, 2010); Alexis Trader, *Ancient Christian Wisdom and Aaron Beck's Cognitive Therapy: A Meeting of Minds*, American University Series (New York: Peter Lang, 2012).

18 Bunge, *Despondency*, 55–56.

19 Bunge, *Despondency*, 55.

20 Bunge, *Despondency*, 57.

21 Feld, *Melancholy and the Otherness of God*, 18.

22 See Peter J. Bellini, *Truth Therapy: Renewing the Mind with the Word of God* (Eugene, Ore.: Wipf and Stock, 2014). *Truth Therapy* is a work in discipleship that employs belief and identity formation integrated with cognitive behavioral theory to create a strategy of spiritual

formation that is based on renewing the mind through basic Christian truth. This text also employs a strategy to identify and modify unwanted thoughts. The author employs an acrostic as a method, M.E.E.T., with M meaning the monitoring of thoughts; the first E meaning the evaluation of thoughts; the second E signifying the expelling of unwanted thinking; and, finally, T standing for the truth (replacing unwanted thoughts with the truth).

23 Feld, *Melancholy and the Otherness of God*, 18.

24 See Rieff, *Triumph of the Therapeutic*.

25 See D. Lynch, K. R. Laws, and P. J. McKenna, "Cognitive Behavioral Therapy for Major Psychiatric Disorder: Does It Really Work? A Meta-analytical Review of Well-Controlled Trials," *Psychological Medicine* 40, no. 1 (2010): 9–24; and Tom J. Johnsen and Oddgeir Friborg, "The Effects of Cognitive Behavioral Therapy as an Anti-depressive Treatment Is Falling: A Meta-analysis," *Psychological Bulletin* 141, no. 4 (2015): 747–68.

26 Bunge, *Despondency*, 94.

27 Bunge, *Despondency*, 107, 137. *Antirrhetikos* was also the title of a work written by Evagrius that addresses the issue of "talking back" to the devil and one's mind in spiritual combat against evil thoughts.

28 Bunge, *Despondency*, 137.

29 See Bellini, *Truth Therapy*. Scriptural names for God, scriptural affirmations, and basic Christian doctrine are used to help the reader renew their mind with the Word of God in order to experience transformation. The Word of God is integral to renewing the mind, a vital process to becoming a new creation.

30 Social organizations such as NAMI and church small groups for those with mental disorders and their families and friends are on the rise in an effort to provide the sociosystemic support needed. Laws such as the Americans with Disabilities Act are working to make changes systemically through legislation to provide advocacy and support.

31 See Bellini, *Unleashed!*

32 Stephen Hawking, *The Grand Design* (New York: Bantam, 2010).

33 For a formidable response to this claim see William Abraham's trilogy *Divine Agency and Divine Action*.

34 The *Internet Encyclopedia of Philosophy* states, "We could say that a property is emergent if it is a novel property of a system or an entity that arises when that system or entity has reached a certain level of complexity and that, even though it exists only insofar as the system or entity exists, it is distinct from the properties of the parts of the system from which it emerges." *Internet Encyclopedia of Philosophy: A Peer-Reviewed Academic Resource*, accessed June 21, 2018, https://www.iep.utm.edu/emergenc/. *The Stanford Encyclopedia of Philosophy* claims that "a property is said to be emergent if it is a new outcome of some other properties of the system and their interaction, while it is itself different from them." Timothy O'Connor and Yu Wong Hong, "Emergent Properties," in *The Stanford Encyclopedia of Philosophy*, ed. Edward N. Zalta, summer 2015 ed., accessed June 20, 2018, https://plato.stanford.edu/archives/sum2015/entries/properties-emergent/.

35 Jaegwon Kim, "Multiple Realization and the Metaphysics of Reduction," in *Philosophy of Mind: A Guide and Anthology*, ed. John Heil (Oxford: Oxford University Press, 2004), 726–48.

36 Paul Churchland, "Eliminative Materialism and the Propositional Attitudes," in Heil, *Philosophy of Mind*, 382–400.

37 See chapters 2 and 3 for detailed analysis of these problems.

38 See some of the integrative work of John Polkinghorne, Philip Clayton, Robert J. Russell, Alexei Nestruk, Arthur Peacocke, and others.

39 The problem of impassibility is addressed in ch. 8.

40 Clayton, *Adventures in the Spirit*, 128.

41 Although I have included and respect the interdisciplinary attempts of open and process theologians at reconciling theology and science, I personally find many problems with both an open and a process view of God. While I respect open and process theologians' attempts at reconciling their faith with science, I think they have compromised classical, orthodox, Nicene Christianity for the sake of congruence with the latest scientific theories and models. I appreciate their sincerity and interest in the coherent and comprehensive nature of truth across disciplines. However, in an effort to work the cosmic puzzle and fit the pieces of Christian dogma and contemporary science together, the teaching of the church gets altered beyond its scriptural and historical recognition, a concession I am not willing to make for a field that is constantly in flux and currently bound by quantum indeterminacy. Also, sound arguments from free will theists like Alvin Plantinga and others have responded responsibly to the challenge of the problem of evil without needing to resort to an open theism. I have included their reconciling attempts to show some of the efforts to move theologically beyond reductive and eliminative physicalism.

42 Clayton, *Adventures in the Spirit*, 14. Spirit reality is seen as an emergent property, like consciousness.

43 "Renewalist" is the singular term used by missiologists to identify the broad-based and highly differentiated Pentecostal-charismatic movements in the global South. Renewalist Christians are those that emphasize primacy of the person and work of the Holy Spirit for faith and practice.

44 E.g., see the work of Pentecostal NT scholar Craig Keener, specifically his comprehensive two-volume set *Miracles: The Credibility of the New Testament Accounts* (Grand Rapids: Baker, 2011) for a biblical, philosophical, religious experience, and testimonial defense of the supernatural that involves divine agency and interaction within a "supernatural" or spirit worldview.

45 As an exception and an example of Pentecostal theology engaging modern science, see James K. A. Smith and Amos Yong, eds., *Science and the Spirit: A Pentecostal Engagement with the Sciences* (Bloomington: Indiana University Press, 2010); Yong, *Spirit of Creation*. However, there have been stinging critiques of Yong and others who have sought to integrate a Pentecostal spirit worldview with emergence, claiming that such moves actually break the laws of emergence and supervenience with property dualist interactionism creating downward causation and thus interdependence, as opposed to supervenience. See Mikael Leidenhag and Joanna Leidenhag, "Science and Spirit: A Critical Examination of Amos Yong's Pneumatological Theology of Emergence," *Open Theology* 1 (October 2015): 425–35, https://doi.org/10.1515/opth-2015-0025. Questions such as whether emergent spirit models contradict the principles of emergence by ultimately claiming downward causation (violating causal closure) and interactionism need to be addressed.

46 See Bellini, *Unleashed!*

47 Bellini, *Unleashed!*

48 Hans Urs von Balthasar, *The Christian and Anxiety* (San Francisco: Ignatius, 2000), 15.

49 Balthasar, *The Christian and Anxiety*, 32.

50 Balthasar, *The Christian and Anxiety*, 32–34.

51 Balthasar, *The Christian and Anxiety*, 141.

52 Balthasar, *The Christian and Anxiety*, 141.

53 Balthasar, *The Christian and Anxiety*, 141.

54 Balthasar, *The Christian and Anxiety*, 142.

55 Balthasar, *The Christian and Anxiety*, 102.

56 Balthasar, *The Christian and Anxiety*, 102. The bracketed insertion is mine, to identify the antecedent used in the prior sentence.

57 Balthasar, *The Christian and Anxiety*, 102–3.

58 Balthasar, *The Christian and Anxiety*, 104.

59 Balthasar, *The Christian and Anxiety*, 40.

60 Balthasar, *The Christian and Anxiety*, 44.

61 Balthasar, *The Christian and Anxiety*, 35–36.

62 Balthasar, *The Christian and Anxiety*, 36.

63 Radden, *Moody Minds Distempered*, 75–94.

64 Balthasar, *The Christian and Anxiety*, 40, 97.

65 As quoted in Timothy J. Yoder, "Hans Urs von Balthasar and Kenosis: The Pathway to Human Agency" (PhD diss., Loyola University Chicago, 2013), *Dissertations*, no. 918, 13, http://ecommons.luc.edu/luc_diss/918.

66 Webb, *Toward a Theology of Psychological Disorder*. Webb makes a case against the consequential model's view that mental distress, according to Scripture, is evidence of selfishness, sin, or the demonic. She cites the Job narrative as an example in which mental distress is not connected to sin, and thus Job becomes an exception to the rule that there is a connection. Webb is merely asserting that one cannot always say in every case that there is a connection, but she does not rule out the connection or a claim to a normative connection. Further, in regard to the demonic she cites that the illnesses relieved by exorcism were more physical than mental, serving as an argument against standardizing the mental distress–demonic connection. However, one example she gives is the narrative of the Gadarene demoniac who, following the exorcism of his legion, was found to be "clothed and in his right mind." Joel Green in his commentary on Luke also notes that the demoniac's "former comportment as a maniac has been replaced by self-discipline and meritorious dignity," and gives a reference to the word *sophroneo*, "reasonable or sound mind." Green, *The Gospel of Luke*, in *The New International Commentary of the New Testament* (Grand Rapids: Eerdmans, 1997), 340.

67 Balthasar, *The Christian and Anxiety*, 48.

68 Balthasar, *The Christian and Anxiety*, 59.

69 Balthasar, *The Christian and Anxiety*, 63.

70 For a thorough treatment of the problems related to disability and divine providence, see Reinders, *Disability, Providence, and Ethics*, 14–16.

71 Balthasar, *The Christian and Anxiety*, 64–65.

72 Balthasar, *The Christian and Anxiety*, 72–73.

73 Balthasar, *The Christian and Anxiety*, 73.

74 Balthasar, *The Christian and Anxiety*, 58, 83.

75 Balthasar, *The Christian and Anxiety*, 74.

76 Balthasar, *The Christian and Anxiety*, 75.

77 Balthasar, *The Christian and Anxiety*, 75.

78 Balthasar, *The Christian and Anxiety*, 86.

79 Balthasar, *The Christian and Anxiety*, 97.

80 Reinders, *Disability, Providence, and Ethics*, 9.

81 Our interpretation of mental disorder can easily be driven by a lurking will to power, as Foucault has demonstrated so well in his *Madness and Civilization*.

CHAPTER 7: THEOLOGICAL TYPE 3—THE PURGATIVE

1 Gerald G. May, *The Dark Night of the Soul: A Psychiatrist Explores the Connection between Darkness and Spiritual Growth* (New York: HarperCollins, 2003), 4.

2 See popular writer Eckhart Tolle as an example of one who uses the term to describe any experience of meaninglessness triggered by an event, external or internal, in which the breakdown of reason occurs (https://www.eckharttolle.com). Another example is the best-selling self-help book entitled *Dark Nights of the Soul: A Guide to Finding Your Way through Life's Ordeals* by Thomas Moore. The title is telling.

3 Examples such as Paul of the Cross or Mother Teresa of Calcutta illustrate the dark night of St. John but through different patterns and lengths of time. In many cases, such as Mother Teresa's, the dark night is not resolved in illumination and union with God. In this tradition, examples from Scripture, like the experience of Job, David, or even Christ in the garden of Gethsemane, may be read into the tradition preceding and anticipating what St. John of the Cross would later codify.

4 Mother Teresa and Brian Kolodiejchuk, *Come Be My Light: The Private Writings of Mother Teresa* (New York: Image, 2009); David Scott, *The Love That Made Mother Teresa: How Her Secret Visions and Dark Night Can Help You Conquer the Slums of Your Heart* (Manchester, N.H.: Sophia Institute, 2016).

5 Rubin, *Religious Melancholy and Protestant Experience in America*. Rubin thoroughly covers the landscape of Western Protestant evangelicalism, its pursuit of salvation, and the melancholy that emerged out of its excesses. Comparison can be made to the Catholic DN tradition, but Rubin sees a distinction because "no amount of obsessively pursued practical devotions could remit the stain of sin and the terror attendant to the conviction of desertion by God" (5). In this sense, I would compare it to the depression attendant with the DN that St. John identifies and that is described below in this work. The DN can go awry and lead to pathological depression. Thus, I would not distinguish the religious melancholy of evangelical Protestantism from the DN. Of course, many of the accounts of religious melancholy and their manifestations, such as those of Luther, Calvin, or those sitting on Finney's anxious bench, show relief and peace in salvation—not ongoing symptoms that lead to irreparable pathology.

6 St. John of the Cross, *Dark Night of the Soul*, trans. and ed. by E. Allison Peers (New York: Doubleday, 1990), 64.

7 St. John of the Cross, *Dark Night*, 64.

8 St. John of the Cross, *Dark Night*, 64.

9 St. John of the Cross, *Dark Night*, 64.

10 St. John of the Cross, *Dark Night*, 64.

11 St. John of the Cross, *Dark Night*, 65.

12 St. John of the Cross, *Dark Night*, 65.

13 St. John of the Cross, *Dark Night*, 65.

14 St. John of the Cross, *Dark Night*, 65.

15 St. John of the Cross, *Dark Night*, 67.

16 St. John of the Cross, *Dark Night*, 68.

17 Kevin Culligan, "The Dark Night and Depression," in *Carmelite Prayer*, ed. Keith J. Egan (New York: Paulist, 2003).

18 Culligan, "Dark Night and Depression," in Egan, *Carmelite Prayer*, 124.

19 Culligan, "Dark Night and Depression," in Egan, *Carmelite Prayer*, 120–21.

20 Culligan, "Dark Night and Depression," in Egan, *Carmelite Prayer*, 122.

21 Culligan, "Dark Night and Depression," in Egan, *Carmelite Prayer*, 122.

22 Culligan, "Dark Night and Depression," in Egan, *Carmelite Prayer*, 122.

23 Culligan, "Dark Night and Depression," in Egan, *Carmelite Prayer*, 125.

24 Culligan, "Dark Night and Depression," in Egan, *Carmelite Prayer*, 126.

25 Culligan, "Dark Night and Depression," in Egan, *Carmelite Prayer*, 130.

26 Culligan, "Dark Night and Depression," in Egan, *Carmelite Prayer*, 130.

27 Culligan, "Dark Night and Depression," in Egan, *Carmelite Prayer*, 131.

28 May, *Dark Night of the Soul*, 156.

29 May, *Dark Night of the Soul*, 156.

30 May, *Dark Night of the Soul*, 156.

31 May, *Dark Night of the Soul*, 157.

32 May, *Dark Night of the Soul*, 157.

33 Culligan, "Dark Night and Depression," in Egan, *Carmelite Prayer*, 134–35.

34 May, *Dark Night of the Soul*, 157–58.

35 Culligan, "Dark Night and Depression," in Egan, *Carmelite Prayer*, 132.

36 Culligan, "Dark Night and Depression," in Egan, *Carmelite Prayer*, 132. May, *Dark Night of the Soul*, 158. Both authors dispel in detail the erroneous mutual exclusion of faith and treatment and such misconceptions that stem from it.

37 Glòria Durà-Vilà, Simon Dein, Roland Littlewood, and Gerard Leavey, "The Dark Night of the Soul: Causes and Resolution of Emotional Distress among Contemplative Nuns," *Transcultural Psychiatry* 47, no. 4 (2010): 548–70, doi: 10.1177/1363461510374899.

38 Durà-Vilà, Dein, Littlewood, and Leavey, "Dark Night of the Soul," 545.

39 Anastasia Philippa Scrutton, "Two Christian Theologies of Depression: An Evaluation and Discussion of Clinical Implications," *Philosophy, Psychiatry, & Psychology* 22, no. 4 (2015): 275–89 (275).

40 Scrutton, "Two Christian Theologies of Depression," 275.

41 Scrutton, "Two Christian Theologies of Depression," 275.

42 Scrutton, "Two Christian Theologies of Depression," 277, 279.

43 Scrutton, "Two Christian Theologies of Depression," 279.

44 Scrutton, "Two Christian Theologies of Depression," 279.

45 Scrutton, "Two Christian Theologies of Depression," 277.

46 Scrutton, "Two Christian Theologies of Depression," 279.

47 Scrutton, "Two Christian Theologies of Depression," 279.

48 This is Scrutton's difficulty with the Durà-Vilà et al. study.

49 Scrutton, "Two Christian Theologies of Depression," 282.

50 Scrutton, "Two Christian Theologies of Depression," 280.

51 Often such a move ends up deflating one's view of God. After making concessions and attributing suffering to free will and natural causes and identifying suffering as evil, something has to compensate on the other end of the equation. Usually, one resorts to open theism or some other nonorthodox construct of the divine that is often deflationary.

52 Culligan, "Dark Night and Depression," in Egan, *Carmelite Prayer*, 136.

53 Culligan, "Dark Night and Depression," in Egan, *Carmelite Prayer*, 136.

54 Culligan, "Dark Night and Depression," in Egan, *Carmelite Prayer*, 136.

55 Culligan, "Dark Night and Depression," in Egan, *Carmelite Prayer*, 136.

56 May, *Dark Night of the Soul*, 2–3.

57 May, *Dark Night of the Soul*, 4–5.

58 I. J. Kidd, "Transformative Suffering and the Cultivation of Virtue," *Philosophy, Psychiatry, & Psychology* 22, no. 4 (2015): 291–94.

59 Kidd, "Transformative Suffering," 281.

60 Kidd, "Transformative Suffering," 287. Yet, there are even those who have survived the Holocaust or childhood sexual abuse, for example, who have, remarkably, spiritually grown as a result of their struggle, i.e., Frankl, *Man's Search for Meaning*. Nonetheless, although there are miraculous cases of those who have overcome such horrendous evil, this type of suffering should never be idealized, exemplified (i.e., seen as an example to encourage those who have not suffered the same), objectified, or commodified in any instance.

61 Otto, *Idea of the Holy*, 21.

62 Scrutton, "Two Christian Theologies of Depression," 281.

63 Swinton, "Theology or Therapy?" 296.

64 Swinton, "Theology or Therapy?" 296.

65 Swinton, "Theology or Therapy?" 296.

66 Swinton, "Theology or Therapy?" 297.

CHAPTER 8: THE MELANCHOLIC GOD

1 For an analytical and practical exposition of Romans 6 from the standpoint of our identification and union with Christ on the cross, see D. Martyn Lloyd-Jones, *Romans: The New Man, an Exposition of Chapter 6* (Grand Rapids: Zondervan, 1972), 73.

2 Gordon Fee, "The New Testament and Kenosis Christology," in Evans, *Exploring Kenotic Christology*, 29.

3 Fee, "The New Testament and Kenosis Christology," in Evans, *Exploring Kenotic Christology*, 33.

4 Fee, "The New Testament and Kenosis Christology," in Evans, *Exploring Kenotic Christology*, 34.

5 In 451 CE the Ecumenical Council of Chalcedon was convened to work out some of these controversies surrounding the divine and human natures of Christ as related to his person, responding to the claims of Nestorianism and Eutyches (monophysitism), who was reacting against the Nestorian heresy that denied the unity of the two natures in one person. The council confirmed the unity of the two distinct natures (divine and human) in the one person Jesus Christ.

The Chalcedonian Definition
Therefore, following the holy fathers, we all with one accord teach men to acknowledge one and the same Son, our Lord Jesus Christ, at once complete in Godhead and complete in manhood, truly God and truly man, consisting also of a reasonable soul and body; of one substance with the Father as regards his Godhead, and at the same time of one substance with us as regards his manhood; like us in all respects, apart from sin; as regards his Godhead, begotten of the Father before the ages, but yet as regards his manhood begotten, for us men and for our salvation, of Mary the Virgin, the God-bearer; one and the same Christ, Son, Lord, Only-begotten, recognized in two natures, without confusion, without change, without division, without separation; the distinction of natures being in no way annulled by the union, but rather the characteristics of each nature being preserved and coming together to form one person and subsistence, not as parted or separated into two persons, but one and the same Son and Only-begotten God the Word, Lord Jesus Christ; even as the prophets from earliest times spoke of him, and our Lord Jesus Christ himself taught us, and the creed of the fathers has handed down to us.

6 Thomas R. Thompson, "Nineteenth Century Kenotic Christology," in Evans, *Exploring Kenotic Christology*, 79.

7 Thompson, "Nineteenth Century Kenotic Christology," in Evans, *Exploring Kenotic Christology*, 82.

8 Thompson, "Nineteenth Century Kenotic Christology," in Evans, *Exploring Kenotic Christology*, 82–83.

9 For an insightful introduction to seventeenth-century kenotic responses to Lutheran Scholasticism on overdivinizing the human nature of Christ via the *communication idiomaticum* and the beginnings of modern British kenotic Christology, see Adrian Giorgiov, "The Kenotic Christology of Charles Gore, P. T. Forsyth, and H. R. Mackintosh," *Perichoresis* 2, no. 1 (2004): 47–66.

10 Thomas J. J. Altizer, *The Gospel of Christian Atheism* (Philadelphia: Westminster, 1966). See also Thomas J. J. Altizer and William Hamilton, eds., *Radical Theology and the Death of God* (Indianapolis: Merrill, 1966).

11 Balthasar's eternal kenosis in the Trinity draws heavily from the Russian theologian Sergei Bulgakov.

12 Hans Urs von Balthasar, *Mysterium Paschale* (1970; San Francisco: Ignatius, 2000). See also Edward T. Oakes, "'He Descended into Hell': The Depths of God's Self-Emptying Love on Holy Saturday in the Thought of Hans Urs von Balthasar," in Evans, *Exploring Kenotic Christology*, 218–45.

13 Stephen T. Davis, "Is Kenosis Orthodox?" in Evans, *Exploring Kenotic Christology*, 113.

14 I.e., claims to the Hellenization of early Christianity from Harnack, Ritschl, and others. See Paul Gavrilyuk's *Suffering of the Impassible God: The Dialectics of Patristic Thought*, Oxford Early Christian Studies (Oxford: Oxford University Press, 2006) for a thorough refutation of the claim that the theology of the early church was unduly influenced by Hellenization, especially in terms of the notion of divine impassibility.

15 The growing influence of higher criticism and also the preoccupation with the historical Jesus.

16 I.e., the day and hour of Christ's return, the assumption that David wrote Psalm 110, or Christ grew in wisdom and stature, while still claiming divinity.

17 Davis, "Is Kenosis Orthodox?" in Evans, *Exploring Kenotic Christology*, 115–22.

18 I.e., growing in wisdom, suffering, not knowing the day and hour of his return.

19 Davis, "Is Kenosis Orthodox?" in Evans, *Exploring Kenotic Christology*, 115. Stephen Davis claims that many kenotic theories attempt to replace the Chalcedonian definition; he affirms Chalcedon but supplies a kenotic interpretation of the traditional definition.

20 Here I am building on Morris, who developed his argument from Anselm. See Thomas V. Morris, *The Logic of God Incarnate* (Ithaca, N.Y.: Cornell University Press, 1986), 89–102.

21 For a critical examination of the doctrine of divine simplicity and its defense in a constituent approach to ontology, see William F. Vallicella, "Divine Simplicity," in *The Stanford Encyclopedia of Philosophy*, ed. Edward N. Zalta, spring 2019 ed., accessed October 27, 2019, https://plato.stanford.edu/archives/spr2019/entries/divine-simplicity/.

22 See Sarah Coakley, "Does Kenosis Rest on a Mistake?" and Edwin Chr. van Driel, "The Logic of Assumption," in Evans, *Exploring Kenotic Christology*, 249–50, 275–76. Coakley looks at Cyril of Alexandria and Gregory of Nyssa and their reading of the Philippian hymn and their respective notions of the *communicatio*, what Coakley calls "assumption" and "progressive transfusion." For extensive examination of Aquinas' view on kenosis see Gregorio Montejo, "Truly Human, Fully Divine: The Kenotic Christ of Thomas Aquinas" (PhD diss., Marquette University, 2016), accessed October 25, 2019, https://epublications.marquette.edu/cgi/viewcontent.cgi?article=1694&context=dissertations_mu. Aquinas understands the communication of attributes "not as eschewal of the divine nature, but rather the assumption of humanity" (134).

23 The Lutheran Scholastic theologian Martin Chemnitz is responsible for the meticulous working out of three of the *genera*; these do not include the genus of humility, which is picked up in the kenotic theories of the nineteenth century. Chemnitz and other Lutheran Scholastics opposed this view. See his *The Two Natures of Christ*, trans. J. Preus (St. Louis: Concordia, 1971). There are two *genera* besides majesty and humility: the *genus idiomaticum* that is the communicating of the properties of one nature to the one person, and the *genus apotelesmoticum* that the soteriological actions of the one person are only ascribed to one of the other nature.

24 For an analysis of the various *genera* of the *communicatio idiomatum* from a Lutheran perspective, see David W. Congdon, "*Nova Lingua Dei*: The Problem of Chalcedonian Metaphysics and the Promise of the *Genus Tapeinoticon* in Luther's Late Theology" (PhD diss., Princeton Theological Seminary, 2011), accessed October 26, 2019, https://www.academia .edu/586346/Nova_Lingua_Dei_The_Problem_of_Chalcedonian_Metaphysics_and_the _Promise_of_the_Genus_Tapeinoticon_in_Luthers_Later_Theology. This essay locates the problem of the *genus kenoticum* in Luther himself, his view of Chalcedon prioritizing person over natures in thought and speech, and attributing the passible attributes of humanity to the divine nature, not just the person of Christ (47–53). According to Congdon's interpretation of Luther, Luther clearly goes beyond Chalcedon almost to monophysitism.

25 For a thorough philosophical treatment of the logical consistency and coherence of the Christology of the first seven Ecumenical Councils, specifically the seeming contradiction of how one person can be divine and human and have the respective attributes of each, see Timothy Pawl, *In Defense of Conciliar Christology: A Philosophical Essay* (Oxford: Oxford University Press, 2016). Also see his *In Defense of Extended Conciliar Christology* (Oxford: Oxford University Press, 2019).

26 While much of patristic, medieval, and Reformation(s) Christianity has espoused divine immutability and impassibility (the two are not mutually inclusive), recently many well-known so-called orthodox or conservative theologians and philosophers, including Barth, Balthasar, Bonhoeffer, Moltmann, Jenson, Plantinga, Swinburne, Torrance, and others, have questioned, modified, or denied divine immutability and impassibility. For further discussion from both sides of this complex argument on impassibility and immutability, see the following works: Jeffrey Brower, "Making Sense of Divine Simplicity," *Faith and Philosophy* 25, no. 1 (2008): 3–30; Richard Creel, *Divine Impassibility* (Cambridge: Cambridge University Press, 1986); James E. Dolezal, *All That Is in God: Evangelical Theology and the Challenge of Classical Theism* (Grand Rapids: Reformation Heritage, 2017); Gavrilyuk, *Suffering of the Impassible God*; Gerard Hanlon, *The Immutability of God in the Theology of Hans Urs von Balthasar* (Cambridge: Cambridge University Press, 1990); James Keating and Thomas White, *Divine Impassibility and the Mystery of Human Suffering* (Grand Rapids: Eerdmans, 2009); Brian Leftow, "Eternity and Immutability," in *The Blackwell Guide to Philosophy of Religion*, ed. William E. Mann (Malden, Mass.: Blackwell, 2004); Brian Leftow, "Immutability," in *The Stanford Encyclopedia of Philosophy*, ed. Edward N. Zalta, fall 2008 ed.; Alvin Plantinga, "On Ockham's Way Out," *Faith and Philosophy* 3, no. 3 (1986): 235–69; Richard Swinburne, *The Coherence of Theism* (Oxford: Clarendon Press, 1993); Thomas G. Weinandy, *Does God Change?* (Still River: St. Bede's, 1985).

27 As noted in Webb, *Toward a Theology of Psychological Disorder*, 96.

28 I recommend the following texts as a good place to start: Keating and White, *Divine Impassibility*; Rob Lister, *God Is Impassible and Impassioned: Toward a Theology of Divine Emotion* (Wheaton, Ill.: Crossway, 2013); Robert J. Matz and A. Chadwick Thornhill, eds., *Divine Impassibility: Four Views of God's Emotions and Suffering* (Downers Grove, Ill.: IVP Academic, 2019); Weinandy, *Does God Change?*

29 Rob Lister offers the provisional definition of J. I. Packer that impassibility is not impassivity, unconcern, or impersonal detachment in the face of creation: not insensitivity and indifference to the distresses of a fallen world; not inability or unwillingness to empathize with human pain and grief; but simply that God's experiences do not come upon him as ours come upon us, for his are foreknown, willed, and chosen by him, and are not involuntary surprises forced on him from outside, apart from his own decision, in the way that ours regularly are. J. I. Packer, "Theism for Our Time," in *God Who Is Rich in Mercy*, ed. Peter T. O'Brien and David G. Peterson (Grand Rapids: Baker, 1986), 17, cited by Lister, *God Is Impassible and Impassioned*, 33. Put simply, the question of divine impassibility is, Does God experience passion (*pathos*), emotion, and hence suffering? Why or why not?

30 Thomas Blair Speed Mount, "Existential Dimensions of the Contemporary Impassibility Debate: A Pastoral Approach to the Question of Divine Suffering within the Context of Conservative Evangelicalism" (research proposal for the Doctor of Philosophy Programme, South African Theological Seminary, 2015), 30–32, https://portfolios.sats.edu .za/cgi-bin/koha/opac-detail.pl?biblionumber=14676. Mount's work is an overview of the historical arguments for and against divine impassibility and its bearing on contemporary evangelical issues.

31 Gilles Emery, "The Immutability of the God of Love," in Keating and White, *Divine Impassibility*, 32.

32 Aquinas, *Summa Theologiae* 1.3.

33 Emery, "Immutability of the God of Love," in Keating and White, *Divine Impassibility*, 59.

34 Aquinas, *Summa Theologiae* 1.8.1.

35 For Aquinas' treatise on the notion of essence, see Thomas Aquinas, *De Ente et Essentia*, trans. George G. Leckie (New York: D. Appleton–Century, 1937).

36 The God of becoming or self-actualization is a God who is not simple or immutable but is in process, working out the divine destiny, usually through mutual interaction with the created order, implying *causa sui* and *creatio continua*. We find such a construct of the divine in Hegel, Whitehead, process theology, Moltmann, and others.

37 Aquinas, *De Ente et Essentia* 28.

38 Duns Scotus argued for formal distinction within the divine essence, distinction that is irreducibly distinct and logically inseparable. See Thomas H. McCall, "Trinity Doctrine: Plain and Simple," in *Advancing Trinitarian Theology: Exploration in Constructive Dogmatics*, ed. Oliver D. Crisp and Fred Sanders (Grand Rapids: Zondervan, 2014), 51–57.

39 Aquinas, *Summa Theologiae* 1.9. For an opposing view concerning the nature of God, see process theology and its main proponents, such as Alfred North Whitehead, Charles Hartshorne, and John Cobb. Panentheism, which is often linked to process theology, does not understand God in necessary, immutable, impassible, and absolute terms in its relationship with creation.

40 Aquinas, *Summa Theologiae* 1.9.1.

41 Emery, "Immutability of the God of Love," in Keating and White, *Divine Impassibility*, 64. Impassibility is also due to God's incorporeality.

42 Perfection and love being properties joined in the nature of God, with love an immanent procession of divine will revealed in God's acts of creation, incarnation, and new creation.

43 For a thorough and sound treatment of Aquinas' theology of divine immutability and its relation to the love of God, see Michael J. Dodds, *The Unchanging God of Love: Thomas Aquinas and Contemporary Theologians on Divine Immutability*, 2nd ed. (Washington, D.C.: Catholic University of America Press, 2008).

44 I.e., as in Moltmann, whose statement "If God cannot suffer, then he cannot love and is unworthy of our worship" sums up Moltmann's assertion of a crucified God. In reaction

to what he believes to be a Greek pagan, philosophical, impassible construct of the divine, Moltmann's own *theologia crucis* holds that in order for God to be truly God (love), God must be so in human terms by fully embracing the human condition and suffering and dying as God both as the Logos on the cross and through the separation of Father and Son. Thus, the (Trinitarian) event of the cross is the place and time in which God truly fulfills his end and becomes truly God. God is a triune event, not a divine being or nature, of love and liberation revealed on the cross. Moltmann proposes a staurocentric Trinitarianism. The suffering in the event of the cross, for Moltmann, has Trinitarian consequences, that is, the undoing of the Trinity with the kenosis of the Son and the Spirit, beginning with the incarnation, and the rejection of the Son by the Father. Jürgen Moltmann, *The Crucified God* (New York: Harper & Row, 1974). See also the position of Jenson, whereby God ontologically actualizes himself and becomes truly divine by entering the world process and human history and taking on and overcoming suffering and evil. Robert Jenson, *"Ipse Pater Non Est Impassibilis,"* in Keating and White, *Divine Impassibility*.

45 For a conversation among the four positions, see Robert J. Matz and A. Chadwick Thornhill, eds., *Divine Impassibility: Four Views of God's Emotions and Suffering* (Downers Grove, Ill.: IVP Academic, 2019). For an overview of the various position on divine impassibility and a history of the development of the doctrine, see Lister, *God Is Impassible and Impassioned*.

46 For a historical overview of the doctrine of divine impassibility, see the classic by J. K. Mozley, *The Impassibility of God: A Survey of Christian Thought* (1926; Cambridge: Cambridge University Press, 2014).

47 Irenaeus demonstrated this balance by opposing the gnostic creation myth with its passible Aeons, but also opposing the Marcionites for their refusal to acknowledge the wrath of God in the Old Testament. Cited in Lister, *God Is Impassible and Impassioned*, 67–69.

48 Although holding to divine otherness, Tertullian also points out the analogical language in Scripture that is used to portray the relational nature of God's dealing with creation. Cited in Lister, *God Is Impassible and Impassioned*, 71–74.

49 Often polemical and open to multivalent interpretation, Origen works out a stasis of divine impassibility and divine passion through his notion of God's love that suffers metaphorically and thus immutably. Lister, *God Is Impassible and Impassioned*, 78, citing Thomas G. Weinandy, *Does God Suffer?* (Notre Dame, Ind.: University of Notre Dame Press, 2000), 99–100.

50 A student of Origen, Gregory sought to balance divine impassibility with divine passion in his work *Ad Theopompum de passibili et impassibili in Deo*, as cited in Lister, *God Is Impassible and Impassioned*, 78–79.

51 For Lactantius, divine anger was viewed as compatible with impassibility because it was necessary for divine perfection, providence, and justice. Cited in Lister, *God Is Impassible and Impassioned*, 79–81.

52 Athanasius, along with the First Ecumenical Council, rejected the idea of temporality and mutability in the second person of the Trinity.

53 Gregory of Nazianzus sums up his view of the impassible divine nature and the passible human nature of Christ in these words: "What is lofty, you are to attribute to the divinity, to that nature in Him which transcends sufferings and the body; but all that is humble, you are to attribute to the composite condition of Him who for your sakes emptied himself and became flesh—yes, it is no worse to say, was made human and afterwards was also exalted." Gregory of Nazianzus, "Oration 29," in *The Five Theological Orations*, trans. Stephen Reynolds (estate of Stephen Reynolds, 2011), 64, http://hdl.handle.net/1807/36303.

54 Within his view of divine impassibility, St. Augustine recognized the compatibility of divine emotions that were analogically expressed in Scripture. For example, in *Contra*

adversarium legis et prophetarum, he writes, "By the repentance of God is meant the change of things which lie within His power, unexpected by man: the anger of God is His vengeance upon sin; the pity of God is the goodness of His help; the jealousy of God is that providence whereby He does not allow those whom He has in subjection to Himself to love with impunity what He forbids." As cited in Lister, *God Is Impassible and Impassioned*, 89.

55 Cyril's opponent Nestorius held the two natures apart, seeking to preserve the ontological distance between the divine and human. However, Nestorius radically separates the natures, even denying a rational soul to the man Jesus Christ. For Nestorius, there is a clear distinction between the eternal *Logos* and the human Jesus. There are two persons or subjects that have predication and attribution. On the other hand, Cyril understood the two natures as, though distinct, yet joined together in unity in one subject. Thus, what can be said of either nature can be said of the person due to the hypostatic union. Cyril critiqued Nestorius' Logos-Jesus connection as no different than hypercharged prophet. Cyril of Alexandria, *On the Unity of Christ*, ed. John Anthony McGuckin, Popular Patristic Series (Crestwood, N.Y.: St. Vladimir's Seminary Press, 2015), 65, 90–98, 107–18, and 129–33.

56 St. Leo's *Tome* was heavily debated at Chalcedon and had an immense influence on the formulation of the definition of two natures in one person and the classical construal of the communication of properties of both natures in the one subject, Jesus Christ. Thus, suffering can be ascribed to the *Logos* but only through the human nature of Jesus Christ.

57 Lister, *God Is Impassible and Impassioned*, 66–94.

58 Cited in Lister, *God Is Impassible and Impassioned*, 71–74.

59 Cyril of Alexandria, *On the Unity of Christ*, 107.

60 Charles A. Heurtley, trans., *St. Leo's Epistle to Flavian* (London: Parker, 1885), 13.

61 Heurtley, *St. Leo's Epistle to Flavian*, 23.

62 From the Second Ecumenical Council of Constantinople, Canon 10.

63 Cyril of Alexandria, "Council of Ephesus, Second Letter of Cyril to Nestorius," in *Decrees of the Ecumenical Councils*, vol. 1, ed. Norman P. Tanner (Washington, D.C.: Georgetown University Press, 2017), 42.

64 Luther's position on divine impassibility seems ambiguous. In places he embraces the traditional view, and at other times seems to hold the view that the two natures can exchange predicates and properties, resulting in a communication of properties as *genus maiestaticum* and *genus tapeinoticum*. For a passibilist reading of Luther, see David J. Luy, *Dominus Mortis: Martin Luther on the Incorruptibility of God in Christ* (Minneapolis: Fortress, 2014). See also Dennis Ngien, *The Suffering of God: According to Martin Luther's "Theologica Crucis"* (Vancouver, B.C.: Regent College, 2005).

65 We note this in key figures such as Bulgakov, Barth, Moltmann, Torrance, and Jenson, among others. Tracing the contemporary transition, Gavrilyuk makes the poignant distinction between the patristic (and traditional) notion of impassibility and the modern passible construal. The former is metaphysical, radically distinguishing God from the created order. The latter is psychological and empathic, claiming God is capable of experiencing human emotions and suffering. Paul Gavrilyuk, "God's Impassible Suffering in the Flesh: The Promise of Paradoxical Christology," in Keating and White, *Divine Impassibility*, 139. Mount also identifies the traditional view as addressing metaphysical concerns, while recognizing the modern passibilist perspective in terms of addressing existential concerns.

66 Shoah is Hebrew for the Holocaust.

67 Some late eighteenth- and nineteenth-century attempts at genocide include those in the Congo (Belgian conquest), Ethiopia, Algeria (French conquest), Namibia, Argentina (an indigenous population), Canada (First Nations tribes), Haiti, and Armenia (Ottoman massacre).

68 Jürgen Moltmann (1926–) best expresses this view in his groundbreaking work *The Crucified God*, 222, 225, 230.

69 Moltmann, *Crucified God*, 222.

70 Disputing a Hellenization hypothesis, Gavrilyuk asserts a stark contrast between patristic ideas of divine *apatheia* and those of paganism. His work has been integral in demonstrating that Hellenization did not speak with a unified voice concerning divine (im)passibility. He meticulously argues that Hellenization offered no single theory or view of divine *apatheia* that the fathers could have adopted unanimously. In other words, there is no one Hellenized idea of *apatheia*. Not only did the fathers not rely on pagan constructs of the divine, specifically regarding immutability, what they purposefully crafted was in part a reaction to pagan anthropomorphisms.

Rob Lister devotes an entire chapter to respond negatively, in similar fashion as Gavrilyuk, to the claim of Hellenization. Lister acknowledges patristic borrowing from Greek concepts. However, he makes a case that such borrowing was critically contextualized (my language) for communication to the prevailing culture (61). Within the Hellenization hypothesis is the contention that the Fathers chose pagan constructs and language over against biblical ideas and expressions. Lister mounts a weighty case against such an indictment by citing patristic deference to Scripture, specifically in terms of the development of the doctrines of the Trinity, a personal deity, creation, and the incarnation (62). Lister, *God Is Impassible and Impassioned*, 41–63.

Intensely focusing on the radical transcendence and otherness of God, patristic attempts were categorically intentional in distinguishing theological impassibility from anthropomorphic expressions of the divine. Pagan attributes, such as excessive immanence and mutability, easily led to manipulation of the divine and were to be avoided. Gavrilyuk, *Suffering of the Impassible God*, 5. Impassibility as an "apophatic qualifier" and corrective assisted in safeguarding divine transcendence not only against Greek philosophical influence but also against heresies that penetrated the church, including Gnosticism (opposed by Irenaeus), Marcionism (opposed by both Irenaeus and Tertullian), Sabellianism/patripassianism (opposed by Tertullian), and monophysitism (opposed by Cyril of Alexandria).

71 Moltmann, *Crucified God*, 273–74, quoting Elie Wiesel, *Night* (1969), 75.

72 This is a term strongly used by Polish-born and Jewish-American scholar and rabbi Abraham Heschel in his book *The Prophets*. The claim is that the function and experience of a prophet in the Hebrew Bible is to be in touch with the emotional life of God. The prophet feels and experiences what God experiences in God's relationship (i.e., love and anger) with God's people. From this shared emotional life with the divine, the prophet communicates the divine *pathos* in his prophetic message. Abraham Joshua Heschel, *The Prophets: Two Volumes in One* (Peabody, Mass.: Hendrickson, 2007), 126.

73 Moltmann, *Crucified God*, 249–52.

74 Moltmann, *Crucified God*, 246.

75 Moltmann, *Crucified God*, 246.

76 Moltmann, *Crucified God*, 243.

77 Moltmann, *Crucified God*, 243–45.

78 Bruce D. Marshall, "Dereliction of Christ," in Keating and White, *Divine Impassibility*, 250.

79 Marshall, "Dereliction of Christ," in Keating and White, *Divine Impassibility*, 251–52.

80 "Theopanism" is a term used by Erich Przywara in his *Analogia Entis* for expressing a univocal understanding of God in the world.

81 Moltmann, *Crucified God*, 7.

82 Moltmann, *Crucified God*, 65.

83 Moltmann, *Crucified God*, 207–19.

84 Moltmann, *Crucified God*, 241.

85 Moltmann, *Crucified God*, 212.

86 Any strict reading of Rahner's Rule that the immanent Trinity fully exhausts the economic Trinity, or of LaCugna's Corollary that there is no knowledge or speech of the so-called immanent Trinity, but all we have is the *economia*, is reductive, anthropological, and can lead to nihilism. See Peter Bellini, "The *Processio-Missio* Connection: A Starting Point in *Missio Trinitatis* or Overcoming the Immanent-Economic Divide in a *Missio Trinitatis*," *Wesleyan Theological Journal* 49, no. 2 (2014): 7–23.

87 Moltmann, *Crucified God*, 246.

88 Weinandy argues similarly concerning the relationship between sin and suffering, that in this sense God cannot suffer. Weinandy, *Does God Suffer?* 147–57.

89 Marshall, "Dereliction of Christ," in Keating and White, *Divine Impassibility*, 285.

90 Emery, "Immutability of the God of Love," in Keating and White, *Divine Impassibility*, 43–44.

91 Barth espoused a modified and limited view of divine passibility that is internal and voluntary, as illustrated in this passage:

> The personal God has a heart. He can feel and be affected. He is not impassible. He cannot be moved from outside by an extraneous power. But this does not mean that He is not capable of moving Himself. No, God is moved and stirred, yet not like ourselves in powerlessness, but in His own free power, in His innermost being: moved and touched by Himself, i.e., open, ready, inclined (*propensus*) to compassion to another's suffering and therefore to assistance, impelled to take the initiative to relieve this distress. It can only be a question of compassion, free sympathy, with another's suffering. God finds no suffering in Himself. And no cause outside God can cause Him suffering if He does not will it so. But it is, in fact, a question of sympathy with the suffering of another in the full scope of God's own personal freedom. This is the essential point if we are really thinking of the God attested by Scripture and speaking only of Him. Everything that God is and does is determined and characterized by the fact that there is rooted in Him, that He Himself is, the original free powerful compassion, that from the outset He is open and ready and inclined to the need and distress and torment of another, that His compassionate words and deeds are not grounded in a subsequent change, in a mere approximation to certain conditions in the creature which is distinct from Himself, but are rooted in His heart, in His very life and being as God. (Karl Barth, *Church Dogmatics* II/1, 370)

For Barth's understanding of divine passibility, see Bruce L. McCormack, "Divine Impassibility or Simple Divine Constancy? Implications of Karl Barth's Later Christology for Debates over Impassibility," in Keating and White, *Divine Impassibility*, 150–86.

92 The Swiss theologian Hans Urs von Balthasar's position can be summarized in his own words:

> We shall never know how to express the abyss-like depths of the Father's self-giving, that Father who, in an eternal "super-kenosis," makes himself "destitute" of all that he is and can be so as to bring forth a consubstantial divinity, the Son. Everything that can be thought and imagined where God is concerned is, in advance, included and transcended in this self-destitution which constitutes the person of the Father, and, at the same time, those of the Son and the Spirit. God as the "gulf" (Eckhart: *Un-Grund*) of absolute Love contains in advance, eternally,

all the modalities of love, of compassion and even of a "separation" motivated by love and founded on the infinite distinction between the hypostases—modalities which may manifest themselves in the course of a history of salvation involving sinful humankind. (Balthasar, *Mysterium Paschale*, viii–ix)

Balthasar attempts to draw a causal parallel for the *oikonomia* in the immanent processions of the Trinity, including his view of the kenosis of the second person of the Trinity. He claims a kenosis of the Son that originates in the Trinity, as the Father empties (superkenosis) himself in divine love toward the Son and ultimately toward the Spirit, creating an infinite *diastasis* that accounts for all difference and separation in creation. Trinitarian superkenosis and incarnation, which is centered on the cross, culminates with the descent of the Son from the cross into hell (Holy Saturday) to assume and suffer the death and punishment for all humanity. His controversial conception of the descent into hell is not reduced to the narrow "paradise" of the Old Testament faithful of latter Judaism. Instead, Christ experiences solidarity with the dead in general and overcomes the punishment of hell for all. Not that hell is emptied but that salvation is offered to all and that all must respond to that offer (177–78). In terms of the suffering of God, for Balthasar it is not ontological but a relational suffering of absence, unlike Moltmann's that asserts a disruption in the nature of God.

I concur with Balthasar, who is citing Aquinas in *Summa Theologiae* 1.45.6.1: "processiones divinarum personarum sunt causa creationis," that the eternal immanent processions of the divine persons are the cause and reason (*causa et ratio*) of creation and created effects. However, cause and reason do not entail a parallel, let alone an exact parallel. The processions are eternal. The missions are temporal. The incarnation, which involves laying aside divine privilege and incorporating human nature, does not necessitate a superkenosis in the Trinity as a causal explanation. As stated above, divine love does not separate or nihilate. In terms of the incarnation, all created being, including human nature, is ultimately derived ex nihilo and not as an extension of divine being. With the divine mission of the sending of the Son, the eternal takes on a new mode (humanity) that is temporal, so that humanity may be sanctified. Thus, the Word taking on human nature in temporal mission is not an exact parallel with the divine processions and relations from their eternal origin in the Father (see *Summa Theologiae*, q. 43), not repeated or paralleled in the Trinity, i.e., a superkenosis. Gilles Emery retorts, "Aquinas's doctrine of the missions maintains the essential difference between God and his created effects, with no danger of confusing the Trinity and his created gifts. The issue at stake is not just the foundation of the missions in the eternal processions, or the missions as a manifestation of the inmost life of the Trinity, but a fuller understanding of the Trinitarian nature of revelation and salvation, and of the Trinity itself." Emery, "The Vision of the Mystery of the Trinity in Thomas Aquinas," *Credere, amare e vivere la verità / Believing, Loving and Living Truth: The Proceedings of the XIII Plenary Session in the Year of the Faith*, June 21–23, 2013, accessed September 15, 2020, http://www.past.va/content/dam/past/pdf/dc_2014/doctor_communis_2014.pdf.

Thus, the eternal love of the Father infinitely given and poured out ("emptied") in the Son and the intrapersonal trinitarian mutual giving and receiving of divine love does not entail a diminishing or losing of that attribute, perfection, such that the nature is changed or lost, whether it is in creation, incarnation, or the passion, but it reveals externally the eternal quality of perfect love. The infinite love revealing the distinction of the persons does not effect a separation within the divine nature, as Balthasar seems to suggest, and thus ground all temporal separation. The infinite love revealed in the distinction of the eternal generation of the Son and the spiration of the Spirit is analogically reflected in the distinction of created being and the further distinctions within created being. Yet, the infinite self-giving and pouring out of divine love by nature does not diminish the love or change, alter, exhaust, separate, or annihilate the divine nature. The nature of such love by definition cannot change. One can claim the same infinite self-giving love of the Father in the eternal generation of the Son revealed in the mission of the incarnation without resorting to kenosis in the Trinity and divine mutability and passibility in the incarnation and the passion.

For a critique of Balthasar's superkenosis and impassibility in general, see Marshall, "Dereliction of Christ," in Keating and White, *Divine Impassibility*, 246–99; and "The Unity of the Triune God: Reviving an Ancient Question," *Thomist: A Speculative Quarterly Review* 74, no. 1 (2010): 1–32, https://doi.org/10.1353/tho.2010.0000. Marshall's argument is that the identity of God is found in the immanent Trinity apart from the *economia*. Economic workings, i.e., kenosis, which Marshall does not admit either, should not define the nature of God. Thus, an assertion of economic kenosis should not define the immanent Trinity and necessitate a superkenosis to ground the kenosis of the Son (17–32).

Also for a thorough treatment of Balthasar's understanding of divine immutability and passibility in the superkenosis, the kenosis of the incarnation, and the kenosis of Holy Saturday or the descent of the Son in hell, see Gerard F. O'Hanlon, *The Immutability of God in the Theology of Hans Urs von Balthasar* (New York: Cambridge University Press, 1990).

93 Jenson, "*Ipse Pater Non Est Impassibilis*," in Keating and White, *Divine Impassibility*, 117–26.

94 Richard Bauckham, "'Only the Suffering God Can Help': Divine Passibility in Modern Theology," *Themelios* 9, no. 3 (April 1984): 6–12, among others.

95 Abraham Heschel, among others. For a scriptural and theological analysis of divine impassibility that incorporates theopathetic language and actions, see chapters 3 and 4 in Weinandy, *Does God Suffer?*

96 Namely Barth, Moltmann, Balthasar, and Jenson as well as what is seen in process theology and open theism.

97 These arguments and strategies, as well as others, have been debated in the texts and footnotes cited throughout this chapter. Again, for an in-depth treatment of divine (im)passibility from various perspectives, see Keating and White, *Divine Impassibility*. And for a historical survey of the subject, see Lister, *God Is Impassible and Impassioned*. See also Mozley, *Impassibility of God*.

98 Weinandy, in chapters 8 and 9 of *Does God Suffer?* makes a similar argument for the need of Christ's suffering and death as a human suffering and death and that suffering in the divine nature as opposed to the human nature would leave God untouched by human suffering.

99 Marshall, "Dereliction of Christ," in Keating and White, *Divine Impassibility*, 281–83.

100 There are some who hold to the classical two-natures-in-one-person hypostasis and an "impassioned" impassibility. Rob Lister holds to a modified view of impassibility while maintaining Chalcedonian Christology. With Lister's view, God is impassible but not passionless. He chooses voluntarily, not under compulsion, to express a full range of divine emotions (i.e., love, joy, wrath, jealousy) in harmony with his ontological transcendence, perfection, foreknowledge, and sovereignty, which in this sense are unlike human emotions. Thus, God can freely choose to experience divine pathos but is not acted upon involuntarily. Lister, *God Is Impassible and Impassioned*.

101 Gavrilyuk, Lister, Weinandy, and others acknowledge that the church fathers recogonize some qualified notion of theopathic capacity.

102 See chaper 6 in Weinandy, *Does God Suffer?*

103 With reductive physicalism, consciousness is ultimately somatic in origin. Nonreductive physicalism identifies consciousness as a property of the brain and hence ultimately somatic. In interactive substance dualism, the mind and body dialectically suffer, whereas, in noninteractive substance dualism, the body and mind suffer separately. Hence in most cases, the body is involved in suffering and often is the source.

104 Aquinas makes a distinction between love and sacrifice with self-service involved as some ends (love of concupiscence) and disinterested, unconditional love in which the motive or the end does not involve self-benefit (love of friendship, divine friendship). Michael Dodds examines Aquinas' work on this distinction as well as the distinction between the limits of human sympathetic suffering and empathy, and the transcendence and perfection of divine compassion. See Dodds, *Unchanging God of Love*, 207–38.

105 Lister, *God Is Impassible and Impassioned*, 259.

106 Lister, *God Is Impassible and Impassioned*, 199.

107 Anastasia Philippa Scrutton, "Emotion in Augustine of Hippo and Thomas Aquinas: A Way Forward for the Im/passibility Debate?" *International Journal of Systematic Theology* 7, no. 2 (2005): 170–76. From Scrutton, see also *Thinking through Feeling: God, Emotion and Possibility* (New York: Bloomsbury Academic, 2013).

108 For Aquinas, fruits such as love, joy, and the like, are of the intellectual appetite and not a passion of the sensitive appetite. Aquinas, *Summa Theologiae* 2.1.22.3.

109 As unpacked above, the analogical interval between divine and created being expresses a similitude and even greater dissimilitude between the analogates of the subject and the analogue. In this same sense, the relational language of created being used to speak of uncreated being in Scripture reflects both a similitude and a greater dissimilitude. Scripture, at times, employs an anthropomorphic literary style to describe divine agency and action in contingent terms.

110 Lister, *God Is Impassible and Impassioned*, 199.

CHAPTER 9: TOWARD A TRINITARIAN THEOLOGY OF DEPRESSION

1 Gaventa, *Disability and Spirituality*, 3.

2 Gaventa, *Disability and Spirituality*, 3.

3 Fiona A. Kumari Campbell, "Exploring Internalized Ableism Using Critical Race Theory," *Disability & Society* 23 (2008): 5–6, https://doi.org/10.1080/09687590701841190.

4 An insider and inclusive term referring to the intersection of disability studies and status with the studies and status of gender, sex, race, and socioeconomic class and how they relate.

5 Robert McRuer, "Compulsory Able-Bodiness and Queer/Disabled Existence," in *Disability Studies: Enabling the Humanities*, ed. Sharon L. Snyder, Brenda Jo Brueggemann, and Rosemarie Garland-Thomson (New York: Modern Language Association, 2002), 88–99 (96).

6 Nitsan Almog, "'Everyone Is Normal, and Everyone Has a Disability': Narratives of University Students with Visual Impairment," *Social Inclusion* 6, no. 4 (2018): 218–29 (224), doi: 10.17645/si.v6i4.1697.

7 Frankl created a form of therapy around meaning making called *Logotherapy*. As depicted in *The Gulag Archipelago*, Aleksandr Solzhenitsyn similarly faced horror and meaninglessness in the Soviet gulags and found meaning in personal responsibility and truth telling that enabled him to survive.

8 Frankl, *Man's Search for Meaning*.

9 Swinton, *Spirituality and Mental Health Care*, 122–28.

10 Eastern Orthodoxy often understands theological anthropology in terms of catholic or universal community as opposed to individual human personhood. For example, see Lossky, *In the Image and Likeness of God*, 169–94.

11 For the origins and early development of Christology in its multifacets, including a *Logos* Christology, see James D. G. Dunn, *Christology in the Making: A New Testament Inquiry into the Origins of the Doctrine of the Incarnation* (Grand Rapids: Eerdmans, 1996). For a historical and theological overview of Spirit Christologies, see Herschel O. Bryant, *Spirit Christology in the Christian Tradition: From the Patristic Period to the Rise of Pentecostalism in the Twentieth Century* (Cleveland, Tenn.: CPT Press, 2019). For the relation of the missions of the Son and the Spirit, see Balthasar, *Theo-drama*, vol. 3. For more on Christ as baptizer in the Spirit, see Frank D. Macchia, *Jesus the Spirit Baptizer: Christology in the Light of Pentecost* (Grand Rapids: Eerdmans, 2018).

12 Lossky, *In the Image and Likeness of God*, 135.

13 Lossky, *In the Image and Likeness of God*, 136, 153–55.

14 Swinton, *Spirituality and Mental Health Care*, 112–22.

15 Swinton, *Spirituality and Mental Health Care*, 131.

16 Swinton, *Spirituality and Mental Health Care*, 131.

17 Thunberg, *Microcosm and Mediator*, 32.

18 From the title *The Word Made Strange*, by John Milbank.

19 Balthasar, *Theo-drama*, 3:222.

20 I am echoing the theme of Balthasar who identified Christ's Sonship in the *oikonomia* with his consciousness of mission. The two became inseparable. The person and his work, Trinitarian and soteriological aspects, coincide and are intertwined in the God-man. The Son of God and the sending of the Son (see sending formula in John's Gospel) into the world to bring salvation are joined. Further, his mission was that we would believe in him and be given the right to become sons and daughters of God. Balthasar, *Theo-drama*, 3:149–250.

21 *The Matrix Reloaded*, dir. the Wachowskis (Burbank, Calif.: Warner Bros. Pictures, 2003).

22 What I am presenting is just a surface-level plain reading of the account of Mephibosheth. Of course, he figures profoundly into disability studies and the Hebrew Bible. The Mephibosheth narrative can be construed as a figure used to explain the complex transition from the line of (unfit rule) Saul to the establishment and legitimizing of the Davidic reign and ensuing nationalism, utilizing the trope of disability. See Jeremy Schipper, *Disability Studies and the Hebrew Bible: Figuring Mephibosheth in the David Story* (New York: T&T Clark, 2006), 20, 25.

23 There are actually several variations of his name in the Hebrew text.

24 LifeWay Research, an evangelical Christian think tank, did a study on mental health issues and Christianity entitled "Study of Acute Mental Illness and Christian Faith." One of the main findings is that churches are ill equipped to minister to persons with mental health issues. A common misconception is that believers in Christ do not get depressed, resulting in stigma and shame, as well as underdiagnosis and undertreatment in some cases. See the report online at http://lifewayresearch.com/wp-content/uploads/2014/09/Acute-Mental-Illness-and-Christian-Faith-Research-Report-1.pdf.

25 I am defining humanity in terms of the analogical interval of difference in opposition to divine being. Humanity is known by its imperfection, limitations, finitude, and susceptibility. We observe humanity in its weakness and passibility. Thus, extreme forms of human

weakness, such as so-called disability (differently abled) and mental disorder are examples of hyperhuman expressions, which do not dehumanize but reveal our humanity in its contingency. These true revelations of humanity pierce our thinly veneered, feeble constructs of human ability.

26 For a liberation view on God as disabled, see Eiesland, *Disabled God*, 98–105.

27 One Old Testament image saw the sacrifice as scapegoat. The sin, guilt, and shame of the people were transmitted to the scapegoat through the high priest.

28 It seems, at least temporarily, that Christ experiences depression symptomatically indicated in the phrase, "My heart is exceedingly sorrowful even unto death." He is overwhelmed with sadness and despondency to the point where he feels approached by death. This trauma seems to have come on him for at least two reasons. The first is his personal experience of having to face death. The second is his personal experience of having the sin and death of the human race placed upon him. Marcia Webb makes an insightful distinction between distress and disorder. The former is faced with the right coping and genetic background that prevents the latter from occurring. So for Webb, "Jesus Christ himself experienced extreme suffering, with great distress, but with no apparent indication of disorder." Webb, *Toward a Theology of Psychological Disorder*, 97. Also, though Christ carries our stigma, the world is often not so kind. The stigma around mental health abounds cross-culturally. The church led by the Spirit needs to advocate for those with mental disabilities through education and just legislation. The church also needs to make space and empower those with disabilities to fulfill their purpose in the kingdom as ministers, witnesses, healers, and teachers. We need to allow their gift to make room for them at the table (Proverbs 18:16).

29 This was the mantra of LSD guru Timothy Leary that inspired an entire youth-led counterculture to experiment with free sex, drugs, and whichever path led to leaving behind one's hang-ups and pursuing a higher consciousness of happiness. A professor and psychologist, Leary proclaimed this message at the 1967 "Human Be-In" in San Francisco. He basically meant to turn on to drugs as performance enhancers to higher consciousness. Tune in to yourself, your brothers and sisters, and the new message of love being promoted. And drop out of conformity—out of school and out of the over-thirty-year-old society of "the man," "big brother" (the government), and the Johnson-Nixon war machine.

30 LSD was not declared illegal until 1966.

31 There have been several biographies written about Barrett. A few examples are Rob Chapman, *A Very Irregular Head: The Life of Syd Barrett* (Cambridge, Mass.: Da Capo, 2012); Mike Watkinson and Pete Anderson, *Crazy Diamond: Syd Barrett and the Dawn of Pink Floyd*, rev. ed. (London: Omnibus, 2007); and Tim Willis, *Madcap: The Half-Life of Syd Barrett, Pink Floyd's Lost Genius* (London: Short, 2003).

32 For example, listen to the tracks "Brain Damage" and "Eclipse," among others.

33 For example, see Webb, *Toward a Theology of Psychological Disorder*, chapters 3–7, where she makes a case against causally identifying psychological distress with sin, and against any causal connection between personal sin and mental disorder.

34 For example, works such as Peter Bellini's *Truth Therapy* propose a healing strategy that integrates Christian doctrinal formation, discipleship, and sanctification with cognitive behavioral therapy and the neuroscientific dynamics of neurogenesis and neuroplasticity. Spiritual, mental, and physical renewal transpires through meditation on the Word of God that utilizes cognitive behavioral hermeneutics and strategies of restructuring to impact the rerouting of neural pathways for healing and even the emerging of new neurons with new assignments for reinvention and renovation.

35 For a simple and clear overview of Eastern Orthodox thinking that draws from the *Philo-kalia* on salvation as healing, see Father George Morelli, "Healing the Infirmity of Sin: A Spiritual Nutshell," accessed December 16, 2019, http://ww1.antiochian.org/content/healing-infirmity-sin-spiritual-nutshell.

36 For a thorough account of the healing movement in the nineteenth century that impacted the Holiness movement, the Keswick movement, and other traditions, see the trilogy *Divine Healing* from James Robinson (Eugene, Ore.: Wipf and Stock, 2011–2014).

37 There are many excellent works that capture the Pentecostal-Charismatic movement and divine healing. Two highly regarded historical accounts are Anderson, *Introduction to Pentecostalism*; and Synan, *Holiness-Pentecostal Tradition*. For a theological understanding of Pentecostalism and healing, see Dayton, *Theological Roots of Pentecostalism*. For an integrative approach to divine healing and science, see Candy Gunther Brown, *Testing Prayer: Science and Healing* (Cambridge, Mass.: Harvard University Press, 2012). For a practical and influential work on divine healing, see Francis MacNutt, *Healing* (Notre Dame, Ind.: Ave Maria, 1999).

38 Many of the traditions that allow for healing through the Eucharist and/or the anointing of the sick expand the range of healing to include physical, mental, and emotional healing.

39 The Book of Common Prayer of the Anglican Church includes prayer for the anointing of the sick. For the Eastern Orthodox, holy unction is ministered in a sacramental service in public rather than in private. For Roman Catholics, the sacrament of healing was called extreme unction until 1972, then named anointing of the sick. See the Catechism of the Catholic Church, 1499–1532. Pope Francis often claims the Eucharist is "not a prize for the perfect but a powerful medicine and nourishment for the weak." The Eucharist in Roman Catholic and Anglican traditions is often thought of as "spiritual food" and "spiritual medicine" that we feed upon in our hearts by faith. See the Church of England's web-page "Wholeness and Healing," https://www.churchofengland.org/prayer-and-worship/worship-texts-and-resources/common-worship/wholeness-and-healing/wholeness-and-healing.

40 As a popular, and for some a controversial, example of this, see Bill Johnson and Beni Johnson, *The Power of Communion: Accessing Miracles through the Body and Blood of Jesus* (Shippenberg, Penn.: Destiny Image, 2019). Most of these renewalist groups will not hold to the sacramental realism of the Roman Catholic, Eastern Orthodox, or Lutheran communions but will at least embrace some version of spiritual presence in the elements following the *epiclesis*.

41 In sacramental traditions, healing through the Eucharist and anointing of the sick is not understood dogmatically or normatively as it often is in more charismatic traditions. For example, the Roman Catholic anointing of the sick for centuries was performed primarily as a last rite along with the Viaticum. Here, healing is seen as more an occasional practice rather than normative, and in this case it is not curative but rather is spiritual preparation for dying and resurrection.

42 These healings have often occurred alongside the gifts of medical science and at times without the use or effects of medicine.

43 For example, because of an accident, my daughter broke her humerus in half and experienced severe nerve damage that paralyzed her left arm and hand. She could slightly lift her arm at the shoulder but had no movement in her wrist, hand, and fingers. The doctors said that after three months, if the nerves did not begin to recover, as evident through some movement, most likely they would never be restored, and she would need a transplant. After three months, she had no movement. After five months, with still no movement, she was willing to receive prayer and anointing for healing. At that time in her life, she

was extremely averse to having any conversation about the Christian God, let alone receiving anointing and prayer. However, after anointing, the laying on of hands, and receiving
prayer, she immediately felt electricity and a power go into her hand, enabling her to begin
to move her fingers, which she could not do before. She also heard an inward voice say that
God was going to heal her. Every day for the next few weeks she gained more and more
movement and dexterity in her left arm, hand, and fingers until within a month she was
completely healed. The doctors were startled. They were planning for the surgery but did
say that recovery was not unheard of, though very rare.

44 For example, see Larry Dossey, *Healing Words: The Power of Prayer and The Practice of
Medicine* (San Francisco: HarperCollins, 1993), and Gunther Brown, *Testing Prayer*.

45 "Divine healing is an integral part of the gospel. Deliverance from sickness is provided for
in the Atonement, and is the privilege of all believers (Isaiah 53:4, 5; Matthew 8:16, 17; James
5:14-16)." This statement is from the Assemblies of God official position paper entitled
"Divine Healing," accessed February 6, 2020, https://ag.org/Beliefs/Position-Papers/Divine
-Healing. Both the Holiness and Pentecostal movements derive their emphasis on healing
from the nineteenth-century healing revival. One stream of the nineteenth-century healing revival came out of the Faith-Cure movement, featuring the writings and ministry of
Charles Cullis, and William Boardman, who influenced the writings and ministry of A. B.
Simpson, Andrew Murray, A. J. Gordon, Carrie Judd Montgomery, Robert Kelso Carter,
and others who held to the doctrine of healing in the atonement. This stream flowed into
the theology of the Keswick and Holiness movements and ultimately Pentecostalism and
the Charismatic movement, becoming a cardinal doctrine of so-called Spirit-filled Christianity. See Dayton, *Theological Roots of Pentecostalism*, 115–41; Nancy A. Hardesty, *Faith
Cure: Divine Healing in the Holiness and Pentecostal Movements* (Grand Rapids: Baker, 2003).

46 See chapter 5, "An Integrative Approach to Healing and Deliverance," in Bellini, *Unleashed!*
An important reminder from the first chapter is that medical science in all of its successes is
limited and fallible and at times can contribute to the disease, disability, and disorder that it
claims to treat and cure. Medicalization, like any process in society, can become hegemonic
and exclude those who need healing the most.

47 For critiques of the health and wealth movement, see Gordon Fee, *The Diseases of the
Health and Wealth Gospels* (Vancouver, B.C.: Regent College, 2006); Bruce Barron, *The
Health and Wealth Gospel* (Downers Grove, Ill.: IVP, 1987).

48 Yong, *Theology and Down Syndrome*, 242–45. It is important to note that Yong makes a
distinction between disability and illness, sickness, or disease. He states, "The latter can be
improved while the former cannot" (245). Thus healing and restoration for the disabled
look different in the new creation than they do for someone with depression. Disability
is central to the identity of the disabled, which is not the case for the depressed. Disability
is constitutive and not accidental to personal identity. For Yong, disabled persons can be
whole in their disability.

49 Resurrection is both healing and cure. It is the healing that cures, and the cure that heals.

50 John W. Oliver, *Giver of Life: The Holy Spirit in the Orthodox Tradition* (Brewster, Mass.:
Paraclete, 2011), 27–33. Oliver makes this poignant distinction that relief, the case in this
text being relief from depression symptoms, is not always the best solution if it does not
address what may be a deeper problem.

51 *Anomalisa*, dir. Charlie Kaufman and Duke Johnson (Los Angeles: Paramount Pictures,
2015).

52 For an intersectional perspective on these and other issues as they relate to the church,
see Grace Ji-Sun Kim and Susan M. Shaw, *Intersectional Theology: An Introductory Guide*
(Minneapolis: Fortress, 2018). For a view on how the church exploits those it serves, see

Steve Corbett and Brian Fikkert, *When Helping Hurts: How to Alleviate Poverty without Hurting the Poor and Yourself* (Chicago: Moody, 2009), and Robert Lupton, *Toxic Charity: How the Church Hurts Those They Help and How to Reverse It* (San Francisco: Harper-Collins, 2011). For a systems approach on how the church can exacerbate or mitigate anxiety, see Peter L. Steinke, *Healthy Congregations: A Systems Approach* (Herndon, Va.: Albin Institute, 2006). For a view on racism within Christianity, see Jeannine Fletcher Hill, *The Sin of White Supremacy: Christianity, Racism, and Religious Diversity in America* (Maryknoll, N.Y.: Orbis Books, 2017). These texts are a sampling and a segue into further conversations and perspectives on these issues and are not meant to be prescriptive or exhaustive.

53 The healing of the person in terms of one's integrative constitution, which is the spiritual, physical, emotional, and relational dimensions, is a function of expressing the image of God in Christ. The wisdom of God defines, manifests, and times healing as it facilitates holiness along an eschatological trajectory of glorification.

54 Suicide is always a possibility lurking in the shadows of mental disorders. Hands-off approaches that refuse to work toward amelioration or healing for fear of being labeled ableist cannot be entertained when working with mental disorders. We need to be aware of and to educate those around us about suicidal wishes, ideation, triggers, warning signs, and plans. In too many cases, those struggling with mental disorders, including depression, die by suicide. This is the harsh reality. There are no words or theology that can bring immediate consolation or hope to the friends and family of the deceased. The proclamation of the gospel or theology surrounding and expounding it, such as this study, is not meant to demean the experience of the sufferer or provide any absolute guarantee of "victory" or false sense of triumphalism over life-threatening symptoms in this life. Many self-professing Christians with mental health struggles have committed suicide as a result of their battle with mental disorders. Even though it is not consoling at the moment, or for quite some time, the good news of healing in the resurrection is the beginning and end of our healing in Christ. Even in death, we may find life. The church needs to be educated on the risks of mental health symptoms and the possibility, warning signs, and ideation of suicide, which can always be a reality. On the other hand, the church should not address the symptoms of mental disorders hopelessly, as if the good news of Christ does not offer God's presence and comfort and at times relief from such symptoms, especially when coupled with proper medical treatment. Why some experience healing as alleviation or relief of symptoms more than others may be related to many variables, known and unknown, the greatest being the mystery of God's providence. So much is unknown when considering these aspects of mental disorders. We are often left silent or in lament as we consider the mystery of suffering in our world.

55 Ecological and cosmic healing.

56 On the other hand, chaos theory would grant that disorder is a natural part of the greater order. Harmonizing with science, we may want to qualify disorder in the case of the fall as moral and relational disorder with God and each other.

57 Amos Yong in *Theology and Down Syndrome* offers Theo-Econo-Politics of Disability as an example of the church addressing the larger sociostructural issues that create or perpetuate disease, disability, and disorder and announcing and embodying the liberating mission and power of the kingdom (253–58).

58 World Health Organization, "Gender and Women's Mental Health." For thorough and extensive data on mental disorder and social factors, see Hannah Ritchie and Max Roser, "Mental Health," from *Our World in Data*, April 2018, accessed December 26, 2019,

https://ourworldindata.org/mental-health. For a study on the relationship between mental health, race, and ethnicity, see U.S. Department of Health and Human Services, *Mental Health: Culture, Race, and Ethnicity: A Supplement to Mental Health: A Report of the Surgeon General* (Rockville, Md.: U.S. Department of Health and Human Services, Substance Abuse and Mental Health Services Administration, Center for Mental Health Services, 2001), accessed September 15, 2020, https://www.ncbi.nlm.nih.gov/books/NBK44243/. See also Fernando, *Mental Health, Race and Culture*.

59 For select reading on the connection between forgiveness and mental health, see Robert Enright, "A New Approach to Reducing Depression," *Psychology Today*, April 6, 2017; Mayo Clinic Staff, "Forgiveness: Letting Go of Grudges and Bitterness," November 4, 2017, accessed September 15, 2020, https://www.mayoclinic.org/healthy-lifestyle/adult -health/in-depth/forgiveness/art-20047692; "Forgiveness," in *Integrative Medicine*, ed. David Rakel, 4th ed. (Philadelphia, Pa.: Elsevier, 2018); Kirsten Weir, "Forgiveness Can Improve Mental and Physical Health," *American Psychological Association CE Corner* 48, no. 1 (2017): 30, http://www.apa.org/monitor/2017/01/ce-corner.aspx; S. Akhtar et al., "Understanding the Relationship between State Forgiveness and Psychological Wellbeing: A Qualitative Study," *Journal of Religion and Health* 56 (2017): 450; Loren L. Toussaint, Everett L. Worthington, and David R. Williams, eds., *Forgiveness and Health: Scientific Evidence and Theories Relating Forgiveness to Better Health* (New York: Springer, 2015); Everett L. Worthington Jr., *Dimensions of Forgiveness: Psychological Research and Theological Perspectives* (Radnor, Penn.: Templeton, 1998); Everett L. Worthington Jr. and Steven J. Sandage, *Forgiveness and Spirituality in Psychotherapy: A Relational Approach* (Washington, D.C.: American Psychological Association, 2015); David W. Augsburger, *Helping People Forgive* (Louisville, Ky.: Westminster John Knox, 1996); Gregory L. Jones, *Embodying Forgiveness: A Theological Analysis* (Grand Rapids: Eerdmans, 1995).

60 See some of the sources, including the work of Everett Worthington, listed above for an integrative approach.

61 There are various theories of the atonement and how they relate to forgiveness of sin: penal satisfaction, substitutionary theories, *Christus Victor* and the related ransom theory, the moral government theory, and moral example, among others, i.e., James Beilby, ed., *The Nature of the Atonement: Four Views* (Downers Grove, Ill.: IVP, 2006). I am not endorsing any one theory here. It seems the portrait painted in Scripture of the atonement is not limited to any one dimension offered by the various theories. However, Scripture is simply clear that God forgives sin based on the work of Jesus Christ at the cross.

62 Some studies have linked lack of self-compassion, or what I would call self-forgiveness, with depression, as tests indicate that lack of self-compassion predicts subsequent depressive symptoms, i.e., Tobias Krieger, Thomas Berger, and Martin grosse Holtforth, "The Relationship of Self-Compassion and Depression: Cross-Lagged Panel Analyses in Depressed Patients after Outpatient Therapy," *Journal of Affective Disorders* 202 (September 15, 2016): 39–45, https://doi.org/10.1016/j.jad.2016.05.032.

63 See Augsburger, *Helping People Forgive*; and Jones, *Embodying Forgiveness*.

64 The reference and usage of *therapeia* is being employed in the Eastern Christian sense of healing soul sickness en route to theosis through repentance and sanctification, as opposed to the commercial view of therapy and self-help that has inundated the church at a popular level, i.e., such as through moral therapeutic deism.

65 For a well-sourced investigation of the meaning and background of Paraclete, see Cornelius Bennema, *The Power of Saving Wisdom: An Investigation of Spirit and Wisdom in Relation to the Soteriology of the Fourth Gospel* (Eugene, Ore.: Wipf and Stock, 2012), 216–21. See also

Ben Witherington III, *Jesus the Sage: The Pilgrimage of Wisdom* (Minneapolis: Augsburg Fortress, 2000); and *John's Wisdom: A Commentary on the Fourth Gospel* (Louisville, Ky.: Westminster John Knox, 1995).

66 Cornelius Bennema in *Power of Saving Wisdom*, 216, cites various translations from various interpreters: "Helper" (Bultmann), "Representative" (George Johnston), "Supporter/ Sponsor" (K. Grayston), "Exhorter/Comforter/Consoler" (J. G. Davies), "Counsellor" (James Dunn), "Teacher/Preacher" (E. Franck), "Paraclete," and "Advocate" (Raymond Brown).

67 See the Chalcedonian Definition with its four borders placed around the assertion of two natures in one person, discussed in chapter 8. Christianity shares a common apophatic heritage in the early church fathers—works of Clement of Alexandria, Origen, the Cappadocian fathers, Augustine, Pseudo-Dionysius, Maximus the Confessor, and Symeon the New Theologian. Though understood differently between the East (Gregory Palamas) and the West (Thomas Aquinas' *via eminentiae*, Meister Eckhart, and the Catholic mystics such as St. John of the Cross), both traditions have utilized apophatic theology to understand the unknowable God.

68 St. John, in chapters 5–10 of book 2 of *Dark Night of the Soul*, describes in detail the affliction of the soul passing through purgation. See St. John of the Cross, *Dark Night of the Soul*.

69 Aaron T. Beck, *Depression: Causes and Treatment* (Philadelphia: University of Pennsylvania Press, 1967), 14.

70 Yong, *Theology and Down Syndrome*, 253–58.

71 Depersonalization and derealization are reported experiences from depressed persons but not official *DSM-5* symptoms that could diagnose depression. However, Depersonalization/ Derealization Disorder is classified in the *DSM-5*.

72 Jim Morrison, vocalist, "People Are Strange," 1967, by Jim Morrison and Robbie Krieger (lyricists), the Doors (composers), side B, track 1 on *Strange Days* (New York: Elektra Records, 1967). One wonders how much of the lyrics were autobiographical for Morrison, who seemed to struggle with depression.

73 Not only those mentally estranged but also those socially and politically estranged— migrants, immigrants, asylum seekers, and refugees.

74 Jean Vanier, *Befriending the Stranger* (Mahwah, N.J.: Paulist, 2004). Although Vanier's work is marred by his moral failure, others share from L'Arche, Vanier's ministry, how Christ befriends us in our weakness and calls us to do the same in building authentic, loving communities.

75 For more on this notion of Christian hospitality, see Christine Pohl, *Making Room: Recovering Hospitality as a Christian Tradition* (Grand Rapids: Eerdmans, 1999).

76 Years after its numerous awards, high accolades, and acclaimed reviews, the film has received stinging criticism for how it "whitewashes and dumbs down American history at every turn," and how it lacks critical awareness of racial issues and oversimplifies complex social and political issues; I do not disagree that a viewing now and perhaps even in 1994 warrants such criticism. However, critics are missing the point of the film, which is the narrator's point of view: a narrator who most likely is on the autism spectrum. Although the film lightheartedly and almost comically employs a highlight reel of social and political events from our baby boomer memory, it does not signify that the film was intended to be viewed seriously from either perspective. Critics, such as the one quoted, need perhaps to pay attention to the ableist language of "dumbing down" to describe the perspective of one with intellectual disabilities. See Eric Kohn, "*Forrest Gump*, 25 Years Later: A Bad Movie

That Gets Worse with Age," *IndieWire*, July 4, 2019, accessed May 17, 2020, https://www
.indiewire.com/2019/07/forrest-gump-bad-movie-25-anniversary-1202154214/.

77 Bennema, *Power of Saving Wisdom*, 225.

78 Aquinas, *Summa Theologiae* 1.2.26.4.

79 Dodds, *Unchanging God of Love*, 208–9.

80 Dodds, *Unchanging God of Love*, 210.

81 Dodds, *Unchanging God of Love*, 217–25.

82 Dodds, *Unchanging God of Love*, 217, referencing Thomas Aquinas.

83 The marred work of the late Jean Vanier (1928–2019) through L'Arche, which globally
established communities of friendship for those with intellectual and developmental disabilities, attempted to exemplify such an effort to minister healing through belonging.
Although later discoveries of Vanier's patterns of abuse in ministry nullify his personal
witness, the ministry of L'Arche and the work of others remain a faithful model of Christian friendship. L'Arche valued the potential of all persons to live and grow together and
experience fulfillment, by not only seeing their value as persons but also by seeing them
as teachers and not burdens because of their challenges. Our need to be taught by the
weak helps to liberate us to become truly human (https://www.larcheusa.org/about/). See
Jean Vanier, *Becoming Human*, 2nd ed. (Toronto: House of Anansi, 2008); Stanley Hauerwas and Jean Vanier, *Living Gently in a Violent World: The Prophetic Witness of Weakness*
(Downers Grove, Ill.: IVP, 2018); Anne-Sophie Constant, *Jean Vanier: Portrait of a Free
Man* (Walden, N.Y.: Plough, 2019).

Bibliography

Abraham, William J. *Divine Agency and Divine Action*. 3 vols. Oxford: Oxford University Press, 2017–2018.

Akhtar, S., et al. "Understanding the Relationship between State Forgiveness and Psychological Wellbeing: A Qualitative Study." *Journal of Religion and Health* 56 (2017): 450.

Allan, Kenneth. "The Postmodern Self: A Theoretical Consideration." *Quarterly Journal of Ideology* 20, nos. 1–2 (1997): 3–24.

Almog, Nitsan. "'Everyone Is Normal, and Everyone Has a Disability': Narratives of University Students with Visual Impairment." *Social Inclusion* 6, no. 4 (2018): 218–29. doi: 10.17645/si.v6i4.1697.

Altizer, Thomas J. J. *The Gospel of Christian Atheism*. Philadelphia: Westminster, 1966.

Altizer, Thomas J. J., and William Hamilton, eds. *Radical Theology and the Death of God*. Indianapolis: Merrill, 1966.

American Psychiatric Association. *Diagnostic and Statistical Manual of Mental Disorders*. 4th ed. Washington, D.C.: American Psychiatric Association, 1994. Cited in the text and notes as *DSM-4*.

———. *Diagnostic and Statistical Manual of Mental Disorders*. 5th ed. Arlington, Va.: American Psychiatric Association, 2013. Cited in the text and notes as *DSM-5*.

Anderson, Allan Heaton. *An Introduction to Pentecostalism: Global Charismatic Christianity*. 2nd ed. Cambridge: Cambridge University Press, 2014.

Anomalisa. Dir. Charlie Kaufman and Duke Johnson. Los Angeles: Paramount Pictures, 2015.

Aquinas, Thomas. *De Ente et Essentia*. Translated by George G. Leckie. New York: D. Appleton–Century, 1937.

———. *Summa Theologica of St. Thomas Aquinas: English Dominican Province Translation*. Notre Dame, Ind.: Christian Classics, 1981.

Aristotle. *Aristotle: Problems*. Vol. 16. Translated by W. S. Hett. Loeb Classical Library. Cambridge, Mass.: Harvard University Press, 1957.

———. *De Anima (On the Soul)*. Translated by Hugh Lawson-Tancred. London: Penguin Classics, 1987.

Assemblies of God. "Divine Healing." Accessed February 6, 2020. https://ag.org/Beliefs/Position
-Papers/Divine-Healing.

Athanasius. *On the Incarnation*. Yonkers, N.Y.: St. Vladimir's Seminary Press, 1993.

Augsburger, David W. *Helping People Forgive*. Louisville, Ky.: Westminster John Knox, 1996.

Augustine. *Confessions and Enchiridion*. Translated by Albert C. Outler. Philadelphia: Westminster, 1955.

———. *Contra adversarium legis et prophetarum*. Edited by Klaus D. Daur. Corpus Christianorium: Series Latina 49. Turnhout: Brepols, 1985.

Balthasar, Hans Urs von. *The Christian and Anxiety*. San Francisco: Ignatius, 2000.

———. *Mysterium Paschale*. 1970; San Francisco: Ignatius, 2000.

———. *Theo-drama: Theological Dramatic Theory*. Vol. 3, *Dramatis Personae: Persons in Christ*. San Francisco: Ignatius, 1992.

Barbour, Ian G. *Religion and Science: Historical and Contemporary Issues*. San Francisco: Harper-Collins, 1997.

Barron, Bruce. *The Health and Wealth Gospel*. Downers Grove, Ill.: IVP, 1987.

Barth, Karl. *Church Dogmatics*. Edinburgh: T&T Clark, 1936–1969.

Bauckham, Richard. "'Only the Suffering God Can Help': Divine Passibility in Modern Theology." *Themelios* 9, no. 3 (April 1984): 6–12.

Beck, Aaron T. *Cognitive Theory of Depression*. New York: Guilford, 1987.

———. *Depression: Causes and Treatment*. Philadelphia: University of Pennsylvania Press, 1967.

Beckett, Samuel. *Endgame: A Play in One Act, Followed by Act without Words, a Mime for One Player*. Translated by the author. New York: Grove Press, 1958.

———. *Three Novels: Molloy, Malone Dies, The Unnamable*. New York: Grove, 2009.

———. *Waiting for Godot: A Tragicomedy in Two Acts*. New York: Grove, 2011.

Beilby, James, ed. *The Nature of the Atonement: Four Views*. Downers Grove, Ill.: IVP, 2006.

Bellini, Peter J. *Participation: Epistemology and Mission Theology*. Lexington, Ky.: Emeth, 2010.

———. "The *Processio-Missio* Connection: A Starting Point in *Missio Trinitatis* or Overcoming the Immanent-Economic Divide in a *Missio Trinitatis*." *Wesleyan Theological Journal* 49, no. 2 (2014): 7–23.

———. *Truth Therapy: Renewing the Mind with the Word of God*. Eugene, Ore.: Wipf and Stock, 2014.

———. *Unleashed! The C1-13 Integrative Deliverance Needs Assessment: A Qualitative and Quantitative Probability Indicator*. Eugene, Ore.: Wipf and Stock, 2018.

Bengt, Brülde. "Wakefield's Hybrid Account of Mental Disorder." *World Psychiatry* 6, no. 3 (2007): 163–64.

Bennema, Cornelius. *The Power of Saving Wisdom: An Investigation of Spirit and Wisdom in Relation to the Soteriology of the Fourth Gospel*. Eugene, Ore.: Wipf and Stock, 2012.

Berger, Peter. *A Rumor of Angels: Modern Society and the Rediscovery of the Supernatural*. New York: Anchor, 1970.

Bergstrom, Carl T., and Frazer Meacham. "Depression and Anxiety: Maladaptive Byproducts of Adaptive Mechanisms." *Evolution, Medicine, and Public Health* 2016, no. 1 (2016): 214.

Betz, John. "After Barth: A New Introduction to Erich Przywara's *Analogia Entis*." In White, *Analogy of Being*.

Bhaskar, Roy. *A Realist Theory of Science*. New York: Routledge, 2008.

Blazer, Dan G. *The Age of Melancholy: Major Depression and Its Social Origins*. New York: Routledge, 2005.

Boethius. *Liber De Persona et Duabus Naturis Contra Eutychen et Nestorium*. *Patrologia Latina*, edited by J. P. Migne. Paris, 1878–1890.

Brower, Jeffrey. "Making Sense of Divine Simplicity." *Faith and Philosophy* 25, no. 1 (2008): 3–30.

Brown, Candy Gunther. *Testing Prayer: Science and Healing*. Cambridge, Mass.: Harvard University Press, 2012.

Brown, George W., and Tirril Harris. *Social Origins of Depression*. London, UK: Routledge, 1978.

Brunner, Emil, and Karl Barth. *Natural Theology*. Eugene, Ore.: Wipf and Stock, 2002.

Bryant, Herschel O. *Spirit Christology in the Christian Tradition: From the Patristic Period to the Rise of Pentecostalism in the Twentieth Century*. Cleveland, Tenn.: CPT Press, 2019.

Buber, Martin. *I and Thou*. Translated by Walter Kaufmann. New York: Touchstone, 1971.

Bunge, Gabriel. *Despondency: The Spiritual Teaching of Evagrius Ponticus on Acedia*. Yonkers, N.Y.: St. Vladimir's Seminary Press, 2011.

Burton, Robert. *The Anatomy of Melancholy*. Introduction by William H. Gass. Edited by Holbrook Jackson. New York: New York Review Books, 2001.

Cairns, David. *The Image of God in Man*. New York: Philosophical Library, 1953.

Campbell, Fiona A. Kumari. "Exploring Internalized Ableism Using Critical Race Theory." *Disability & Society* 23 (2008): 5–6. https://doi.org/10.1080/09687590701841190.

Camus, Albert. *The Myth of Sisyphus*. New York: Vintage, 2018.

———. *The Stranger*. New York: Vintage, 1989.

Caputo, John D., and Michael J. Scanlon, eds. *Transcendence and Beyond: A Postmodern Inquiry*. Bloomington: Indiana University Press, 2007.

Carlton, Clark. *The Faith: Understanding Orthodox Christianity, an Orthodox Catechism*. Salisbury, Mass.: Regina Orthodox Press, 1997.

Cassian, John. *The Conferences*. Translated by Boniface Ramsey. New York: Paulist, 1997.

Cavanaugh, William T., and James K. A. Smith, eds. *Evolution and the Fall*. Grand Rapids: Eerdmans, 2017.

Chakravartty, Anjan. "Scientific Realism." In *The Stanford Encyclopedia of Philosophy*, ed. Edward N. Zalta, summer 2017 ed. https://plato.stanford.edu/archives/sum2017/entries/scientific-realism/.

Chapman, Rob. *A Very Irregular Head: The Life of Syd Barrett*. Cambridge, Mass.: Da Capo, 2012.

Chemnitz, Martin. *The Two Natures of Christ*. Translated by J. Preus. St. Louis: Concordia, 1971.

Churchland, Paul. "Eliminative Materialism and the Propositional Attitudes." In Heil, *Philosophy of Mind*.

Church of England. "Wholeness and Healing." https://www.churchofengland.org/prayer-and-worship/worship-texts-and-resources/common-worship/wholeness-and-healing/wholeness-and-healing.

Clayton, Philip. *Adventures in the Spirit: God, World, and Divine Action*. Minneapolis: Fortress, 2008.

———. "Kenotic Trinitarian Panentheism." *Dialog* 44, no. 3 (2005): 250–55. https://doi.org/10.1111/j.0012-2033.2005.00265.x.

Clayton, Philip, and Arthur Peacocke, eds. *In Whom We Live and Move and Have Our Being: Panentheistic Reflections on God's Presence in a Scientific World*. Grand Rapids: Eerdmans, 2004.

"Clinical Characteristics of Intellectual Disabilities." In *Mental Disorders and Disabilities among Low-Income Children*, by the Committee to Evaluate the Supplemental Security Income Disability Program for Children with Mental Disorders; Board on the Health of Select Populations; Board on Children, Youth, and Families; Institute of Medicine; Division of

Behavioral and Social Sciences and Education; National Academies of Sciences, Engineering, and Medicine, edited by Thomas F. Boat and Joel T. Wu. Washington, D.C.: National Academies Press, 2015, accessed September 21, 2020. https://www.ncbi.nlm.nih.gov/books/NBK332877/table/tab_9-1/?report=objectonly.

Coakley, Sarah. "Does Kenosis Rest on a Mistake?" In Evans, *Exploring Kenotic Christology*.

Coffey, David. *Deus Trinitas: The Doctrine of the Triune God*. New York: Oxford University Press, 1999.

Collins, Kenneth, and John Tyson, eds. *Conversion in the Wesleyan Tradition*. Nashville, Tenn.: Abingdon, 2001.

Cone, James. *A Black Theology of Liberation*. Maryknoll, N.Y.: Orbis Books, 2010.

———. *The Cross and the Lynching Tree*. Maryknoll, N.Y.: Orbis Books, 2013.

Congdon, David W. "*Nova Lingua Dei*: The Problem of Chalcedonian Metaphysics and the Promise of the *Genus Tapeinoticon* in Luther's Late Theology." PhD diss., Princeton Theological Seminary, 2011, accessed October 26, 2019. https://www.academia.edu/586346/Nova_Lingua_Dei_The_Problem_of_Chalcedonian_Metaphysics_and_the_Promise_of_the_Genus_Tapeinoticon_in_Luthers_Later_Theology.

Constant, Anne-Sophie. *Jean Vanier: Portrait of a Free Man*. Walden, N.Y.: Plough, 2019.

Corbett, Steve, and Brian Fikkert. *When Helping Hurts: How to Alleviate Poverty without Hurting the Poor and Yourself*. Chicago: Moody, 2009.

Coulter, Dale M., and Amos Yong, eds. *The Spirit, the Affections, and the Christian Tradition*. Notre Dame, Ind.: University of Notre Dame Press, 2016.

Craig, William Lane. "Religious Epistemology." In *Philosophical Foundations for a Christian Worldview*, by J. P. Moreland and William Lane Craig, 2nd ed. Downers Grove, Ill.: IVP Academic, 2017.

Creel, Richard. *Divine Impassibility*. Cambridge: Cambridge University Press, 1986.

Culligan, Kevin. "The Dark Night and Depression." In *Carmelite Prayer*, edited by Keith J. Egan. New York: Paulist, 2003.

Cunningham, Conor. *Genealogy of Nihilism: Philosophies of Nothing and the Difference of Theology*. New York: Routledge, 2002.

Cyril of Alexandria. "Council of Ephesus, Second Letter of Cyril to Nestorius." In *Decrees of the Ecumenical Councils*, vol. 1, ed. Norman P. Tanner. Washington, D.C.: Georgetown University Press, 2017.

———. *On the Unity of Christ*. Edited by John Anthony McGuckin. Popular Patristic Series. Crestwood, N.Y.: St. Vladimir's Seminary Press, 2015.

Damasio, Antonio R. *Descartes' Error: Emotion, Reason, and the Human Brain*. New York: Avon Books, 1994.

———. *The Feeling of What Happens: Body and Emotion in the Making of Consciousness*. San Diego: Harcourt, 1999.

Davis, Stephen T. "Is Kenosis Orthodox?" In Evans, *Exploring Kenotic Christology*, 113.

Dayton, Donald W. *The Theological Roots of Pentecostalism*. Grand Rapids: Baker Academic, 1987.

de Duve, Christian, and Neil Patterson. *Genetics of Original Sin: The Impact of Natural Selection on the Future of Humanity*. New Haven, Conn.: Yale University Press, 2012.

"Depression: A Global Public Health Concern," World Health Organization, 2012, accessed January 20, 2016. http://www.who.int/mental_health/management/depression/en.

Descartes, René. *Meditations on First Philosophy*. Indianapolis: Hackett, 1993.

Dodds, Michael J. *The Unchanging God of Love: Thomas Aquinas and Contemporary Theologians on Divine Immutability*, 2nd ed. Washington, D.C.: Catholic University of America Press, 2008.

———. *Unlocking Divine Action: Contemporary Science and Thomas Aquinas*. Washington, D.C.: Catholic University of America Press, 2012.

Dolezal, James E. *All That Is in God: Evangelical Theology and the Challenge of Classical Theism*. Grand Rapids: Reformation Heritage, 2017.

Dossey, Larry. *Healing Words: The Power of Prayer and The Practice of Medicine*. San Francisco: HarperCollins, 1993.

Douglas, Kelly Brown. *The Black Christ*. Maryknoll, N.Y.: Orbis Books, 1993.

"Driven by New Therapeutic Drug Classes, Depression Drug Market to Grow to $7.3 Billion by 2024." Pharmaprojects: Track pharma R&D. *Pharma Intelligence*, October 8, 2017, accessed September 16, 2020. https://pharmaintelligence.informa.com/resources/product-content/depression-drug-market-to-grow.

Dunn, James D. G. *Christology in the Making: A New Testament Inquiry into the Origins of the Doctrine of the Incarnation*. Grand Rapids: Eerdmans, 1996.

Durà-Vilà, Glòria, Simon Dein, Roland Littlewood, and Gerard Leavey. "The Dark Night of the Soul: Causes and Resolution of Emotional Distress among Contemplative Nuns." *Transcultural Psychiatry* 47, no. 4 (2010): 548–70. doi: 10.1177/1363461510374899.

Eiesland, Nancy L. *The Disabled God: Toward a Liberation Theology of Disability*. Nashville, Tenn.: Abingdon, 1994.

Elden, Stuart. "To Say Nothing of God: Heidegger's Holy Atheism." *Heythrop Journal* 45, no. 3 (2004): 344–48. https://doi.org/10.1111/j.1468-2265.2004.00259.x.

Ellis, Albert. *A Guide to Rational Living*. Englewood Cliffs, N.J.: Prentice Hall, 1961.

Emerson, Eric. "Poverty and People with Intellectual Disabilities." *Mental Retardation and Developmental Disabilities Research Reviews* 13, no. 2 (2007): 107–13, Special Issue: Public Policy Aspects of the Developmental Disabilities. https://doi.org/10.1002/mrdd.20144.

Emery, Gilles. "The Immutability of the God of Love." In Keating and White, *Divine Impassibility*, 32.

———. "The Vision of the Mystery of the Trinity in Thomas Aquinas." *Credere, amare e vivere la verità / Believing, Loving and Living Truth: The Proceedings of the XIII Plenary Session in the Year of the Faith*, June 21–23, 2013. Accessed September 15, 2020, http://www.past.va/content/dam/past/pdf/dc_2014/doctor_communis_2014.pdf.

Enright, Robert. "A New Approach to Reducing Depression." *Psychology Today*, April 6, 2017.

Evagrius of Pontus (Evagrius Ponticus). *The Praktikos and Chapters on Prayer*. Translated by John Eudes Bamberger. 2nd ed. Kalamazoo, Mich.: Cistercian, 1972.

———. *Talking Back [Antirrhetikos]: A Monastic Handbook for Combating Demons*. Translated by David Brakke. Trappist, Ky.: Cistercian, 2009.

Evans, C. Stephen, ed. *Exploring Kenotic Christology: The Self-Emptying of God*. Vancouver, B.C.: Regent College, 2010.

Fee, Gordon. *The Diseases of the Health and Wealth Gospels*. Vancouver, B.C.: Regent College, 2006.

———. "The New Testament and Kenosis Christology." In Evans, *Exploring Kenotic Christology*.

Feld, Alina. *Melancholy and the Otherness of God: A Study of the Hermeneutics of Depression*. Plymouth, UK: Lexington Books, 2011.

Fernando, Suman. *Mental Health, Race and Culture*. 3rd ed. London: Springer Nature, 2010.

Ficino, Marsilio. *Three Books on Life*. Translated by Carol V. Kaske and John R. Clark. New York: Medieval and Renaissance Texts and Studies, 1989.

"Forgiveness." In *Integrative Medicine*, ed. David Rakel. 4th ed. Philadelphia.: Elsevier, 2018.

Frankl, Viktor E. *Man's Search for Meaning*. New York: Simon & Schuster, 1959.

Freud, Sigmund. *On Freud's "Mourning and Melancholia."* Edited by Thierry Bokanowski, Leticia Gloser Fiorini, and Sergio Lewkowicz. New York: Routledge, 2010.

Gałecki, Piotr, and Monika Talarowska. "The Evolutionary Theory of Depression." *Medical Science Monitor* 23 (2017): 2267–74. doi: 10.12659/MSM.901240.

Galen. *On the Affected Parts*. Edited and translated by Rudolph Siegel. Basel: Karger, 1976.

Gaventa, William C. *Disability and Spirituality: Recovering Wholeness*. Studies in Religion, Theology, and Disability. Waco, Tex.: Baylor University Press, 2018.

Gaventa, William C., Jr., and David L. Coulter. *Spirituality and Intellectual Disability: International Perspectives on the Effect of Culture and Religion on Healing Body, Mind, and Soul*. New York: Routledge, 2014.

Gavrilyuk, Paul. "God's Impassible Suffering in the Flesh: The Promise of Paradoxical Christology." In Keating and White, *Divine Impassibility*.

———. *Suffering of the Impassible God: The Dialectics of Patristic Thought*. Oxford Early Christian Studies. Oxford: Oxford University Press, 2006.

Gergen, Kenneth J. *The Saturated Self: Dilemmas of Identity in Contemporary Life*. New York: Basic Books, 1991.

Giorgiov, Adrian. "The Kenotic Christology of Charles Gore, P. T. Forsyth, and H. R. Mackintosh." *Perichoresis* 2, no. 1 (2004): 47–66.

Giroux, Élodie. *Naturalism in the Philosophy of Health: Issues and Implications*. History, Philosophy, and Theory of the Life Sciences. New York: Springer, 2016.

Goering, Sara. "Rethinking Disability: The Social Model of Disability and Chronic Disease." *Current Reviews in Musculoskeletal Medicine* 8, no. 2 (2015): 134–38, doi: 10.1007/s12178-015-9273-z.

Goetz, Stewart, and Charles Taliaferro. *Naturalism*. Grand Rapids: Eerdmans, 2008.

Good, Byron J. *Medicine, Rationality, and Experience: An Anthropological Perspective*. Cambridge: Cambridge University Press, 1994.

Green, Joel B. *Body, Soul, and Human Life: The Nature of Humanity in the Bible*. Grand Rapids: Baker, 2008.

———. *The Gospel of Luke*. In *The New International Commentary of the New Testament*. Grand Rapids: Eerdmans, 1997.

———, ed. *In Search of the Soul: Perspectives on the Mind-Body Problem*. 2nd ed. Eugene, Ore.: Wipf and Stock, 2005.

Greenberg, Paul E. "The Growing Economic Burden of Depression in the U.S." MIND Guest Blog, *Scientific American*, February 25, 2015. https://blogs.scientificamerican.com/mind-guest-blog/the-growing-economic-burden-of-depression-in-the-u-s/.

Gregory of Nazianzus. *Epistle 101*. In *On God and Christ: The Five Theological Orations and Two Letters to Cledonius*. Popular Patristics Series. Yonkers, N.Y.: St. Vladimir's Seminary Press, 2002.

———. "Oration 29." In *The Five Theological Orations*, trans. Stephen Reynolds. Estate of Stephen Reynolds, 2011. http://hdl.handle.net/1807/36303.

Grenz, Stanley J. *The Social God and the Relational Self: A Trinitarian Theology of the Imago Dei*. Louisville, Ky.: Westminster John Knox, 2001.

———. *Theology for the Community of God*. Grand Rapids: Eerdmans, 2000.

Grohol, John. "Overdiagnosis, Mental Disorders and the DSM-5." *PsychCentral*, July 8, 2018. Accessed September 16, 2020, https://psychcentral.com/blog/overdiagnosis-mental-disorders-and-the-dsm-5/.

Gunther Brown, Candy. *Testing Prayer: Science and Healing*. Cambridge, Mass.: Harvard University Press, 2012.

Hall, Melinda C. "Critical Disability Theory." In *The Stanford Encyclopedia of Philosophy*, ed. Edward N. Zalta, winter 2019 ed. https://plato.stanford.edu/archives/win2019/entries/disability-critical/.

Hanlon, Gerard. *The Immutability of God in the Theology of Hans Urs von Balthasar*. Cambridge: Cambridge University Press, 1990.

Hardesty, Nancy A. *Faith Cure: Divine Healing in the Holiness and Pentecostal Movements*. Grand Rapids: Baker, 2003.

Hart, David Bentley. *The Beauty of the Infinite: The Aesthetics of Christian Truth*. Grand Rapids: Eerdmans, 2002.

Hauerwas, Stanley, and Jean Vanier. *Living Gently in a Violent World: The Prophetic Witness of Weakness*. Downers Grove, Ill.: IVP, 2018.

Hawking, Stephen. *The Grand Design*. New York: Bantam, 2010.

Heschel, Abraham Joshua. *The Prophets: Two Volumes in One*. Peabody, Mass.: Hendrickson, 2007.

Heurtley, Charles A., trans. *St. Leo's Epistle to Flavian*. London: Parker, 1885.

Heil, John, ed. *Philosophy of Mind: A Guide and Anthology*. Oxford: Oxford University Press, 2004.

Hiebert, Paul. *Anthropological Insights for Missionaries*. 17th ed. Grand Rapids: Baker Academic, 1986.

———. *The Missiological Implications of Epistemological Shifts: Affirming Truth in a Modern/Postmodern World*. Harrisburg, Penn.: Trinity, 1999.

———. *Transforming Worldviews: An Anthropological Understanding of How People Change*. Grand Rapids: Baker Academic, 2008.

Hill, Jeannine Fletcher. *The Sin of White Supremacy: Christianity, Racism, and Religious Diversity in America*. Maryknoll, N.Y.: Orbis Books, 2017.

Hippocrates. *Works of Hippocrates*. Translated and edited by W. Jones and E. Witherington. 4 vols. Cambridge, Mass.: Harvard University Press, 1923–1931.

Horowitz, Allan V., and Jerome C. Wakefield. *All We Have to Fear: Psychiatry's Transformation of Natural Anxieties into Mental Disorders*. Oxford: Oxford University Press, 2012.

Iacovu, Susan. "What Is the Difference between Existential Anxiety and So-Called Neurotic Anxiety?" *Existential Analysis: Journal of the Society for Existential Analysis* 22, no. 2 (2011): 356–67.

Internet Encyclopedia of Philosophy: A Peer-Reviewed Academic Resource. Accessed June 21, 2018, https://www.iep.utm.edu/emergenc/.

Jaarsma, Pier, and Stellan Welin. "Autism as a Natural Human Variation: Reflections on the Claims of the Neurodiversity Movement." *Health Care Analysis* 20, no. 1 (2012): 20–30, doi: 10.1007/s10728-011-0169-9.

Jackson, Stanley W. *Melancholia and Depression: From Hippocratic Times to Modern Times*. New Haven, Conn.: Yale University Press, 1986.

Jeeves, Malcolm, and Warren S. Brown. *Neuroscience, Psychology, and Religion: Illusions, Delusions, and Realities about Human Nature*. West Conshohocken, Penn.: Templeton, 2009.

Jenson, Robert. "*Ipse Pater Non Est Impassibilis*." In Keating and White, *Divine Impassibility*.

Johnsen, Tom J., and Oddgeir Friborg. "The Effects of Cognitive Behavioral Therapy as an Anti-depressive Treatment Is Falling: A Meta-analysis." *Psychological Bulletin* 141, no. 4 (2015): 747–68.

Johnson, Bill, and Beni Johnson. *The Power of Communion: Accessing Miracles through the Body and Blood of Jesus*. Shippenberg, Penn.: Destiny Image, 2019.

Jones, Gregory L. *Embodying Forgiveness: A Theological Analysis*. Grand Rapids: Eerdmans, 1995.

Kafka, Franz. *The Castle*. Translated by Mark Harman. New York: Schocken, 1998.

———. *Metamorphosis*. Translated by Susan Bernofsky. New York: Norton, 2014.

Keating, James, and Thomas White. *Divine Impassibility and the Mystery of Human Suffering*. Grand Rapids: Eerdmans, 2009.

Kee, Alistair. *Constantine versus Christ: The Triumph of an Ideology*. Eugene, Ore.: Wipf and Stock, 2016.

Keener, Craig. *The Mind of the Spirit: Paul's Approach to Transformed Thinking*. Grand Rapids: Baker, 2016.

———. *Miracles: The Credibility of the New Testament Accounts*. 2 vols. Grand Rapids: Baker, 2011.

Keith, Heather E., and Kenneth D. Keith. *Intellectual Disability: Ethics, Dehumanization and a New Moral Community*. West Sussex, UK: Wiley, 2013.

Kidd, I. J. "Transformative Suffering and the Cultivation of Virtue." *Philosophy, Psychiatry, & Psychology* 22, no. 4 (2015): 291–94.

Kierkegaard, Søren. *The Concept of Anxiety*. Edited and translated by Reidar Thomte. Princeton, N.J.: Princeton University Press, 1980.

Kim, Grace Ji-Sun, and Susan M. Shaw. *Intersectional Theology: An Introductory Guide*. Minneapolis: Fortress, 2018.

Kim, Jaegwon. "Multiple Realization and the Metaphysics of Reduction." In Heil, *Philosophy of Mind*.

———. *Supervenience and Mind: Selected Philosophical Essays*. Cambridge: Cambridge University Press, 1993.

Kingma, Elselijn. "What Is It to Be Healthy?" *Analysis* 67, no. 294 (2007): 128–33.

Kleinman, Arthur. *The Illness Narratives: Suffering, Healing, and the Human Condition*. New York: Basic Books, 1988.

———. *Patients and Healers in the Context of Culture: An Exploration of the Borderland between Anthropology, Medicine, and Psychiatry*. Berkeley: University of California Press, 1980.

———. *Rethinking Psychiatry: From Cultural Category to Personal Experience*. New York: Simon & Schuster, 1981.

———. *Social Origins of Distress and Diseases: Depression, Neurasthenia, and Pain in Modern China*. New Haven, Conn.: Yale University Press, 1986.

Kleinman, Arthur, and Byron Good, "Introduction: Culture and Depression." In *Culture and Depression: Studies in the Anthropology and Cross-cultural Psychiatry of Affect and Disorder*. Berkeley: University of California Press, 1985.

Koch, T. "Disability and Difference: Balancing Social and Physical Constructions." *Journal of Medical Ethics* 27, no. 6 (2001): 370–76.

Kohn, Eric. "*Forrest Gump*, 25 Years Later: A Bad Movie That Gets Worse with Age." *IndieWire*, July 4, 2019. Accessed May 17, 2020, https://www.indiewire.com/2019/07/forrest-gump -bad-movie-25-anniversary-1202154214/.

Kraepelin, Emil. *Psychiatrie: Ein kurzes Lehrbuch für Stuirende und Aerzte.* 2nd ed. Leipzig: Abel, 1887. English translation: *Textbook of Psychiatry.* Edited by George M. Robinson. Edinburgh: E. & S. Livingstone, 1920.

Kretschmer, Madeline, and Lance Storm. "The Relationships of the Five Existential Concerns with Depression and Existential Thinking." *International Journal of Existential Psychology & Psychotherapy* 7, no. 1 (2017).

Krieger, Tobias, Thomas Berger, and Martin grosse Holtforth. "The Relationship of Self-Compassion and Depression: Cross-lagged Panel Analyses in Depressed Patients after Outpatient Therapy." *Journal of Affective Disorders* 202 (September 15, 2016): 39–45. https://doi.org/10.1016/j.jad.2016.05.032.

Krishnan, V., and E. J. Nestler. "Animal Models of Depression: Molecular Perspectives." In *Molecular and Functional Models in Neuropsychiatry*, ed. Jim J. Hagan. Current Topics in Behavioral Neurosciences 7. Berlin: Springer, 2011. https://doi.org/10.1007/7854_2010_108.

Kristeva, Julia. *Black Sun.* New York: Columbia University Press, 1987.

Kumari Campbell, Fiona A. "Ability." In *Keywords for Disability Studies*, edited by Rachel Adams, Benjamin Reiss, and David Serlin, 12–14. New York: New York University Press, 2015.

———. "Exploring Internalized Ableism Using Critical Race Theory." *Disability & Society* 23 (2008): 5–6. https://doi.org/10.1080/09687590701841190.

———. "Inciting Legal Fictions: 'Disability's' Date with Ontology and the Ableist Body of Law." *Griffith Law Review* 10 (2001): 42–62.

Lakhan, Ram. "Profile of Social, Environmental and Biological Correlates in Intellectual Disability in a Resource-Poor Setting in India." *Indian Journal of Psychological Medicine* 37, no. 3 (2015): 311–16. doi: 10.4103/0253-7176.162957.

Lane, William L. *The Gospel of Mark.* New International Commentary on the New Testament. Grand Rapids: Eerdmans, 1974.

Lasch, Christopher. *The Culture of Narcissism: American Life in an Age of Diminishing Expectations.* New York: Norton, 1979.

———. *The Minimal Self: Psychic Survival in Troubled Times.* New York: W. W. Norton, 1984.

Lasch-Quinn, Elisabeth. Introduction to Rieff, *Triumph of the Therapeutic.*

Lawlor, Clark. *From Melancholia to Prozac.* Oxford: Oxford University Press, 2012.

Lawson, Stephen. "The Incarnation in the Theology of Maximus the Confessor." Paper given at the Stone-Campbell Journal Conference, April 14, 2012. https://www.academia.edu/1964198/The_Incarnation_in_the_Theology_of_Maximus_the_Confessor.

Lee, Hong. "Biological Functionalism and Mental Disorder." PhD diss., Bowling Green State University, 2012. https://scholarworks.bgsu.edu/philosophy_diss/22/.

Leftow, Brian. "Eternity and Immutability." In *The Blackwell Guide to Philosophy of Religion*, ed. William E. Mann. Malden, Mass.: Blackwell, 2004.

———. "Immutability." In *The Stanford Encyclopedia of Philosophy*, ed. Edward N. Zalta, fall 2008 ed.

Leidenhag, Mikael, and Joanna Leidenhag. "Science and Spirit: A Critical Examination of Amos Yong's Pneumatological Theology of Emergence." *Open Theology* 1 (October 2015): 425–35. https://doi.org/10.1515/opth-2015-0025.

Levinas, Emmanuel. *Alterity and Transcendence.* Translated by Michael B. Smith. New York: Columbia University Press, 1999.

———. *Otherwise Than Being or Beyond Essence.* Translated by Alphonso Lingis. Pittsburgh: Duquesne University Press, 1981.

Lewis, C. S. *The Problem of Pain*. San Francisco: HarperCollins, 1940.

LifeWay Research. "Study of Acute Mental Illness and Christian Faith." http://lifewayresearch .com/wp-content/uploads/2014/09/Acute-Mental-Illness-and-Christian-Faith-Research -Report-1.pdf.

Lifton, Jay. *The Protean Self: Human Resilience in an Age of Fragmentation*. Chicago: University of Chicago Press, 1993.

Lindstrom, Fredrick. *Suffering and Sin: Interpretations of Illness in the Individual Complaint Psalms*. Uppsala: Almqvist & Wiksell, 1994.

Lister, Rob. *God Is Impassible and Impassioned: Toward a Theology of Divine Emotion*. Wheaton, Ill.: Crossway, 2013.

Lloyd-Jones, D. Martyn. *Romans: The New Man, an Exposition of Chapter 6*. Grand Rapids: Zondervan, 1972.

Lossky, Vladimir. *In the Image and Likeness of God*. Crestwood, N.Y.: St. Vladimir's Seminary Press, 1985.

Louth, Andrew. *Maximus the Confessor*. New York: Routledge, 1996, *Ambiguum* 41, 155–62;

Lupton, Robert. *Toxic Charity: How the Church Hurts Those They Help and How to Reverse It*. San Francisco: HarperCollins, 2011.

Luy, David J. *Dominus Mortis: Martin Luther on the Incorruptibility of God in Christ*. Minneapolis: Fortress, 2014.

Lynch, D., K. R. Laws, and P. J. McKenna. "Cognitive Behavioral Therapy for Major Psychiatric Disorder: Does It Really Work? A Meta-analytical Review of Well-Controlled Trials." *Psychological Medicine* 40, no. 1 (2010): 9–24.

Macchia, Frank D. *Jesus the Spirit Baptizer: Christology in the Light of Pentecost*. Grand Rapids: Eerdmans, 2018.

MacNutt, Francis. *Healing*. Notre Dame, Ind.: Ave Maria, 1999.

Marion, Jean-Luc. *Being Given: Toward a Phenomenology of Givenness*. Stanford, Calif.: Stanford University Press, 2002.

——. *In Excess: Studies of Saturated Phenomena*. New York: Fordham University Press, 2004.

Marshall, Bruce D. "Dereliction of Christ." In Keating and White, *Divine Impassibility*.

——. "The Unity of the Triune God: Reviving an Ancient Question." *Thomist: A Speculative Quarterly Review* 74, no. 1 (2010): 1–32. https://doi.org/10.1353/tho.2010.0000.

The Matrix Reloaded. Dir. the Wachowskis. Burbank, Calif.: Warner Bros. Pictures, 2003.

Matz, Robert J., and A. Chadwick Thornhill, eds. *Divine Impassibility: Four Views of God's Emotions and Suffering*. Downers Grove, Ill.: IVP Academic, 2019.

Maximus the Confessor. *On Difficulties in the Church Fathers: The Ambigua: Volume II, Maximos the Confessor*. Edited and translated by Nicholas Constas. London: Harvard University Press, 2014.

——. *On Difficulties in Sacred Scripture: The Responses to Thalassios (Quaest. ad. Thal.)*. Translated by Fr. Maximos Constas. Washington, D.C.: Catholic University of America Press, 2018.

May, Gerald G. *The Dark Night of the Soul: A Psychiatrist Explores the Connection between Darkness and Spiritual Growth*. New York: HarperCollins, 2003.

May, Rollo. *Man's Search for Himself*. New York: Norton, 1953.

——. *The Meaning of Anxiety*. Rev. ed. New York: W. W. Norton, 2015.

Mayo Clinic Staff. "Forgiveness: Letting Go of Grudges and Bitterness." November 4, 2017, accessed September 15, 2020. https://www.mayoclinic.org/healthy-lifestyle/adult-health/in -depth/forgiveness/art-20047692.

McCall, Thomas H. "Trinity Doctrine: Plain and Simple." In *Advancing Trinitarian Theology: Exploration in Constructive Dogmatics*, ed. Oliver D. Crisp and Fred Sanders. Grand Rapids: Zondervan, 2014.

McCormack, Bruce L. "Divine Impassibility or Simple Divine Constancy? Implications of Karl Barth's Later Christology for Debates over Impassibility." In Keating and White, *Divine Impassibility*, 150–86.

McRuer, Robert. "Compulsory Able-Bodiness and Queer/Disabled Existence." In *Disability Studies: Enabling the Humanities*, ed. Sharon L. Snyder, Brenda Jo Brueggemann, and Rosemarie Garland-Thomson. New York: Modern Language Association, 2002.

Mead, George Herbert. *Mind, Self and Society*. Edited by C. Morris. Chicago, Ill.: University of Chicago Press, 1934.

Meynen, Gerben. "Free Will and Mental Disorder: Exploring the Relationship." *Theoretical Medicine and Bioethics* 31 (2010): 429–43. doi: 10.1007/s11017-010-9158-5.

Middleton, J. Richard. *The Liberating Image: The Imago Dei in Genesis 1*. Grand Rapids: Baker, 2005.

Milbank, John. *Theology and Social Theory: Beyond Secular Reason*. 2nd ed. Malden, Mass.: Blackwell, 2006.

Moltmann, Jürgen. *The Crucified God*. New York: Harper & Row, 1974.

———. *God in Creation: A Theology of Creation and the Spirit of God*. New York: Harper & Row, 1991.

Montejo, Gregorio. "Truly Human, Fully Divine: The Kenotic Christ of Thomas Aquinas." PhD diss., Marquette University, 2016, accessed October 25, 2019. https://epublications .marquette.edu/cgi/viewcontent.cgi?article=1694&context=dissertations_mu.

Moore, Thomas. *Dark Nights of the Soul: A Guide to Finding Your Way through Life's Ordeals*.

Morelli, Father George. "Healing the Infirmity of Sin: A Spiritual Nutshell." Accessed December 16, 2019, http://ww1.antiochian.org/content/healing-infirmity-sin-spiritual-nutshell.

Morris, Thomas V. *The Logic of God Incarnate*. Ithaca, N.Y.: Cornell University Press, 1986.

Morrison, Jim. Vocalist, "People Are Strange," 1967, by Jim Morrison and Robbie Krieger (lyricists), the Doors (composers), side B, track 1 on *Strange Days*. New York: Elektra Records, 1967.

Mount, Thomas Blair Speed. "Existential Dimensions of the Contemporary Impassibility Debate: A Pastoral Approach to the Question of Divine Suffering within the Context of Conservative Evangelicalism." Research proposal for the Doctor of Philosophy Programme, South African Theological Seminary, 2015. https://portfolios.sats.edu.za/cgi-bin/ koha/opac-detail.pl?biblionumber=14676.

Mozley, J. K. *The Impassibility of God: A Survey of Christian Thought*. 1926; Cambridge: Cambridge University Press, 2014.

Myers, Benjamin. "A Tale of Two Gardens: Augustine's Narrative Interpretation of Romans 5." In *Apocalyptic Paul: Cosmos and Anthropos in Romans 5–8*, ed. Beverly Roberts Gaventa. Waco, Tex.: Baylor University Press, 2013.

National Disability Navigator. Population Specific Fact Sheet. Accessed May 25, 2020, https:// nationaldisabilitynavigator.org/ndnrc-materials/fact-sheets/population-specific-fact-sheet -intellectual-disability/.

Nestruk, Alexi. "The Universe as Hypostatic Inherence in the Logos of God." In Clayton and Peacocke, *In Whom We Live and Move and Have Our Being*.

Ngien, Dennis. *The Suffering of God: According to Martin Luther's "Theologica Crucis."* Vancouver, B.C.: Regent College, 2005.

Niebuhr, H. Richard. *Christ and Culture*. New York: Harper & Row, 1975.

Northoff, Georg. "Brain and Self: A Neurophilosophical Account." *Child Adolescent Psychiatry Mental Health* 7, art. 28 (2013), doi: 10.1186/1753-2000-7-28.

O'Connor, Timothy, and Yu Wong Hong. "Emergent Properties." In *The Stanford Encyclopedia of Philosophy*, edited by Edward N. Zalta, summer 2015 ed. Accessed June 20, 2018, https://plato.stanford.edu/archives/sum2015/entries/properties-emergent/.

O'Hanlon, Gerard F. *The Immutability of God in the Theology of Hans Urs von Balthasar*. New York: Cambridge University Press, 1990.

O'Meara, Thomas F., O.P. "Tillich and Heidegger: A Structural Relationship." *Harvard Theological Review* 61, no 2 (1968).

Oakes, Edward T. "'He Descended into Hell': The Depths of God's Self-Emptying Love on Holy Saturday in the Thought of Hans Urs von Balthasar." In Evans, *Exploring Kenotic Christology*.

Oliver, John W. *Giver of Life: The Holy Spirit in the Orthodox Tradition*. Brewster, Mass.: Paraclete, 2011.

Oord, Thomas ed. *Theologies of Creation: Creatio Ex Nihilo and Its New Rivals*. New York: Routledge, 2015.

Otto, Randall E. "The *Imago Dei* as *Familitas*." *Journal of the Evangelical Theological Society* 35, no. 4 (1992): 503–13.

Otto, Rudolf. *The Idea of the Holy*. Oxford: Oxford University Press, 1923.

Packer, J. I. "Theism for Our Time." In *God Who Is Rich in Mercy*, ed. Peter T. O'Brien and David G. Peterson. Grand Rapids: Baker, 1986.

Parker, Gordon, Georgia McClure, and Amelia Paterson. "Melancholia and Catatonia: Disorders or Specifiers?" *Current Psychiatry Reports* 17 (2015): 536. https://doi.org/10.1007/s11920-014-0536-y.

Pascal, Blaise. *Pensées*. Translated by W. F. Trotter. New York: Random House, 1941.

Pawl, Timothy. *In Defense of Conciliar Christology: A Philosophical Essay*. Oxford: Oxford University Press, 2016.

———. *In Defense of Extended Conciliar Christology*. Oxford: Oxford University Press, 2019.

Peters, John L. *Christian Perfection and American Methodism*. Nashville, Tenn.: Abingdon, 1956.

Pilgrim, David, and Richard Bentall. "The Medicalisation of Misery: A Critical Realist Analysis of the Concept of Depression." *Journal of Mental Health* 8, no. 3 (1999): 261–74.

Plantinga, Alvin. "On Ockham's Way Out." *Faith and Philosophy* 3, no. 3 (1986): 235–69.

———. *Warrant: The Current Debate*. Oxford: Oxford University Press, 1993.

———. *Warrant and Proper Function*. Oxford: Oxford University Press, 1993.

———. *Warranted Christian Belief*. Oxford: Oxford University Press, 2000.

Plato. *Phaedo*. In *Plato: Complete Works*, edited by John M. Cooper and Associate Editor D. S. Hutchinson. Indianapolis: Hackett, 1997.

Pohl, Christine. *Making Room: Recovering Hospitality as a Christian Tradition*. Grand Rapids: Eerdmans, 1999.

Polanyi, Michael. *Personal Knowledge: Towards a Post-critical Philosophy*. Chicago: University of Chicago Press, 1958, 1962.

Popper, Karl. *Objective Knowledge: An Evolutionary Approach*. Oxford: Oxford University Press, 1972.

———. "Three Worlds." Tanner Lecture on Human Values, University of Michigan, 1978. https://tannerlectures.utah.edu/_documents/a-to-z/p/popper80.pdf.

Przywara, Eric. *Analogia Entis*. Translated by John R. Betz and David Bentley Hart. Grand Rapids: Eerdmans, 2014.

Radden, Jennifer. *Moody Minds Distempered: Essays on Melancholy and Depression*. Oxford: Oxford University Press, 2009.

———. *The Nature of Melancholy: From Aristotle to Kristeva*. Oxford: Oxford University Press, 2000.

Ramirez, Erick. "Philosophy of Mental Illness." In *Internet Encyclopedia of Philosophy*. Accessed September 16, 2020, https://www.iep.utm.edu/mental-i/.

Raposa, Michael L. *Boredom and the Religious Imagination*. Charlottesville: University of Virginia Press, 1999.

Reaves, Dylan. "Peter Berger and the Rise and Fall of the Theory of Secularization." *Denison Journal of Religion* 11, art. 3 (2012): 5–8.

Reed, Geoffrey M. "Toward ICD-11: Improving the Clinical Utility of WHO's International Classification of Mental Disorders." *Professional Psychology: Research and Practice* 41, no. 6 (2010): 457–64.

Reinders, Hans S. *Disability, Providence, and Ethics: Bridging Gaps, Transforming Lives*. Waco, Tex.: Baylor University Press, 2014.

———. *Receiving the Gift of Friendship: Profound Disability, Theological Anthropology, and Ethics*. Grand Rapids: Eerdmans, 2008.

Rennó, Joel, Jr., Gislene Valadares, Amaury Cantilino, Jeronimo Mendes-Ribeiro, Renan Rocha, and Antonio Geraldo da Silva, eds. *Women's Mental Health: A Clinical and Evidence-Based Guide*. Cham, Switzerland: Springer Nature Switzerland AG, 2020.

Rieff, Philip. *The Triumph of the Therapeutic: Uses of Faith after Freud*. 40th anniv. ed. Wilmington, Del.: Intercollegiate Studies Institute, 2006.

Ritchie, Hannah, and Max Roser. "Mental Health." *Our World in Data*, April 2018. Accessed December 26, 2019, https://ourworldindata.org/mental-health.

Robinson, James. *Divine Healing*. 3 vols. Eugene, Ore.: Wipf and Stock, 2011–2014.

Romero, Miguel J. "Aquinas on the *Corporis Infirmitas*: Broken Flesh and the Grammar of Grace." In *Disability in the Christian Tradition: A Reader*, edited by Brian Brock and John Swinton, 67–100. Grand Rapids: Eerdmans, 2012.

Rosemann, Philipp W. *Peter Lombard*. Oxford: Oxford University Press, 2004.

Rubin, Julius H. *Religious Melancholy and Protestant Experience in America*. Oxford: Oxford University Press, 1994.

Sartre, Jean-Paul. *Nausea*. New York: New Directions, 2013.

Sattler, J. M. *Assessment of Children: Behavioral and Clinical Applications*. 4th ed. San Diego: J. M. Sattler, 2002.

Schipper, Jeremy. *Disability Studies and the Hebrew Bible: Figuring Mephibosheth in the David Story*. New York: T&T Clark, 2006.

Schlimme, Jann E. "Impairments of Personal Freedom in Mental Disorders." In *Handbook of the Philosophy of Medicine*, edited by T. Schramme and S. Edwards. Dordrecht: Springer, 2016. https://doi.org/10.1007/978-94-017-8706-2_24-1.

———. "Lived Autonomy and Chronic Mental Illness: A Phenomenological Approach." *Theoretical Medicine and Bioethics* 33, no. 6 (2012): 387–404. doi: 10.1007/s11017-012-9235-z.

Schults, F. LeRon. *Reforming Theological Anthropology: After the Philosophical Turn to Relationality*. Grand Rapids: Eerdmans, 2003.

Scott, David. *The Love That Made Mother Teresa: How Her Secret Visions and Dark Night Can Help You Conquer the Slums of Your Heart*. Manchester, N.H.: Sophia Institute, 2016.

Scrutton, Anastasia Philippa. "Emotion in Augustine of Hippo and Thomas Aquinas: A Way Forward for the Im/passibility Debate?" *International Journal of Systematic Theology* 7, no. 2 (2005): 170–76.

————. *Thinking through Feeling: God, Emotion and Possibility*. New York: Bloomsbury Academic, 2013.

————. "Two Christian Theologies of Depression: An Evaluation and Discussion of Clinical Implications." *Philosophy, Psychiatry, & Psychology* 22, no. 4 (2015): 275–89.

Shorter, Edward. *Before Prozac: The Troubled History of Mood Disorders in Psychiatry*. Oxford: Oxford University Press, 2009.

Smith, James K. A., and Amos Yong, eds. *Science and the Spirit: A Pentecostal Engagement with the Sciences*. Bloomington: Indiana University Press, 2010.

Solzhenitsyn, Aleksandr. *The Gulag Archipelago*. London: Vintage Classics, 2018.

St. John of the Cross. *Dark Night of the Soul*. Translated and edited by E. Allison Peers. New York: Doubleday, 1990.

Stainton, Tim. "Reason and Value: The Thought of Plato and Aristotle and the Construction of Intellectual Disability." *Mental Retardation* 39, no. 6 (2001): 452–60.

Stanford, Matthew S. *The Biology of Sin: Grace, Hope, and Healing for Those Who Feel Trapped*. Downers Grove, Ill.: InterVarsity, 2010.

Stein, Edward. *Without Good Reason: The Rationality Debate in Philosophy and Cognitive Science*. New York: Oxford University Press, 1998.

Steinke, Peter L. *Healthy Congregations: A Systems Approach*. Herndon, Va.: Albin Institute, 2006.

Sullivan, Daniel, and Mark Landau. "Toward a Comprehensive Understanding of Existential Threat: Insights from Paul Tillich." *Social Cognition* 30, no. 6 (2012): 734–57.

Swinburne, Richard. *The Coherence of Theism*. Oxford: Clarendon Press, 1993.

Swinton, John. *Spirituality and Mental Health Care: Rediscovering a "Forgotten" Dimension*. London: Jessica Kingsley, 2001.

————. "Theology or Therapy? In What Sense Does Depression Exist?" *Philosophy, Psychiatry, & Psychology* 22, no. 4 (2015): 295–98.

Synan, Vinson. *The Holiness-Pentecostal Tradition: Charismatic Movements in the Twentieth Century*. Grand Rapids: Eerdmans, 1997.

Szasz, Thomas S. *The Myth of Mental Illness: Foundations of a Theory of Personal Conduct*. New York: HarperCollins, 1974.

Taylor, Charles. *A Secular Age*. Cambridge, Mass.: Harvard University Press, 2018.

Teresa of Calcutta [Mother Teresa], and Brian Kolodiejchuk. *Come Be My Light: The Private Writings of Mother Teresa*. New York: Image, 2009.

Thomas, John Christopher. *The Devil, Disease, and Deliverance: Origins of Illness in New Testament Thought*. Sheffield, UK: Sheffield Academic, 1998.

Thompson, Thomas R. "Nineteenth Century Kenotic Christology." In Evans, *Exploring Kenotic Christology*.

Thompson, Thomas R., and Cornelius Plantinga Jr. "Trinity and Kenosis." In *Exploring Kenotic Christology: The Self-Emptying of God*, ed. C. Stephen Evans. Vancouver, B.C.: Regent College, 2010.

Thunberg, Lars. *Microcosm and Mediator: The Theological Anthropology of Maximus the Confessor*. 2nd ed. Chicago: Open Court, 1995.

Tillich, Paul. *The Courage to Be*. New Haven, Conn.: Yale University Press, 1952.

————. *Systematic Theology*, vol. 1. Chicago: University of Chicago Press, 1951.

Tollefsen, Torstein. *The Christocentric Cosmology of Maximus the Confessor*. Oxford: Oxford University Press, 2008.

Toussaint, Loren L., Everett L. Worthington, and David R. Williams, eds. *Forgiveness and Health: Scientific Evidence and Theories Relating Forgiveness to Better Health*. New York: Springer, 2015.

Trader, Alexis. *Ancient Christian Wisdom and Aaron Beck's Cognitive Therapy: A Meeting of Minds*. American University Series. New York: Peter Lang, 2012.

Tsakiridis, George. *Evagrius Ponticus and Cognitive Science: A Look at Moral Evil and the Thoughts*. Eugene, Ore.: Wipf and Stock, 2010.

U.S. Department of Health and Human Services, *Mental Health: Culture, Race, and Ethnicity: A Supplement to Mental Health: A Report of the Surgeon General*. Rockville, Md.: U.S. Department of Health and Human Services, Substance Abuse and Mental Health Services Administration, Center for Mental Health Services, 2001. Accessed September 15, 2020, https://www.ncbi.nlm.nih.gov/books/NBK44243/.

Vallicella, William F. "Divine Simplicity." In *The Stanford Encyclopedia of Philosophy*, edited by Edward N. Zalta, spring 2019 ed. Accessed October 27, 2019, https://plato.stanford.edu/archives/spr2019/entries/divine-simplicity/.

van Driel, Edwin Chr. "The Logic of Assumption." In Evans, *Exploring Kenotic Christology*.

Van Fraassen, Bas. *The Scientific Image*. Oxford: Oxford University Press, 1980.

Vanhoozer, Kevin J. "The Trials of Truth: Mission, Martyrdom, and the Epistemology of the Cross." In *To Stake a Claim: Mission and the Western Crisis of Knowledge*, edited by Kevin J. Vanhoozer and J. Andrew Kirk. Maryknoll, N.Y.: Orbis Books, 1999.

van Huyssteen, J. Wentzel. *The Shaping of Rationality*. Grand Rapids: Eerdmans, 1999.

Vanier, Jean. *Becoming Human*. 2nd ed. Toronto: House of Anansi, 2008.

———. *Befriending the Stranger*. Mahwah, N.J.: Paulist, 2004.

Vatican. *Donum Vitae: Instruction on Respect for Human Life in Its Origin and on the Dignity of Procreation*. London: Publications for the Holy See, 1987.

Venema, Dennis R., and Scot McKnight. *Adam and the Genome: Reading Scripture after Genetic Science*. Grand Rapids: Brazos, 2017.

Wakefield, Jerome C. "The Concept of Mental Disorder: Diagnostic Implications of the Harmful Dysfunction Analysis." *World Psychiatry* 6, no. 3 (2007): 149–56.

———. "Disorder as Harmful Dysfunction: A Conceptual Critique of DSM-III-R's Definition of Mental Disorder," *Psychological Review* 99, no. 2 (1992): 232–47.

Walton, John H. *The Lost World of Adam and Eve*. Downers Grove, Ill.: IVP Academic, 2015.

Ware, Kallistos. "God Immanent yet Transcendent." In Clayton and Peacocke, *In Whom We Live and Move and Have Our Being*.

Wasserman, David, Adrienne Asch, Jeffrey Blustein, and Daniel Putnam. "Disability: Definitions, Models, Experience." In *The Stanford Encyclopedia of Philosophy*, edited by Edward N. Zalta, summer 2016 ed. Accessed November 1, 2019, https://plato.stanford.edu/archives/sum2016/entries/disability/.

Watkinson, Mike, and Pete Anderson. *Crazy Diamond: Syd Barrett and the Dawn of Pink Floyd*. Rev. ed. London: Omnibus, 2007.

Webb, Marcia. *Toward a Theology of Psychological Disorder*. Eugene, Ore.: Wipf and Stock, 2017.

Weems, Carl F., Natalie M. Costa, Christopher Dehon, and Steven L. Berman. "Paul Tillich's Theory of Existential Anxiety: A Preliminary Conceptual and Empirical Examination." *Anxiety, Stress & Coping: An International Journal* 17, no. 4 (2004): 383–99.

Weinandy, Thomas G. *Does God Change?* Still River: St. Bede's, 1985.

———. *Does God Suffer?* Notre Dame, Ind.: University of Notre Dame Press, 2000.

Weir, Kirsten. "Forgiveness Can Improve Mental and Physical Health." *American Psychological Association CE Corner* 48, no. 1 (2017): 30. http://www.apa.org/monitor/2017/01/ce-corner.aspx.

Wesley, John. Sermon 45, "The New Birth." In *The Works of John Wesley*, vol. 6, *Sermons on Several Occasions: First Series Concluded. Second Series*, ed. Thomas Jackson. 14 vols. London: Wesleyan Conference Office, 1872. https://hdl.handle.net/2027/njp.32101075386605.

———. "Treatise on Baptism," "Original Sin" (sermon 44), and *The Doctrine of Original Sin*. In *The Works of the Rev. John Wesley*, edited by Thomas Jackson. 14 vols. London: Wesleyan Conference Office, 1872.

West, Cornel. *Prophesy Deliverance!* Louisville, Ky.: Westminster John Knox, 2012.

"What Causes Depression?" Harvard Health Publishing, Harvard Medical School, June 2009. Accessed June 3, 2020, https://www.health.harvard.edu/mind-and-mood/what-causes-depression.

White, Thomas Joseph, ed. *The Analogy of Being: Invention of the Antichrist or the Wisdom of God?* Grand Rapids: Eerdmans, 2010.

———. "Through Him All Things Were Made (John 1:3)." In White, *Analogy of Being*, 249–50.

Wiley, Tatha. *Original Sin: Origins, Developments, Contemporary Meanings*. Mahwah, N.J.: Paulist, 2002.

Williams, Monnica T., Daniel C. Rosen, and Jonathan W. Kanter, eds. *Eliminating Race-Based Mental Health Disparities: Promoting Equity and Culturally Responsive Care across Settings*. Oakland, Calif.: New Harbinger, 2019.

Willis, Tim. *Madcap: The Half-Life of Syd Barrett, Pink Floyd's Lost Genius*. London: Short, 2003.

Witherington, Ben, III. *Jesus the Sage: The Pilgrimage of Wisdom*. Minneapolis: Augsburg Fortress, 2000.

———. *John's Wisdom: A Commentary on the Fourth Gospel*. Louisville, Ky.: Westminster John Knox, 1995.

Wong, Eunice C., Rebecca L. Collins, Jennifer Cerully, Rachana Seelam, and Beth Roth. "Racial and Ethnic Differences in Mental Illness Stigma and Discrimination among Californians Experiencing Mental Health Challenges." *Rand Health Quarterly* 6, no. 2 (2017): 6.

Wood, Jordan Daniel. "Creation Is Incarnation: The Metaphysical Peculiarity of the *Logoi* in Maximus Confessor." *Modern Theology* 34, no. 1 (2018): 82–102. doi: 10.1111/moth.12382.

World Health Organization. "Gender and Women's Mental Health." Accessed December 26, 2019, https://www.who.int/mental_health/prevention/genderwomen/en/.

Worthington, Everett L., Jr. *Dimensions of Forgiveness: Psychological Research and Theological Perspectives*. Radnor, Penn.: Templeton, 1998.

Worthington, Everett L., Jr., and Steven J. Sandage. *Forgiveness and Spirituality in Psychotherapy: A Relational Approach*. Washington, D.C.: American Psychological Association, 2015.

Yoder, Timothy J. "Hans Urs von Balthasar and Kenosis: The Pathway to Human Agency." PhD diss., Loyola University Chicago, 2013. *Dissertations*, no. 918, 13, http://ecommons.luc.edu/luc_diss/918.

Yong, Amos. *The Spirit of Creation: Modern Science and Divine Action in the Pentecostal-Charismatic Imagination*. Grand Rapids: Eerdmans, 2011.

———. *Theology and Down Syndrome: Reimagining Disability in Late Modernity*. Waco, Tex.: Baylor University Press, 2007.

Zizioulas, John. *Being and Communion*. Yonkers, N.Y.: St. Vladimir's Seminary Press, 1997.

Zohar, Danah, and Ian Marshall. *SQ: Spiritual Intelligence: The Ultimate Intelligence*. New York: Bloomsbury, 2000.

Index

285

Also Available in the SRTD Series

Accessible Atonement: Disability Theology and the Cross of Christ
David McLachlan

Formed Together: Mystery, Narrative, and Virtue in Christian Caregiving
Keith Dow

Wondrously Wounded: Theology, Disability, and the Body of Christ
Brian Brock

Disability and Spirituality: Recovering Wholeness
William C. Gaventa

Crippled Grace: Disability, Virtue Ethics, and the Good Life
Shane Clifton

The Bible and Disability: A Commentary
Edited by Sarah J. Melcher, Mikeal C. Parsons, and Amos Yong

Pastoral Care and Intellectual Disability: A Person-Centered Approach
Anna Katherine Shurley

Becoming Friends of Time: Disability, Timefullness, and Gentle Discipleship
John Swinton

Disability and World Religions: An Introduction
Edited by Darla Y. Schumm and Michael Stoltzfus

Madness: American Protestant Responses to Mental Illness
Heather H. Vacek

Disability, Providence, and Ethics: Bridging Gaps, Transforming Lives
Hans S. Reinders

Flannery O'Connor: Writing a Theology of Disabled Humanity
Timothy J. Basselin

Theology and Down Syndrome: Reimagining Disability in Late Modernity
Amos Yong